Zhuang Medical Culture

(Chinese-English Bilingual Version)

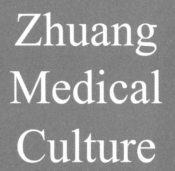

壮医药文化

（中英双语）

庞宇舟　方　刚　主编

谭耿耿　译

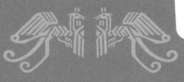

广西科学技术出版社

·南宁·

图书在版编目（CIP）数据

壮医药文化：汉文、英文 / 庞宇舟，方刚主编；
谭耿耿译. —南宁：广西科学技术出版社，2020.8
ISBN 978 - 7 - 5551 - 1280 - 8

Ⅰ. ①壮… Ⅱ. ①庞… ②方… ③谭… Ⅲ. ①壮医—
汉、英 Ⅳ. ①R291.8

中国版本图书馆CIP数据核字（2020）第 166691 号

壮医药文化（中英双语）
ZHUANGYIYAO WENHUA（ZHONG - YING SHUANGYU）

庞宇舟　　方刚　主编
谭耿耿　　译

策　　划：罗煜涛		责任编辑：罗煜涛　韦文印	
特约编辑：曾　静		责任校对：陈剑平	
装帧设计：韦娇林		责任印制：陆　弟	

出 版 人：卢培钊　　　　　　　　　　出版发行：广西科学技术出版社
社　　址：广西南宁市东葛路 66 号　　邮政编码：530023
网　　址：http://www.gxkjs.com

经　　销：全国各地新华书店
印　　刷：广西壮族自治区地质印刷厂
地　　址：南宁市建政东路 88 号　　　邮政编码：530023
开　　本：787 mm×1092 mm　1/16
字　　数：546 千字　　　　　　　　　印　　张：22.75
版　　次：2020 年 8 月第 1 版　　　　印　　次：2020 年 8 月第 1 次印刷
书　　号：ISBN 978 - 7 - 5551 - 1280 - 8
定　　价：128.00 元

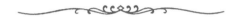

主编简介

庞宇舟，二级教授，博士研究生导师，享受国务院特殊津贴专家，第六批全国老中医药专家学术经验继承工作指导老师，广西优秀专家，广西壮瑶医药与医养结合人才小高地首席专家，广西名中医。现任广西中医药大学党委副书记、国家中医药管理局 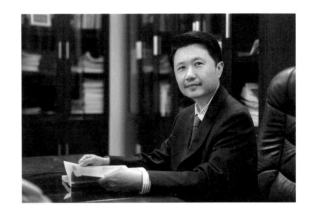 重点学科（壮医学）带头人、广西优势特色重点学科（壮医学）带头人、广西壮瑶药工程技术研究中心主任、广西高校壮医方药基础与应用研究重点实验室主任。兼任中央民族大学客座教授、世界中医药学会联合会药膳食疗研究专业委员会副会长、中国民族医药学会副会长、广西民族医药协会执行会长、广西中医药学会副会长、广西中医药学会中医内科专业委员会副主任委员、广西卫生标准化技术委员会中医壮瑶医专业副主任委员、广西民族医药协会壮医风湿病学专业委员会主任委员。是国家自然科学基金项目评审专家、中华中医药学会科学技术奖励评审专家、广西科技项目评估咨询专家、广西药品审评专家、广西民族药审评专家、广西壮瑶药协同创新中心专家、广西桂学研究会特聘研究员、民族医药博士后合作导师。

长期从事中医内科杂病、风湿病防治以及壮医理论与临床、壮药基础与应用、壮医药文化、壮医高等教育研究。2005 年 10 月创办广西中医学院

（今广西中医药大学）壮医药学院并任首任院长，兼任壮医药研究所所长、民族医药研究与发展中心副主任。率先阐述了壮医毒论核心理论和壮医毒论即"从毒求因、以毒论病、辨毒设法、解毒施治"四位一体应用理论，充实、发展了"毒虚致百病"的壮医病因病机学说，构建了"毒论—毒病—解毒法—解毒药"的壮医学术思想体系，突出了壮医学的特色和优势。临床上善于运用中医临床思维和壮医特色理论诊治风湿病和内科疑难病、常见病、多发病。

近五年来，共主持包括国家自然科学基金课题、国家中医药管理局行业专项等国家和省部级科研项目 10 项，公开发表论文 60 多篇，出版教材、专著 2 部。获广西科学技术进步奖一等奖、二等奖、三等奖各 1 项，中华中医药学会科学技术奖三等奖 1 项，广西医药卫生适宜技术推广一等奖、二等奖各 1 项，广西高等教育自治区级优秀教学成果奖一等奖 1 项、二等奖 2 项，广西高校优秀教材一等奖 1 项。2007 年 6 月被国家中医药管理局、国家民族事务委员会授予首批"全国民族医药工作先进个人"称号。2017 年 11 月获国家中医药管理局、国家民族事务委员会授予"全国少数民族医药工作表现突出个人"称号。

About the Chief Compilers

Pang Yuzhou, the professor level II, a doctoral supervisor and prestigious TCM doctor in Guangxi, has been awarded a special allowance by the State Council, and is a instructor of 6th Inueritance of Academic Experience of National Senior TCM Experts. Pang carries the title of Prestigious Guangxi Expert, and is the chief expert for Guangxi Talent Highland for Zhuang and Yao Medicine and Combination of Medical Care and Elderly Care. Pang is the Deputy Secretary of the Party Committee of Guangxi University of Chinese Medicine, academic leader of key discipline (Zhuang medicine) of State Administration of Traditional Chinese Medicine, academic leader of preponderant, characteristic and key discipline of Guangxi (Zhuang medicine), director of Guangxi Engineering Research Center for Zhuang and Yao Medicine, and director of Key Laboratory of Zhuang Medical Formulae and Applied Research of College and Universities in Guangxi Zhuang Autonomous Region. Also, he holds concurrent posts as visiting professor of Minzu University of China, deputy director of World Federation of Chinese Medicine Societies-Special Committee of Medicated Diet and Dietotherapy, deputy director of China Medical Association of Minorities, executive director of Guangxi Medical Association of Minorities, deputy director of Guangxi TCM Association, vice chairman of Special Committee of TCM Internal Medicine under Guangxi TCM Association, vice chairman of Special Committee of TCM and Zhuang and Yao Medicine under Guangxi Technical Committee for Hygienic Standardization, and chairman of Special Committee of Rheumatology in Zhuang Medicine affiliated with Guangxi Medical Association of Minorities. He holds the position of review expert for National Natural Science Foundation of China, China Association of Chinese Medicine Scientific and Technological Awards, Guangxi drugs and Guangxi ethnic drugs. He is also the consultant and review expert for Guangxi scientific and technological projects, expert of Guangxi Collaborative Innovation Center for Zhuang and Yao Medicine, special-term researcher of Guangxi Seminar for Guangxi Academics, and the post-doctoral co-supervisor in ethnic medicine.

He has long been committed to the study of prevention and treatment of rheumatism and miscellaneous internal medical diseases with TCM, as well as the research of the theory and clinical value, foundation and application, culture, and higher education of Zhuang medicine. In October 2005, he founded the Department of Zhuang Medicine in Guangxi College of Chinese Medicine (the present Guangxi University of Chinese Medicine) and became its first dean. He is also the director of the Institute for Zhuang Medicine and deputy director of the Research and Development Center of Ethnic Medicine. He has taken the lead in elaborating both the core theories and the four-dimensional applied theory (the etiology, pathogenesis, treatment and removal of toxin) of toxic theory in Zhuang medicine. He has enriched and developed the etiological and pathogenetic theory of Zhuang medicine — pathogenicity of toxin and deficiency — and he has also constructed the academic thinking system of Zhuang medicine via the etiology, pathogenesis, treatment and removal of toxin. His efforts have highlighted the characteristics and advantages of Zhuang medicine. He is outstanding at using the clinical method of traditional Chinese medical thought and distinctive Zhuang medical theories to diagnose and treat rheumatism as well as the complicated, common and frequently encountered internal medical diseases.

In the past five years, he has led 10 scientific research projects at national, provincial and ministerial levels, including several subjects of Natural Science Foundation of China, special projects of National Administration of Traditional Chinese Medicine. He published more than 60 publicly available papers, and published 1 textbook and 1 monograph. He won the first, second and third prize of Guangxi Science and Technology Progress Award respectively, the third prize of Science and Technology Award of China Association of Chinese Medicine, the first and second prizes of Prornotion Guangxi Appropriate Health Technology an Medicine respectively, one first and two second prizes of Guangxi Provincial Excellent Teaching Results in Higher Education respectively, and a first prize of Guangxi Superior Teaching Material for Colleges and Universities. In June 2007, he was among the first to be recognized by the State Administration of Traditional Chinese Medicine and the State Ethnic Affairs Commission in the awards as "National Advanced Individuals in Ethnic Medical Work". In November 2017, he was awarded the title of "Nationwide Individual with Outstanding Performance in the Work on Ethnic Medicine" by the National Admdnistration of Tradretanal Chinese Medicine and the National Ethnic Affairs Commission.

壮医学—广西第三批民族院校特色学科建设立项学科
（编号：桂教民教〔2019〕3 号）

Zhuang Medicine as the Discipline under Project-oriented Construction of the Third Lot of Characteristic Disciplines of Institute of Nationalities in Guangxi（No. Gui Jiao Min Jiao〔2019〕3）

相关研究项目：

Related research projects：

1. 中医学（壮医学方向）广西一流学科建设项目（编号：桂教科研〔2018〕12 号）

Traditional Chinese Medicine（Zhuang medicine orientation）on the List of Guangxi First-class Discipline（No. Gui Jiao Ke Yan〔2018〕12）

2. 广西中医药大学岐黄工程高层次人才团队培育项目（编号：2018005）

Development Program of High-level Talent Team under Qihuang Project of Guangxi University of Chinese Medicine（No. 2018005）

3. 广西壮瑶医药与医养结合人才小高地（编号：中共广西区委厅发〔2017〕44 号）

Guangxi Talent Highland for Zhuang and Yao Medicine and Combination of Medical Care and Elderly Care（No. The General office of CPC Guangxi Zhuang Autonomous Region Committee〔2017〕44）

序

　　壮族是我国少数民族中人口最多的一个民族，主要聚居在东起广东省连山壮族瑶族自治县，西至云南省文山壮族苗族自治州，南至北部湾，北达贵州省从江县，西南至中越边境的广大区域。

　　壮族历史悠久，源远流长。考古研究表明，距今 50000～10000 年的"柳江人""麒麟山人""白莲洞人""九头山人""都乐人""甘前人""荔浦人""灵山人""干淹人""九楞山人""隆林人"便是壮族的祖先。早在夏、商、周时代，壮族的先祖就有了专属于他们的称谓——"骆越"和"西瓯"。壮族是古代骆越和西瓯的后裔，系岭南百越民族的一个支系。自古以来，壮族及其先民就在华南-珠江流域生息繁衍。由于地处中原与华南地区、西南地区往来的交会处，长期的多民族杂居、交流与融合，使得其文化具有多元色彩。

　　古老的骆越民族，因其所处的自然环境和特定的生产方式，不仅创造了具有浓厚地域特色的稻作文化、铜鼓文化、干栏文化、山歌文化、崖壁画文化，而且创造了引以为豪的医药文化，它是现代壮医药的重要源头。

　　壮医药是壮族人民在漫长的历史长河中，在日常生活及与疾病做斗争的过程中不断摸索出来的医药经验的总结。壮医药文化作为壮族文化体系中的一种文化形态，虽然以其独特的民族形式和浓厚的地方特色早已客观存在，但是人们对其的认识还处于模糊状态。壮医药虽然在本质上属于医学范畴，但是由于其具有较多的人文因素，因此应从文化学的角度，对壮医药文化进行深入的挖掘和剖析，揭示其概念、发展历程、文化特征、表现形态以及壮族文化对壮医药形成和发展的影响。

　　作者在长期研究的基础上，通过大量的调查和总结，编写了《壮医药文化（中英双语）》这本专著。该专著系统地阐述了壮医药文化的概念、壮医药文化的发展历程、壮医药文化的特征与表现形态以及与壮医药密切相关的壮族哲学宗教信仰文化、壮族稻作文化、壮族习俗文化、壮族歌谣文化、壮族节庆文化、壮族饮食文化、壮族人居文化、壮族舞蹈体育文化，分析了这些壮族文化与壮医药的关系，特别是对壮医药形成与发展的影响。该著作是迄今为止系统研究壮医药文化的第一部专著，对加深人们对壮医药的认识，传承和发展壮医药具有重要意义。

壮医药文化是壮族传统文化的重要组成部分，而壮族传统文化又反映了该民族历史发展的水平。壮族作为岭南地区的土著民族，特殊的自然生态环境和社会环境及由此决定的生产方式，深刻地影响着壮族传统文化的形成和发展，并在很大程度上决定着壮族传统文化本身所具有的特点。正是因为壮族传统文化具有深厚的历史积淀和明显的民族及地域特征，所以它成为民族地区发展的"软实力"，能够在民族地区经济建设和社会发展中发挥自己独特的作用。虽然自 20 世纪以来，我国发生了文化转型的重大历史演进，传统的民族文化受到了严峻的挑战，曾经严重动摇了民族的文化自信心和文化认同感，但是经过一个历史阶段的剧烈动荡和时间淘汰之后，多数人还是清醒地认为，传统的民族文化及其所包含的民族精神，不仅凝结成了它的过去，也可以孕育出新的未来。在历史发展的长河中，民族文化不仅是一个民族的气质所在，而且也是一个民族繁衍与发展的根系所在。壮族传统文化在壮族的发展进程中是根、是魂，更是民族的精神食粮，因此我们必须充分认清文化传承与发展的重要性。近年来，随着经济社会的不断发展进步，人民的物质文化生活得到极大丰富，壮族文化也呈现出前所未有的喜人发展局面。对壮医药文化的研究，不仅有助于促进壮医药事业的发展，而且有助于弘扬中华文化，培养高度的文化自觉和文化自信，增强民族文化自尊心、自信心、自豪感，切实有效地增强壮族的向心力、凝聚力，从而使人们更加自觉地同祖国心连心，同呼吸，共命运，共同推动民族伟大复兴的中国梦早日实现。

值《壮医药文化（中英双语）》出版之际，欣然命笔，是为序。

黄汉儒

2019 年 6 月

（黄汉儒，壮族，著名壮医药学者，壮医学科和壮医理论奠基人，主任医师、教授、博士生导师，中国民族医药学会原副会长，中国民族医药协会原副会长，广西民族医药协会终身名誉会长，第八届全国人大代表，享受国务院特殊津贴专家）

Foreword

The Zhuang nationality is the most populous among China's ethnic minorities, mainly inhabiting the vast region which extends east to west from the Lianshan Zhuang and Yao Autonomous County in Guangdong province to Wenshan Zhuang and Miao Autonomous Prefecture in Yunnan province, south to north from Beibu Gulf to Congjiang County in Guizhou province, and southwest to China-Vietnam border.

The Zhuang nationality has a long history back to ancient times. Archeological study indicates that the ancestors of the Zhuang nationality include "Liujiang Man" "Qilinshan Man" "Bailiandong Man" "Jiutoushan Man" "Dule Man" "Ganqian Man" "Lipu Man" "Lingshan Man" "Ganyan Man" "Jiulengshan Man" and "Longlin Man", all of which are about 10,000 to 50,000 years old. As early as the Xia, Shang and Zhou Dynasties, Zhuang ancestors had tribal titles — "Luoyue" and "Xi'ou". The Zhuang, descendants of Luoyue and Xi'ou, comprises a branch of the Baiyue minority in Lingnan. Since ancient times, the Zhuang nationality and its ancestors have been living and multiplying in the Pearl River Basin in southern China. Located at the confluence of the Central Plains, South China and Southwest China, it has a diversified culture due to long-term multi-ethnic cohabitation, exchanges and fusion.

The ancient Luoyue minority, blessed by its natural environment and unique modes of production, has created not only rice-farming culture, bronze drum culture, Ganlan architecture culture, folk song culture and cliff painting culture with strong regional features, but also proud medical culture constituting an important source of modern Zhuang medicine.

Zhuang medicine is based on the medicinal experience accumulated by Zhuang people in their daily life and the process of struggle against diseases over the course of long history. As one cultural form in Zhuang cultural system, Zhuang medical culture is vaguely understood, although it has been an objective reality with unique ethnic form and strong local characteristics. Essentially, Zhuang medicine belongs to the category of medical science, however, it also has significant dimensions of humanities. Therefore, Zhuang medical culture should be deeply investigated and analyzed from the perspective of culturology to reveal its concepts, course of development, cultural characteristics, manifestations, together with the effect of Zhuang culture on the formation and development of Zhuang medicine.

Based on long-term study, the author has compiled the monograph *Zhuang Medical Culture* (*Chinese-English Bilingual Version*) through extensive research and experience. The monograph systematically elaborates the concepts, course of development, features and manifestations of Zhuang medical culture, as well as other Zhuang cultures closely related to Zhuang medicine (such as Zhuang philosophy, religious beliefs, rice-farming, custom, ballad, festivals, food, dwelling, dance and sports). Also, it analyzes the relationship between those Zhuang cultures and Zhuang medicine, especially their effect on its formation and development of Zhuang medicine. The book, as the first monograph that systematically studies Zhuang medical culture, is of great significance to the deeper understanding, inheritance and development of Zhuang medicine.

Zhuang medicine is an integral part of traditional Zhuang culture, which reflects the historical development of this minority. Zhuang is a native minority of the Lingnan region, where the special natural ecology and social environment and the resulting modes of production have a profound influence on the formation and development of traditional Zhuang culture, and largely determine its features. It is precisely because traditional Zhuang culture has deep historical accumulation and distinctive ethnic and regional features that Zhuang culture is able to become the "soft power" of the development in minority regions, and plays its unique role in their economic construction and social development. During the enormous cultural transformation in China since the 20th century, traditional ethnic culture has been severely challenged, and both the cultural confidence and cultural identity have been seriously shaken. However, after a historical phase of turbulence and rejection, most people still soberly believe that traditional ethnic culture and the underlying ethos have not only formed their past, but will also bring a bright future. Over the long course of history, ethnic culture is something bound up with ethos as well as ethnic reproduction and development. Traditional Zhuang culture is the root and soul of the deve-lopment process of the Zhuang nationality and food for thought for the nation, and so we should fully understand the importance of cultural inheritance and development. With the continuous development and progress of economy and society, people have entered a world of abundant material and cultural life, and the unprecedented development of Zhuang culture has appeared in recent years. Research on Zhuang medical culture can help develop the cause of Zhuang medicine, promote Chinese culture, cultivate high levels of cultural consciousness and confidence, enhance ethnic cultural self-esteem, confidence and pride, and efficiently and effectively strengthen the cohesiveness of the Zhuang nationality. Consequently, people can more consciously dedicate soul and mind to the motherland, and jointly promote the early realization of the Chinese dream — achieving the great rejuvenation of the Chinese nation.

It is my great pleasure to write the foreword for *Zhuang Medical Culture (Chinese-English Bilingual Version)*.

Huang Hanru

June 2019

(Huang Hanru, the Zhuang nationality, distinguished scholar in Zhuang medicine, founder of the discipline and theory of Zhuang medicine, chief physician, professor, doctoral supervisor, former deputy director of China Medical Association of Minorities and former deputy director of China Ethnic Medicine Association, permanent honorary director of Guangxi Medical Association of Minorities, representative of 8th National People's Congress, State Council Expert for Special Allowance)

前言

著名的民俗学者钟敬文说过:"一个民族的文化,是那个民族存在的标志。"与世界上所有智慧民族一样,壮族有着悠久的历史和灿烂的文化。壮族文化从远古走来,到现代仍然闪耀着智慧的光芒。当我们看到朴素的壮族服饰,听到动听的壮话、悠扬的山歌、激昂的铜鼓声,欣赏到欢快的竹杠舞、五彩的壮锦,品尝到美味的五色糯米饭……心中就会涌起一种强烈的自豪感,脑海中就会勾勒出一幅美丽的壮族文化画卷。

壮族文化包含了壮族人民精神生活、物质生活的方方面面,诸如宗教信仰、哲学思想、风俗习惯、医药卫生等。壮医药学的发展,与壮族传统文化也有着千丝万缕的联系。譬如,壮族宗教文化深受道教的影响,因此道教的"道法自然""天人合一"的哲学思想与壮医天、地、人"三气同步"学说有渊源;壮族的"万物波乜观"与壮医"阴阳为本"学说有异曲同工之妙;从壮族稻作文化、"龙王制水"的传统思想当中可以找到壮医"三道两路"学说的影子;从壮族药市、"三月三"歌圩、节日饮食、体育活动等民俗中,更是可以看到壮民族在医疗保健和养生方面的智慧。

我们认为,壮医药文化是壮族传统文化的重要组成部分,壮医药深深根植于壮族传统文化的土壤当中。正如笔者在《壮医药文化概念和内涵初探》一文中指出的:"壮医药文化是壮医药与壮族各种文化交融、结合、渗透形成的产物。"壮族历史上没有规范通行的文字,于是壮医药文化就成了壮医药传承的重要载体之一。

基于以上认识,我们编撰了《壮医药文化(中英双语)》一书。本书共有十二章,主要从宗教信仰文化、稻作文化、民俗文化、歌谣文化、节庆文化、饮食文化、人居文化、舞蹈体育文化等方面，阐述壮族传统文化对壮医药的影响，探究壮族传统文化与壮医药的关系。本书编写分工如下：庞宇舟负责第一章、第二章，蓝毓营负责第三章，薛丽飞负责第四章，曾振东、方刚负责第五章、第七章，莫清莲负责第六章，唐振宇负责第八章，李晶晶负责第九章，宋宁负责第十章，王春玲负责第十一章、第十二章。全书最后由庞宇舟统稿和审定。

　　本书的出版主要面向壮医药爱好者和医学院校的学生。希望读者在学习壮族传统文化的同时，激发对壮医药文化的兴趣和爱好，以提高自己的人文素养，并为进一步研究壮医药的起源、发展，丰富壮医药内容提供资料。

　　壮族文化包罗万象，壮医药文化只是其冰山一角。由于本书篇幅有限，不能面面俱到，加上编者水平有限，难免有不足之处，希望读者在阅读过程中，提出宝贵意见，以便今后进一步补充修改完善。

Preface

Famous folklorist Zhong Jingwen once said, "The culture of a nation is a sign of its existence." The Zhuang nationality has a long history and splendid culture as all wise nationalities do all over the world. The Zhuang culture, coming from the ancient times, still glitters with wisdom in the modern world. When we see plain Zhuang clothing, hear beautiful Zhuang language, melodious mountain songs and passionate beats of bronze drum, appreciate cheerful bamboo pole dance and painted Zhuang brocade, taste delicious five-colored sticky rice... we experience a strong sense of pride and conjure up a great picture of Zhuang culture in our mind.

The Zhuang culture contains every aspect of the spiritual and material life of Zhuang people, such as religious beliefs, philosophical thought, customs, medicine and health. There are inseparable links between the development of Zhuang medicine and traditional Zhuang culture. For example, the religious culture of Zhuang is profoundly influenced by Taoism, therefore philosophic Taoist thought, such as "Tao is nature's way" and "the unity of man and nature", and the theory of "synchrony of triple initial qi (heaven, earth and human qi) " in Zhuang medicine are closely tied to each other. The "pan-boh-meh view" in the Zhuang nationality is similar to the theory of "yin-yang basis" in Zhuang medicine, and the traces of theory of "Sandao lianglu" in Zhuang medicine can be seen in the rice-farming culture and traditional thought such as "the Dragon Kings can control water" in the Zhuang nationality, and the wisdom of Zhuang in healthcare and health maintenance is shown in Zhuang customs, e.g., drug fairs, song fairs in Sanyuesan Festival, festival diet and sports activities.

We believe Zhuang medical culture is an integral part of traditional Zhuang culture, where Zhuang medicine is deeply rooted. As the author pointed out in the article *Primary Study on the Culture Conception and Connotation for the Zhuang Medicine*, "The Zhuang medical culture is the combined result of Zhuang medicine and various Zhuang cultures." Without a generally recognized writing system through its history, the Zhuang nationality still has taken Zhuang medical culture as one of the important carriers of inheritance of Zhuang medicine.

In this light, *Zhuang Medical Culture* (*Chinese-English Bilingual Version*) is compiled. The book consists of twelve chapters, which elaborate the influence of traditional Zhuang culture on Zhuang medicine and explore their relationship from various cultural aspects ranging from religious beliefs, rice-farming, customs, ballads, festivals, food and dwelling to dance and sports. The book is compiled collaboratively: Pang Yuzhou is responsible for Chapters 1 and 2, Lan Yuying for Chapter 3, Xue Lifei for Chapter 4, Zeng Zhendong and Fang Gang for Chapters 5 and 7, Mo Qinglian for Chapter 6, Tang Zhenyu for Chapter 8, Li Jingjing for Chapter 9, Song Ning for Chapter 10, and Wang Chunling for Chapters 11 and 12. Pang Yuzhou is in charge of the final compilation and review of the whole book.

The book is mainly aimed at Zhuang medicine enthusiasts and medical undergraduates, in the hope that readers studying traditional Zhuang culture are able to develop an interest in and a love for Zhuang medical culture, and can improve their own humanistic quality, and can provide materials for the further study of origin and development of Zhuang medicine and its enrichment.

Zhuang medical culture is the tip of the iceberg in front of the all-embracing Zhuang culture. The book cannot cover every aspect and may contain deficiencies due to limited space and limited knowledge of the compilers. Feedback from readers is welcome and valuable for the modification and improvement of the book.

目录

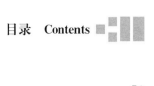

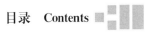

Contents

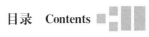

第一章 绪论

第一节 壮医药文化的诠释

一、文化的含义

"文化"一词，应该说是当今世界上使用频率最高的词之一。"文化"一词源于拉丁语的"colere"，最初是指土地的耕耘和改良，后来逐步扩大，包含加工、修养、教育和礼貌等多种含义。17世纪，德国法学家普芬多夫提出："文化是人的活动所创造的东西和有赖于人的社会生活而存在的东西的总和。"19世纪中叶是第一次文化热的时代，英国人类学家泰勒被公认为现代文化学的鼻祖。他在其著作《原始文化》中给文化下了定义："所谓文化或文明，乃是包括知识、信仰、艺术、道德、法律、习俗以及包括作为社会成员的个人而获得的其他任何能力、习惯在内的综合体。"

20世纪，各国关于文化的定义趋于多元。《法国大百科全书》认为，"文化是社会群体所特有的文明现象的总和""文化是一个复合体，它包括知识、信仰、艺术、道德、法律、习俗，以及包括作为社会成员的人所共有的一切其他规范和习惯"。德国1971年出版的《迈尔百科辞典》认为，文化是"人类社会在征服自然和自我发展中所创造的物质和思想财富"。1973年出版的《苏联大百科全书》认为，广义的文化"是社会和人在历史上一定的发展水平，它表现为人们进行生活和活动的种种类型和形式，以及人们所创造的物质和精神财富"，而狭义的文化"仅指人们的精神生活领域"。

我国著名学者梁漱溟先生在《中国文化要义》中说："文化之本义，应在经济、政治，乃至一切无所不包。"由此可见，文化的含义在本质上是比较宽泛的。目前，在我国对于文化有两种比较流行的定义：一是《辞海》的解释，广义指人类社会历史实践过程中所获得的物质、精神的生产能力和创造的物质财富、精神财富的总和，狭义指精神生产能力和精神产品，包括一切社会意识形式，如自然科学、技术科学、社会意识形态。二是《现代汉语词典》的解释，文化是"人类在社会历史发展过程中所创造的物质财富和精神财富的总和，特指精神财富，如文学、艺术、教育、科学等"。

二、壮医药文化的概念

伟大的医学家巴甫洛夫曾经说过："有了人类，就有医疗活动。"医药是人类与生俱来的需求，每个民族在历史上都有自己的医学创造和医药积累。壮族是一个具有悠久历史和灿烂文化的民族，它源于我国南方古百越族的西瓯、骆越部族。考古发现，早在旧石器时代，壮族地区就有古人类活动。远古时期，壮族地区生存条件恶劣。唐代刘恂的《岭表录异》记载："岭表山川，盘郁结聚，不易疏泄，故多岚雾作瘴。人感之多病，腹胀成蛊。"在与疾病做斗争的过程中，壮族先民逐步积累了丰富的医药知识和经验，形成了独特的壮医药文化体系。

壮医药文化是壮族传统文化中与医药相关的精神文化、组织制度文化和物质文化的总和，是壮族先民的生理病理观、病因病机论、诊疗方法和与之相关的心理指向、符号标记、民风民俗和药物器具等物质或非物质的表现形态，是壮医药与壮族各种文化交融、结合、渗透形成的产物。

一方面，壮医药文化是壮民族在历史上创造的医药文化，它对人体生命现象进行了观察和追踪，对人与自然的关系进行了思考与总结，本质上属于医学范畴，对本民族的生存繁衍做出了不可磨灭的贡献；另一方面，壮医药文化又蕴含了民族智慧、精神价值和思维方式等无形的内容，因而又具有较丰富的人文因素。总之，壮医药文化既有自然文化，又有人文文化；既有物质文化，又有非物质文化，还有非物质文化寓于物质文化之中难以分割的双重文化。

壮医药文化是壮民族创造的物质财富和精神财富之一，因此无疑也是人类文化特别是壮族文化的重要组成部分。

三、壮医药文化的基本类型

1. 精神文化

壮医药精神文化是壮医药哲学基础、生理病理观、治疗理念的反映，其核心部分是壮医药理论体系。

壮医药精神文化总的来说是唯物辩证的。

首先，就壮医对自然与人的认识而言，壮族先民认为，宇宙由天空、地面和水域"三界"组成，是客观物质的，而不是虚无缥缈的意识状态。人体相应地分为三部，人气与天地之气息息相通，"人不得逆天地"，人的生命周期受天地之气涵养和制约，天地之气是不断变化的，人作为万物之灵，对天地之气的变化有一定的主动适应能力。

其次，就壮医对人体生理病理认识而言，壮医认为，内脏、气、血、骨、肉是构成人体的主要物质基础。位于颅内和胸腔、腹腔内相对独立的实体都称为脏腑，没有很明确的"脏"和"腑"的区分观念。颅内容物壮语称为"坞",含有统筹、思考和主宰精神活动的意思。如精神病出现精神症状,壮医统称为"坞乱"或"巧坞乱",即总指挥部功能紊乱的意思。壮语称心脏为"咪心头",有脏腑之首的意思。壮语称肺为"咪钵",肝为"咪叠",胆为"咪背",肾为"咪腰",胰为"咪曼",脾为"咪隆",胃为"咪胴",肠为"咪虽",膀胱为"咪小肚",妇女胞宫为"咪花肠"。这些内脏各有自己的功能,共同维持人体的正常生理状态。当内脏实体受损伤或其他原因引起功能失调时,就会引起疾病。骨(壮语称为"夺")和肉(壮语称为"诺")构成人体的框架和形态,并保护人体内的脏器在一般情况下不受外部伤害。骨、肉还是人体的运动器官。壮医认为,血液(壮语称为"勒")是营养全身骨肉脏腑、四肢百骸的极为重要的物质,得天地之气而化生,赖天地之气以运行。壮医对气(壮语称为"嘘")极为重视。气是动力,是功能,是人体生命活动力的表现。气虽然肉眼看不见,但是可以感觉得到。

壮族是我国最早种植水稻的民族之一,知道五谷禀天地之气以生长,赖天地之气以收藏,得天地之气以滋养人体。其进入人体得以消化吸收的通道称为"谷道"(壮语称为"条根埃"),主要是指食管和胃肠。水为生命之源,人体由水道进水、出水,与大自然发生最直接、最密切的联系。水道与谷道同源而分流,在吸取水谷精微营养物质后,由谷道排出粪便,水道则主要排出汗、尿。气道是人体与大自然之气相互交换的通道,进出于口、鼻。三道畅通,调节有度,人体之气就能与天地之气保持同步协调平衡,即保持健康状态。三道阻塞或调节失度,则三气不能同步而疾病丛生。

壮医称龙路与火路是人体内虽未直接与大自然相通,但却能维持人体生机和反映疾病动态的两条极为重要的内封闭通路。壮族传统认为龙是制水的,龙路在人体内即是血液的通道(故有些壮医又称之为血脉、龙脉),功能主要是为内脏、骨、肉输送营养。龙路有干线及网络,遍布全身,循环往来,中枢在心脏。火为触发之物,其性迅速("火速"之谓),感之灼热。壮医认为,火路在人体内为传感之道,即现代语言所说的"信息通道"。其中枢在"巧坞"。火路同龙路一样,有干线及网络,遍布全身,使正常人体能在极短的时间内感受外界的各种信息和刺激,并经中枢"巧坞"的处理,迅速做出反应,以此来适应外界的各种变化,实现"三气同步"的生理平衡。

壮族地区位于亚热带,山林茂盛,气候湿热,动植物腐败产生瘴毒,野生有毒的动植物和其他毒物尤多,如毒草、毒树、毒虫、毒蛇、毒水、毒矿等。无数中毒致病甚至死亡的实例和教训,使壮族先民对毒有着特别直接和深刻的感受。邪毒、毒物进入人体后,是否发病取决于人体对毒的抵抗力和自身解毒功能的强弱,即取决于人体内正气的强弱。另外,壮医认为虚是两大致病因素之一,虚即正气虚或气血虚，虚既是致病的原因，同时也是病态的反映。毒和虚使人体失去常度而表现为病态。

最后，就壮医的治疗观念而言，在原始社会至封建社会时期，壮族先民不能对一些疾病进行合理解释，认为是鬼神作祟或受了毒咒，通过实施巫术可以驱邪除恶，这是客观唯心主义的反映。随着壮医对人体生理病理和病因病机认识的进一步深入，壮医对疾病的治疗逐步形成了"调气、解毒、补虚"的治疗原则，并有效地指导了临床诊疗疾病。

2. 制度文化

壮医药制度文化主要包括壮医诊治方法、用药规则以及一些医药卫生习俗。

壮医诊治方法多样且富有特色。壮医认为，人体是一个高度协调的生命体，除病灶异常外，在身体的任何部分发生病变，都会在体表有所表征，通过观察体表和一些简单的测试可以推断疾病。壮医诊术可以分为望诊、闻诊、询诊、按诊、探诊等五大类以及目诊、脉诊、甲诊、指诊、腹诊、野芋头试诊、石灰水试诊等数十种具体诊法。壮医治疗方法可以分为草药内服、外洗、熏蒸、敷贴、佩药、骨刮、角疗、灸法、挑针等几十种方法。

壮族地区地处亚热带，气候温和，雨量丰沛，草木生长茂盛，四季常青，药物资源十分丰富。壮医喜欢就地取材，逐渐形成喜用鲜药的习惯，如仙人掌、蒲公英、鲜生地、鲜芦根、鲜石斛、鲜藿香等，这些药既可用于内服，又可用于外敷。壮医在长期的临床实践中，积累了对药物功效的认识并编成广为流传的歌诀："辛行气血能解表，跌打风湿并散寒。酸主固涩能收敛，止泻固精疗虚汗。苦寒祛湿能攻下，治疗实热排便难。麻能镇痛散痈疖，并疗舌伤与顽痰。涩主收敛能抗菌，止血烧伤能消炎。咸味化痞散瘰疬，通便泻下可软坚。甘味和中亦滋补，调和百药能矫味。淡味祛湿亦利水，镇静除烦且安眠。"壮医还总结出药物形态与功用关系的歌诀："有毛能祛风，浆液可拔脓。中空能利水，方茎发散功。毛刺多消肿，蔓藤关节通。对枝又对叶，跌打风湿痛。叶梗都有毛，止血烧伤用。诸花能发散，凡子沉降宏。方梗开白花，寒性皆相同。红花又圆梗，性味多辛温。"壮医还把药物分为公药、母药以及主药、帮药、引药，根据需要进行药物配伍，以提高药物治疗的效果。

壮医药卫生习俗丰富多彩。在生活卫生方面，壮族人民喜断发，服饰尚青黑色，居干栏建筑。在防病保健习俗方面，佩药、赶药市、悬艾虎。在饮食养生习俗方面，讲究岁时饮食，如农历正月底采白头翁、艾叶和米为粽；农历三月初三采金银花、青艾等制成糯米糍粑；农历四月初八为浴佛节，炊乌米饭，食之以辟疫；农历五月初五，老少饮菖蒲酒、雄黄酒以辟疠疫。壮族人民善于制作药膳，如龙虎（蛇、猫）斗、龙凤（蛇、鸡）会、三蛇（眼镜蛇、金环蛇、灰鼠蛇）酒等。

3. 物质文化

壮医药物质文化也可称为有形文化，是指与医药相关的有形之物，主要包括诊

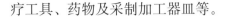

疗工具、药物及采制加工器皿等。

由于壮族历史上没有统一的语言文字，医药知识主要靠民间的口耳相传，而口耳相传的知识在每个时代或在不同的个体身上都会有不同的理解和诠释，从今天民间流传的神话故事、风俗人情来看，我们很难准确地描述壮医药文化发展的历史轨迹。然而，壮医药物质文化却向我们清晰地再现了古代壮族地区的医药卫生情况，广西南宁市武鸣区马头乡西周至春秋时期古墓中出土的青铜针、贵港市西汉古墓出土的铁冬青和银针充分说明壮族地区曾有过先进的医疗卫生水平。壮医广泛使用各种针、药线、瓷碗、骨弓、药锤、牛角、竹罐等医疗工具，相当部分至今仍在沿用。在药物方面，田七（又名三七）、肉桂、八角茴香、薏苡仁、罗汉果、珍珠等主产于壮族地区的名贵药材，早已为壮族群众所了解和广泛应用。如明代李时珍的《本草纲目》记载："田七，生于广西南丹诸州，番峒深山中，为金疮要药。"它们均具有实物的属性，属于壮医药物质文化的主要形式。新中国成立以来，科学技术的普及和发展大大丰富了壮医药物质文化，现代化的制药机械和造型精美、结构科学的诊疗器械正悄然改变着壮医药物质文化的内涵。

第二节 壮医药文化的发展历程

壮医药文化的形成在历史上是一个不断发展和变迁的过程。变迁源于内因和外因，内因的变迁是由于壮族生产力的发展、社会的进步和壮医药水平的提高，从而推动着壮医药文化不断丰富和发展，是一种由简单到复杂的过程，这种变迁是按照壮医药文化自身的规律发展的，是稳定而持续的；外因的变迁是壮医药文化在来自不同形态的其他民族医药文化的冲击和渗透下产生变化的过程，这种变迁是有限的，更多地产生于壮医药文化的物质技术层面或非核心理论层面，这是壮医药文化得以保持自身特色而存在的基础。从纵向历史发展来看，壮医药文化可以分为远古至先秦时期的萌芽阶段、秦代至隋代的初级阶段、唐代至民国时期的丰富发展阶段、新中国成立以来的整合发展阶段。

一、萌芽阶段（远古至先秦时期）

医药文化的产生与人类生产文化的出现相伴相随。距今 50000～20000 年，壮族地区已经有多处人类活动的踪迹。考古发现，在壮族聚居地区已发现的旧石器地点有 100 多处，仅在百色、田阳、田东、平果等 4 个市（县）境内的右江两岸的河流阶地上就发现了 75 处，并采集到各种类型的打制石器 1100 多件。这说明早在旧石器时代，壮族先民就已经会选择大小适中的砾石进行捶击，制造出粗糙的、适用的刃部和尖端，以便在生产和生活中用于砍砸、挖掘。在使用过程中，他们发现这些砾石碰撞人体某些部位可以使某些原有的病痛减轻或消失；他们在劳动及与野兽搏斗中常被石块、碎石击伤，但在碰撞或流血之后，也可使某些原有的病痛减轻或消失。这些出于偶然的生活经验，经过壮族先民若干年类似经历不断重现后，引起了先民的重视，进而反复实践并总结流传下来，成为现在的针刺疗法。

到了新石器时代，随着生产力水平不断提高，壮族先民与大自然、野兽斗争的本领不断增强，生活来源有了保障，经济生活相应地发生了一定的变化。新石器时代文化相比旧石器时代文化，有了明显的进步，同时也大大地促进了医药卫生的发展。这个时期，壮族先民发明了人、畜分居的干栏式建筑，这是壮族先民在恶劣环境下求得生存的重要卫生保健手段。同时，人、畜隔离也体现了壮族先民的卫生保健意识。壮族先民发明了石器的磨光技术及陶器。在桂林甑皮岩、柳州鲤鱼嘴、南宁豹子头等遗址出土了大量丰富多彩的磨光石器。在这些遗址出土的陶器（片），是目前我国发现的年代最为古老的陶器（片）。有了陶器，人们就可以用来煮食物，这利于食物的消化和人体的健康，同时伴随着壮族地区陶瓷文化的崛起，壮医陶针疗法逐渐出现，因其疗效显著，简便易行，至今仍在壮乡民间流传不衰。

周朝末期至春秋时期，壮族地区的社会发展开始步入金属时代，金属的冶炼，不仅使壮族先民的文化生活向前迈进了一步，而且使针刺治疗工具有了改进。广西南宁市武鸣区马头乡的西周至春秋时期古墓中，出土了两枚精致的青铜针。据考证这两枚青铜针是壮族先民的针刺工具，这反映了古代壮族先民在医药方面的成就与社会的发展是密切相关的。

先秦时期，壮族社会还处于部落联盟时代，生产力水平十分低下，壮族先民对自然界的各种现象，如地震、洪水、火山爆发等，甚至最平常的日出、日落、刮风、下雨、雷鸣、闪电等无穷变化的大自然奥秘无法解释，特别是对人在夜间做梦和生老病死更是感到神秘莫测。因此，他们便开始无边无际的幻想，最终臆断世界之外一定存在着某种超自然的力量和神秘的境界主宰自然和社会，于是巫文化产生了。巫文化对壮医产生了重大的影响，如左江花山壁画表现了壮族先民对日、月、星辰的崇拜。有专家认为，除了舞蹈动作，还有些可能是诊疗图，既有施术者和持器（具）者，又有受术者，结合崖壁画的祭祀场面，联系壮族先民的巫文化特点，应当说崖壁画有巫医治病的内容。巫文化对壮医药的影响，首先是"巫""医"合一，然后是"医""巫"并存，最后是"医"盛于"巫"。

二、初级阶段（秦代至隋代）

由于历史和地理条件等方面的原因，壮族地区的社会发展比较缓慢，在商周时期，中原地区已进入奴隶制社会，而地处岭南的壮族地区还属蛮荒之地，处于原始社会末期的部落联盟或军事民主阶段。直到公元前221年秦始皇统一了中国，壮族地区才开始处于中央集权封建王朝的直接统辖之下，经济社会得以快速发展。

秦代至隋代，随着生产力的发展和进步，壮族先民开始有了良好的卫生保健和环保意识，从广西合浦望牛岭西汉晚期墓出土的具有消烟作用的铜凤灯到广西钟山东汉墓出土的陶厕所模型，均反映了壮族先民良好的卫生习惯。另外，一些卫生用具的出土，从另一个角度反映了壮族先民早在 2000 年前就养成了一些良好的卫生习惯，如广西贵港市新村 11 号东汉墓出土的陶虎子（溺器，即现在使用的尿壶）、广西贵港市罗泊湾西汉墓出土的鎏金铜挖耳勺、广西荔浦县兴坪汉墓出土的陶痰盂等。这些对卫生保健的认识，在当时社会发展缓慢、生产力落后、医疗卫生条件差的情况下，是非常难能可贵的。

这一时期壮族先民对于疾病对人体健康的危害已经有了一定的认识。《后汉书·马援传》云："出征交趾，士多瘴气""军吏经瘴疫死者十四五"。隋代巢元方《诸病源候论》指出，瘴气是"杂毒因暖而生""皆由山溪源岭瘴湿毒气故也"。但这一时期人们对于疾病的认识比较笼统，对疾病的类别区分不清，把致病因素统称为"瘴气"，把病名统称为"瘴疫"。晋代葛洪在《肘后方》中记载了壮族先辈治疗脚气病、防治沙虱毒（恙虫病）的经验，对毒、解毒方法也多次提及。

同一时期，壮族地区新的药物品种不断增加，原有的药物也增加了新的用途。在《山海经》《神农本草经》中有不少先秦时期壮族地区的药物和壮族先民用药经验的记载。在秦、汉、魏、晋、南北朝时期，关于壮医药物的记载就更丰富了。晋代嵇含著的《南方草木状》记载了吉利草、薤、豆蔻花等许多壮医用药。晋代葛洪在《诸病源候论》中记载了壮族先民防治瘴、蛊、毒的用药经验。1976 年，在广西贵港市罗泊湾一号汉墓中出土了大批植物种子和果实，经鉴定有不少是药用植物，这说明当时在壮族地区已普遍使用植物药防病治病，药物疗法已有了一定的根基。

秦代至隋代，汉文化对壮族地区产生了重大的影响，由于州学、县学的设立，儒家思想得到了广泛的宣传。随着壮族与中原汉族交流的不断深入，壮族地区的社会、政治、文化、习俗以及医药等情况，通过汉人的著述，得以传播和保留下来，自《山海经》《神农本草经》之后，壮医药见之于文献记载越来越多。

三、丰富发展阶段（唐代至民国时期）

唐代至民国时期，随着壮族地区经济、政治、文化的发展，壮医药从草创走向形成，壮医药文化不断丰富繁荣，达到了鼎盛时期。

唐、宋时代是我国封建社会经济繁荣发展的时期，壮族地区的经济也有了较大的发展，壮医药知识也由零星积累逐渐系统化，壮医理论已处于萌芽状态，壮医对壮族地区常见和多发的瘴、毒、蛊、痧、风、湿等病证的防治达到了相当的水平。唐代文学家、政治家柳宗元被贬到柳州任刺史后，曾亲自收集壮族民间验方，并在自己身上使用，留下了记述疗疮案、脚气案和霍乱案的《柳州救三死方》。宋代范成大的《桂海虞衡志》指出："瘴，二广惟桂林无之。自是而南，皆瘴乡矣。"又说"两江（按：指左江、右江）水土尤恶，一岁无时无瘴""瘴者，山岚水毒与草莽岑气，郁勃蒸熏之所为也，其中人如疟状"，明确指出了瘴气症状如疟疾。宋代周去非的《岭外代答》不仅较为详细地记述了瘴疾的壮医治疗方法，而且还指出了瘴的病因病机："盖天气郁蒸，阳气宣泄，冬不闭藏，草木水泉，皆禀恶气，人生其间，日受其毒，元气不固，发为瘴疾。"这些文献记载虽然不是直接出自壮医之手，但是作者在壮族地区为官多年，对当地风土人情有所了解，反映了当时壮医对瘴病的认识水平，因而是具有参考价值的。与此同时，壮医方药学开始出现雏形，《新修本草》是唐显庆二年（657年）由苏敬等22人编纂，历时2年完成，由朝廷颁发的药典。它是世界上最早的国家药典，共载药850种，其中收载了部分壮族地区药物，如蚺蛇胆、滑石、钓樟根皮、茯苓、桂、蒜、槟榔、白花藤、莎草科、苏方木、狼跋子等。《本草拾遗》也收录了出自壮族地区有名的陈家白药和甘家白药。

元、明、清时期，壮族地区进入了千年土司制度时代。这个漫长的历史阶段，也正是壮医药发展较快的时期。在土司制度下，官方设有医药机构，官方和民间有一定数量的专职医药人员，明代以后广西各地的府、州、县志对此都有明确的记载。据不完全统计，明代嘉靖十年（1531年），广西壮族聚居的40多个府（州、县）土司均设有医学署，如庆远府、思恩县、天河县、武缘县、永淳县、南宁府等（均为壮族聚居地）。特别值得一提的是，这些医学署的医官"本为土人"，即由本民族的医生担任，这对于壮医药的发展是一个促进因素，这也说明土官对本民族的传统医药，相对来说还是比较重视的。

明、清时期，壮医对人体生理病理和本地常见病、多发病已有深刻的认识，根据病证和病因病机把它们区分为痧、瘴、蛊、毒、风、湿等，并总结出了目诊、脉诊、甲诊、指诊、腹诊等诊断方法和草药内服、外洗、熏蒸、敷贴、佩药、骨刮、角疗、灸法、挑针等治疗方法，创制了大量的验方、秘方。壮医药经过漫长的发展历史，到了晚清和民国时期，已初步形成了比较完整的体系，医学著作及名医随之产生，为壮医药的初步形成打下了基础。

从唐代至民国时期的漫长发展历史过程中，伴随着医药知识的积累和应用，人们对壮医药日益重视，与壮医药相关的文化亦日趋繁荣，其突出表现是有关壮医药起源的神话传说"神医三界公""爷奇斗瘟神"开始在壮族地区流传，出现了对名医、神医、药王的崇拜和纪念。清代的《宁明州志·上卷·祠庙》中记载："医灵庙在东门外附近城脚。"清代的《邕宁县志·卷四十三·祠祀志》谓："药王庙，在北门大街，东岳庙左侧。"清代的《柳州县志·卷三》称："药王庙，在西门内。"清代以前，壮族地区基本上没有西医，中医也为数不多。这些被立庙纪念的神医、药王，尽管没有标出姓名，但在很大程度上可以说是民间名医，在壮族地区即是壮医。他们医术高明、医德高尚，能为患者解除疾病痛苦而受到群众的敬仰。又如在忻城土司衙门附近，现仍保存有一座清代修建的三界庙，三界是一位精通治疗内科、外科、五官科等疾病的神医，名气很大，因此得以立庙享受百姓香火。三界庙能修到土司衙门旁边，亦可以从侧面反映出这位神医在壮族人民心目中的崇高形象。这一阶段，赶药市习俗开始形成。壮族地区境内山多林密，百草丛生，药材资源十分丰富。每年农历五月初五，壮乡各村寨的乡民都去赶药市，将自采的各种药材运到圩镇药市出售，或去买药、看药、闻药。壮乡民俗认为，农历五月初五的草药根肥叶茂，药力宏大，疗效最好，这天去药市，饱吸百药之气，就可以预防疾病，全年能少生病或不生病。久而久之，赶药市就成了壮乡民俗，每到农历五月初五这天，即使无药出售的壮族人民，都扶老携幼赶往药市去吸百药之气，这种群防群治的良好风俗，至今仍被壮乡保留。

四、整合发展阶段（新中国成立以来）

壮医药文化虽然有悠久的历史、丰富的内涵，但是在新中国成立前，由于社会上存在对少数民族的偏见和歧视，一直没有得到政府应有的重视。新中国成立以后，在党的民族政策和中医政策的指引下，壮医药文化的发掘、整理和研究工作得到了政府有关部门的重视和支持。特别是从1984年全国民族医药工作会议之后，壮医药的发掘、整理工作在20世纪50～70年代民间中草药调查和个人撰写零星文章的基础上，进入了有组织、大规模的调查研究和全面系统整理阶段。

新中国成立前，虽然在地方志中看到土司衙署内有医药设施的记载，但是至新中国成立前夕，这些机构早已荡然无存。为了继承和弘扬壮医药，1984年广西中医学院（今广西中医药大学）成立了壮医药研究室，首批国医大师班秀文教授被任命为研究室主任。1985年，该研究室招收了我国医史上第一批壮医史硕士研究生。1985年4月，经广西壮族自治区卫生厅批准，我国第一家壮医门诊部在广西中医学院本部正式开诊。著名壮医药线点灸疗法专家龙玉乾、著名壮医挑针疗法专家罗家安、著名壮医杂病专家郭廷璋等应聘到该门诊部工作。

1985年，经国家科委（今科学技术部）和广西壮族自治区人民政府批准，我国首家省区级民族医药科研机构——广西民族医药研究所（今广西民族医学研究院）在南宁市成立。1993年2月，中国中医研究院决定将该所作为研究院的民族医药研究基地，加挂"中国中医研究院广西民族医药研究所"的牌子。

1986年下半年，广西壮族自治区卫生厅成立了少数民族医药古籍普查整理领导小组，全区共抽调200多人组成专业调查队伍。历时6年，调查人员对大量分散在地方志、博物志、正史、野史、中医药著作以及有关民族、民俗、考古等资料中的壮医文献进行了收集整理，对数千名民间壮医进行了造册登记，对大量的民间验方、秘方以及药物标本进行了汇编和收藏。

经过艰苦细致的文献搜集和广泛深入的实地调研考察工作，科研人员从数百种地方志和其他有关汉文资料中，汇集了大量记载壮医药的文字资料，收集了壮医药验方、秘方上万条，发掘整理了多种壮医行之有效的独特诊疗方法，获得了一批壮医药文物和手抄本，对3000多名较有专长的壮医名医进行了造册登记。在此基础上，科研人员发表了《靖西县壮族民间医药情况考察报告》《关于壮族医学史的初步探讨》《壮药源流初探》《壮族先民使用微针考》《广西自然地理与壮族医药》《土司制度下的广西民族医药》《壮医理论体系概述》《浅谈壮医三道两路学说的具体运用》等论文，出版了《发掘整理中的壮医》《广西民族医药验方汇编》《壮药选编》《广西壮药新资源》《壮族医学史》《中国壮医学》等壮医药专著。广西中医学院和广西民族医药研究所的科研人员，运用传统和现代的方法手段，对壮医药线点灸疗法和壮医药罐疗法进行了深入发掘、整理、研究，取得了丰硕的成果，并逐步在临床上推广应用。1995年5月，在国家中医药管理局批准召开的"南宁全国民族医药学术交流会"上，广西民族医药研究所的科研人员做了《壮医基础理论初探》的报告。该报告是在多年调查研究的基础上撰写的，比较全面系统地阐述和论证了壮医的理论体系——"三气同步""三道两路""毒虚致病"等理论。这标志着壮医药的发掘整理研究，已从整体上提高到了一个新的水平。

经过30多年的努力，壮医药在古籍发掘整理、理论体系构建、诊疗方法研究、药物研究、临床应用推广等诸多方面取得了重大成果。同时随着壮族文化与壮医药的关系、壮医药文化价值及其开发利用等方面的研究不断开展和深入，古老的壮医药文化在不断挖掘历史积淀和吸取先进文化精华的整合过程中得到丰富和发展。

参考文献：

[1] 梁庭望. 壮族文化概论 [M]. 南宁：广西教育出版社，2000.

[2] 郭建庆. 中国文化概述 [M]. 2版. 上海：上海交通大学出版社，2005.

[3] 黄汉儒，黄景贤，殷昭红. 壮族医学史 [M]. 南宁：广西科学技术出版社，1998.

[4] 庞宇舟. 壮医药文化概念和内涵初探 [J]. 中国民族民间医药，2007，89（6）：322 - 324.

[5] 庞宇舟，王春玲. 壮医药文化概述 [J]. 中国中医基础医学杂志，2009，15（10）：800 - 802.

第二章　壮医药文化的特征与表现形态

第一节　壮医药文化的特征

一、悠久灿烂的历史

壮医药有着悠久灿烂的历史。作为远古时代就生活在壮族地区的土著民族，壮族先民居住在崇山峻岭地区，这些地区江河纵横、草木茂盛、潮湿多雨、瘴疠横生、毒虫猛兽出没无常。恶劣的自然环境和生存条件，迫使壮族先民创造了原始的医疗手段。可以说，就起源而论，壮医药和华夏其他民族的医药是同时或相继出现的。

从远古时代开始，经过先秦时期以前的草创萌芽，秦汉时期至隋代的实践积累，唐宋时期至民国时期的形成与发展，新中国成立以后的发掘整理和提高，壮医药文化从无到有，从简单到丰富，从零星到系统，走过了漫长辉煌的发展历程。

在不同的历史时期，壮医药文化不论是在物质上还是在精神上，都有自己的独特之处，既丰富了壮族文化内容，又打上了壮族传统文化的烙印。

二、浓厚的地域特色

壮族是中华民族的重要组成部分，其社会历史发展基本上与中原汉族一致，但是由于特殊的地理环境和政治、经济、文化状况等因素，壮族的社会历史发展具有一些明显的特点，这些特点对壮族文化的形成和发展有着重大的影响。

壮族有自己独特的文化，以稻作文化为例，壮族是世界上最早种植稻类的民族之一，也是我国最早创造稻作文明的民族之一，世代以水稻为主食。近年来，国内外学者根据考古资料和史籍有关野生稻分布的记载以及考察研究，认为亚洲栽培稻起源于从中国杭州湾到印度阿萨姆邦这一广阔的半月形地带。壮族所聚居的岭南地区，气候温暖，雨量丰沛，土地肥沃，水源条件好，适宜稻谷生长。壮族先民早在4000年前就会稻作农耕，在广西防城港亚菩山、马兰咀山、杯较山的贝丘遗址发现的磨盘、石器就是壮族先民种植水稻的证据。经过漫长的稻作农耕，壮族形成了由于稻作生产所发生的有关谷物生产发展的一系列问题，以及由于稻作生产影响所及的民间生活方式和种种习俗的稻作文化。稻作文化对壮族的生产、生活、礼仪、民族性格和深层心理，都产生了深刻持久的影响。

　　稻作文化是壮族文化的重要标志，是壮族文化形成的基础，不仅对壮族文化产生了深远的影响，而且还赋予了壮医药文化浓厚的地域特色。稻，根在地，养在天，利于人。稻作文化使壮族先民对阴阳有了较早的认识，形成了阴阳概念。明朝的《广西通志·卷十七》记载壮族民间"笃信阴阳"。壮族称水田为"那"，稻作文化即"那"文化。"那"有最基本的"三横两纵"经纬线，"那"文化是壮医"三道两路"理论的基本定格。壮族先民在日常生活中观察到，水稻禀天地之气以生长，赖天地之气以收藏，得天地之气以滋养人体，而人体则赖"谷物"以养，一日三餐不可或缺，于是将谷物得以进入人体并消化吸收之通道称为"谷道"（壮语称为"条根埃"）。水稻离不开天地之精气涵养和水的滋润，人身亦有与天地进行气和水交换的通道，称为"气道"（壮语称为"条河卡"）和"水道"（壮语称为"条亡林"）。稻作文化离不开水和火，壮族先民崇拜龙，认为龙能制水，而人身有血液运行的通道，壮医称之为"龙路"（壮语称为"条默陆"）。火为触发之物，其性迅速，人身有信息传感通道，其性似火，壮医称之为"火路"（壮语称为"条晕陆"）。壮医"三道两路"理论就源于壮族先民对人与自然的朴素认识和实践经验总结。

　　不仅稻作文化赋予了壮医理论浓厚的地域特色，而且壮族文化中隐含的大量的医疗卫生价值取向的习俗文化、歌谣文化、节庆文化、饮食文化、人居文化、体育文化也具有浓郁的地域民族特色。如在壮族饮食文化中，桂西北地区的壮族人有喝羊糜汤、生羊血的习俗，在外族人看来，实在难以下咽，但对于当地的壮族人来说，羊糜汤清热养胃，生羊血补虚健体，是难得的保健佳肴。

三、丰富的医学内涵

1. 朴素的天人自然观

　　壮族先民在长期的医疗实践中形成了独特的天人自然观。壮医认为，自然界的空间分上、中、下三部，被称为"天、地、人"三部，这三部之气是同步运行的。人体也分为上、中、下三部，上部为天（壮语称为"巧"），下部为地（壮语称为"胴"），中部为人（壮语称为"廊"），人体的天、地、人三部之气也是同步运行的。在生理上，人体的天、地、人三部只有与自然界（上、中、下）同步运行，制约化生，生生不息，人体才能达到健康境界；在病理上，若天、地、人三气不能同步运行，则百病丛生。壮医的天人自然观实际上与中医的天人合一同属"整体观念"范畴，而壮医更加突出人与自然及人体各部位的平衡关系，把"天、地、人三气不同步论"作为病机的重要方面。

2. 独特的生理病理理论

　　（1）阴阳为本理论。壮医认为，万物皆可分阴阳，万变皆由阴阳起，此即阴阳为本理论。壮族先民在生产生活中广泛使用阴阳解释天人关系，说明人体生理病理。

如自然界，天为阳，地为阴；白天为阳，黑夜为阴；火为阳，水为阴。人体，背为阳，腹为阴；外为阳，内为阴。疾病方面，分阳证、阴证。因此，壮医认为大自然的一切变化都是阴阳变化的结果，人体的一切生理病理变化、疾病转归都是阴阳变化的结果。著名壮医罗家安在其所著的《痧证针方图解》一书中，明确以阴盛阳衰、阳盛阴衰、阴盛阳盛对各种痧证进行分类，作为辨证的总纲。

（2）三气同步理论。三气同步是指只有"天、地、人"三气协调平稳运行，才能保证人体的最佳生命状态。"天"指天气，"地"指地气，二者合称天地自然之气。"三气"指天、地、人三气，同步指保持协调平衡。三气同步，即天、地、人三者协调平衡的状态。三气同步理论内涵包括：人禀天地之气而生，为万物之灵；人的生命周期受天地之气的涵养与制约，人气与天地之气相通；天地之气为人体造就了生存和健康的一定"常度"；人本身也是一个小天地，是一个有限的小宇宙单元；人体结构与功能的统一，先天之气与后天之气的协调，使人体具有一定的适应与防卫能力，从而达到天、地、人三气同步的健康境界。三气同步形成了壮医的生理病理观，成为壮医诊断治疗的重要理论依据之一。

（3）"三道两路"理论。三道，是维持人体生命活动的营养物质化生、贮藏、运行以及糟粕排泄输布的通道，即谷道、气道、水道。两路，指龙路与火路，是人体内虽未直接与大自然相通，但却能维持人体生机和反映疾病动态的两条极为重要的内封闭通路。"三道两路"中，谷道是食物消化吸收及精微输布的通道，也是糟粕排泄的通道；气道是人体一身之气化生、输布、贮藏的处所；水道则是人体水液的化生、贮藏、输布、运行的场所；龙路是体内血液运行的场所，也是约束血液运行的通道，其中枢在心脏（咪心头），其功能主要是为内脏、骨肉、官窍输送营养物质；火路是体内传感各种信息，以维持人体内外环境之间的平衡，以及调节体内生理平衡的通路。"三道两路"各司其职，分工合作，生理上互相配合，密切联系；病理上常可相互影响，相互传变。

（4）对脏腑、气血、骨肉和脑的认识。壮医认为，脏腑、气血、骨肉是构成人体的物质基础。其中，位于颅内、胸腔、腹腔内相对独立的实体称脏腑。脏腑各有不同的生理功能，在生命过程中，各负其责，各有所主。气（嘘）是功能，是动力，是生命活力的表现；血（勒）是营养全身脏腑骨肉、四肢百骸的重要物质。骨（夺）肉（诺）构成人体框架和外形，是人体运动器官，保护内脏器官不受伤害，人体的谷道、气道、水道、龙路、火路等运行于其内。骨肉损伤，可导致人体重要通道的损伤，从而引发其他疾病。脑（巧坞），壮医将人的精神活动、语言及思考能力，归结为"巧坞"的功能。"巧坞"是髓汇聚的场所，主精神思维，是精髓和神明高度汇聚之处，如出现精神症状，壮医称为"巧坞乱"。

3. 别具一格的病因病机学说

壮医认为，毒和虚是危害机体健康，导致疾病的重要病因病机。"毒虚致百病"

是壮医主要的病因病机理论。毒邪有广义和狭义之分，广义的毒邪是指一切致病因素的总称；狭义的毒邪是指对机体产生毒性作用的一类致病物质的总称。毒邪种类繁多，但致病机理大都相似，有的损伤皮肉；有的危害脏腑功能和"三道两路"；有的毒性剧烈，人遭受毒邪后立即发病，甚至死亡；有的毒性比较缓和，起缓慢毒性作用。毒邪之所以致病，主要是因为其损害人体正气，危及脏腑功能或损伤形体。各种毒邪由于性质的不同，在临床上表现出各种不同的典型症状和体征。

虚既是发病的原因，也是病理的结果和病态的表现。壮医特别注意"虚"在病因病机中的重要作用。作为病因，虚可以导致脏腑功能减退，也可以导致防卫外邪的能力下降，从而使人体更容易感染外邪和毒邪，进而形成虚、毒并存的局面，病理表现为二者相互影响的恶性循环。正气不足，适应能力和调节能力低下，人体容易对外界的情志刺激产生较为剧烈的反应，从而引发情志病。作为病理结果，虚既可以导致发病，也可以导致死亡。如正气亏虚，"邪气"内生而发病。因为正气不足，正气对脏腑、官窍功能活动的调节能力下降，脏腑、官窍功能失常，由此产生各种病理产物而发病。当正气亏虚到一定程度，失去了对人体的调节能力时，就可能导致死亡。

壮医认为，毒和虚是导致疾病发生的主要原因。毒和虚使人体失去常度而表现为病态，如果这种病态得到适当的治疗，或者人的自我防卫、自我修复能力能够战胜毒邪和虚，则人体常度逐步恢复，疾病趋于好转而痊愈，否则，终因三气不能同步，导致人体气脱、气竭而死亡。

4. 特色鲜明的诊断和辨病方法

壮医对眼睛（勒答）极为重视，认为眼睛是天地赋予人体的窗口，是光明的使者，是天、地、人三气的精华所在。人体脏腑之精上注于目，所以眼睛能包含一切，洞察一切，也能反映百病。同时，眼睛长在头（巧坞）上，直接受头指挥，因此在疾病诊断上，壮医把目诊提到十分重要的地位。壮医目诊是通过观察病人眼睛血管的分布、走向、大小、颜色、弯曲度、斑点等细微变化来诊断全身疾病，正所谓"一目了然"。目诊可以确诊疾病，可以推测预后，也可以确定死亡。对于人体内的脏腑气血、"三道两路""巧坞"功能等，都可以通过目诊而获得相对准确的信息。壮医重视目诊，但并不排斥其他的诊断方法，如问诊、闻诊、脉诊、甲诊、指诊、腹诊等都具有一定的特色。

壮医强调以辨病为主，文献记载和实地调查搜集到的壮医病证名称达数百种之多，其中不少病证名称具有浓厚的岭南地方民族特色。就内科疾病来说，概括起来主要有痧、瘴、蛊、毒、风、湿六大类。壮医的辨病类似于西医的辨病，患什么病就用什么药，故壮医治病常专病专方专药，辨病是决定治疗原则和选方用药的主要依据。

5. 有效指导实践的治疗原则

壮医根据对人体生理病理和病因病机的认识，提出了调气、解毒、补虚的治疗原则，并有效地指导临床实践。

调气，即通过各种治疗方法（多用针灸、刺血、拔罐、引舞气功等非药物疗法），调节、激发或通畅人体之气，使之正常运行，与天地之气保持三气同步。气病在临床上主要表现为疼痛以及其他一些功能障碍性疾病，一般通过针灸、刺血、拔罐和药物调气即可恢复正常。

解毒，即通过内服药物或外治疗法，减少毒邪入体，或加快毒物的排泄，或化解体内之毒，从而达到三气得以恢复同步运行，疾病得以康复的目的。毒病在临床上主要表现为红肿痛热、溃烂、肿瘤、疮疖、黄疸、血液病等急性炎症和器官组织器质性病变以及同时出现的功能改变。通过药物或非药物解毒治疗，有些毒在人体内可以化解，有些毒则需通过"三道"来清除，毒去则正安气复而向愈。

补虚，即通过内服药物或食疗的方法，补充体内亏虚的气血，调整人体内不平衡的三气，以使三气能正常运行，保持人气与天地之气三气同步。以虚为主要临床表现的，多见于慢性病、老年病以及邪毒祛除之后的恢复期，治疗上以补虚为首要任务。壮医重视食疗和使用动物药，认为人应顺其自然，通过食疗来补虚最为常用。因人为灵物，同气相求，壮医认为以血肉有情的动物药来补虚最为有效。

6. 丰富的药物知识、用药习惯和独创的用药配伍

壮医认为，壮药的治疗作用是通过药物的性味，调整人体阴阳偏胜和三气不同步、"三道两路"不通畅等病理状态而实现的。药有动物药、植物药和矿物药，以功用区分为有毒药、解毒药、治瘴气药、治跌打损伤药、清热药、补益药、治痧证药、祛风湿药、杀虫药等。壮族地区的药物品种繁多，有毒的动植物也很多，壮族人民在长期的实践中大胆应用本地出产的毒药治病，并积累了丰富的经验，形成了独特的毒药应用理论。壮医还善于使用解毒药，认为有什么样的邪毒致病，必然有相应的解毒药治病，即所谓"一物降一物"。

壮族地区草木繁茂，四季常青，使壮医形成了喜用鲜药的习惯。壮医在长期的用药实践中发现某一种药配上另一种或几种药使用效果会更好，通过历代不断总结，逐渐形成自己独到的药物配伍方法和方剂。壮医认为，人只有两种病证——阴证和阳证。因此处方中设有公药、母药，相对应用于阴证、阳证。壮医的药物配伍讲求简、便、廉、验，一般由主药、帮（配）药、引药和解毒药组成一个方，各类药物在方中作用明确，主次分明，互相兼顾。一般四五味药即成一方，很少超过十味药。

7. 对针灸形成发展的特殊贡献

进入新石器时代之后，随着壮族地区陶瓷文化的发展，壮族先民的陶针疗法开始出现，到战国时期已较为流行，并对中医"九针"的形成产生了积极影响。据对

现存的壮医陶针的考证，其针形与九针之首——镵（chán）针极为相似。壮医陶针至今仍在壮族民间使用。南宁市武鸣区马头乡西周古墓中出土的 2 枚精细的青铜针，据考证为壮族先民的针刺用具，结合《黄帝内经》中"故九针者，亦从南方来"的论述，说明壮族地区是针刺疗法、九针的发源地之一。2000 多年来，壮族先民不仅具有较高的制针技术，而且从总体上来看，其针刺疗法乃至医药整体水平在当时处于先进行列。

四、多彩的医药习俗

1. 生活卫生习俗

（1）断发。《庄子·内篇·逍遥游》记载，"宋人资章甫而适诸越，越人断发文身，无所用之"，所谓"断发"者，"剪发使短，……而不束发加冠之意也"。根据《汉书·地理志》记载，从吴越到岭南九郡，越人都有"断发"的习俗。从广西宁明花山岩画上的人物像来看，壮族先民——骆越人的发饰确实有"断发"情况存在，不管壮族先民最初基于何种原因而"断发"，由于"断发"后头发易干且利于体温散发，适应于骆越地区湿热为主的气候环境，因此"断发"习俗符合卫生要求。

（2）服饰尚青黑。壮族有植棉纺纱的习惯，用自种自纺的棉纱织出来的布称为"家机"，古代、近代壮族人民多以蓝靛做染料，染成黑色或蓝色，黑色是壮族服饰的主色调。至今，这种主色调仍保留在那坡县与龙州县等地的壮族群体中，如百色市那坡县黑衣壮、崇左市龙州县金龙一带自称"布代"的壮族人民。据记载，蓝靛为十字花科植物菘蓝、草大青，以豆科植物木蓝、爵床科植物马蓝或蓼科植物蓼蓝等叶所制成的染料，具有清热解毒的作用。因此，壮族的青黑色服饰具有解毒作用，可防避蚊虫，适合壮族地区的气候环境。

（3）居干栏建筑。壮族先民根据壮族地区的地理环境和气候条件，很早就发明了干栏建筑，这种建筑的特点是分上、下两层，上层作为人的居所，下层贮放农具或圈养牲畜。《魏书·僚人篇》记载："僚者，盖南蛮之别种……依树积木，以居其上，名曰干栏。"干栏建筑远离地面，既可避虎狼蛇虫侵袭，又可防避毒邪瘴气。干栏建筑使人、畜分离，起到了卫生和保健的作用，不少壮族地区至今仍保留着这种居住习俗。

2. 崇巫尊祖习俗

（1）尚巫术。巫术是原始宗教的一项重要活动内容，先秦时期，骆越人盛行巫术，笃信鬼神。壮族先民由于信仰鬼神而产生了巫文化，古时壮巫分巫婆和魔公，主家有病痛或灾难，请巫婆和神对话，问明病灾的缘由，再择吉日请魔公行法事，杀畜禽敬祭，劝离神仙，禳解厄难，舞刀剑，烧油锅，镇妖赶鬼。直到近现代，壮族地区的巫风仍有所遗存。巫文化对壮医药的影响，首先是"巫""医"合一，然后是"医""巫"并存，最后是"医"盛于"巫"。

（2）文身。壮族先民在史前社会就有文身的习俗，宋代《太平寰宇记》载，邕州左江、右江各州"其百姓悉是雕题、凿齿、画面、文身"。文身习俗的形成最早是出于氏族、部落的图腾标志或图腾徽号，目的是为了求得图腾神的保佑，所谓"以避蛟龙之害"者是也；同时又便于彼此间进行交际和通婚过程中认同和区别。由于文身需用浅刺针具，更重要的是文身活动带有宗教性质，在一定的历史时期会激励壮族人民去效仿，因此文身对壮医浅刺疗法的形成和发展起到一定的促进作用。

（3）捡骨重葬。壮族地区至今流行"二次葬"（捡骨重葬）的习俗。即人死 3 年后，子女将死者遗骨捡出，装入陶罐（壮话叫作"金罐"），选择坟山宝地重新安葬。捡骨重葬体现了壮族人民尊祖和讲究坟山风水的民俗，这一习惯客观上促进了壮医对人体骨骼的正确认识。

3. 防病保健习俗

（1）重预防。壮族地区山高林密，多雨酷热，壮族人民在晨间瘴气雾露弥漫时外出赶路，必口含生姜以辟秽；野外耕作，为防暴雨淋湿后伤风感冒，常取姜葱汤淋浴及热服，以祛寒湿；溽暑天月，高温多雨，对饮用之水，壮族人民必先用白矾过滤，并多吃生大蒜头，以防虫毒在体内滋生；当疬疫流行之时，走村串寨回家，常用草药汤洗澡，以避秽解毒；年老体弱者，常用辟秽解毒或舒筋活络之品垫席而睡；正在发育的儿童，则于胸腹佩戴芳香解毒之品。

（2）赶药市。壮族地区草木繁茂，四季常青，药材资源十分丰富。每年农历五月初五这天，壮乡各村寨的乡民都去赶药市，将自采的各种药材运到圩镇药市出售，或去买药、看药、闻药。当地的习俗认为，端午节的草药根肥叶茂，药力宏大，疗效最好。这天去药市，饱吸百药之气，就可以预防疾病，全年能少生病或不生病。久而久之，赶药市就成了壮乡民俗，其中尤以靖西市的端午药市最为著名。每到端午节，即使无药出售的壮族人民，都扶老携幼赶往药市去吸百药之气。赶药市既是交流药材知识和防治经验的好机会，也是壮族人民崇尚医药的体现。

（3）悬艾虎。悬艾和饮菖蒲酒是壮族端午节非常重要的活动。《靖西县志》记载："五月五日，家家悬艾虎，持蒲剑，饮雄黄酒，以避疠疫。"农历五月初五的清晨，壮族人民在鸡还没有叫之前就要将艾采摘回来，用艾叶、艾根做成人形或老虎的形状（俗称"艾虎"），悬在门楣的中央；将菖蒲制成宝剑挂在屋檐下。这一天还要用艾叶、菖蒲、大蒜烧水洗澡，并将水洒在房前屋后。其实，这样做是非常符合夏季卫生要求的。端午节后，天气转热，正是各种病菌生长繁殖的时期，用中草药煮水喷洒，可有效地遏制病菌的生长乃至消灭病菌，清洁环境卫生。这与在端午节饮菖蒲酒是同一个道理。菖蒲性温和，可以化痰、祛湿、润肺、祛风寒，对预防夏季外感病有一定的作用。

4. 防疫防毒习俗

（1）佩药。壮族聚居地地处岭南，属于亚热带地区，山峦起伏，江河溪沟密布，林木茂盛，加之气候多雨潮湿，空气中湿热交蒸，酿成瘴毒。因感受瘴毒而发的疾病称之为"瘴气"，是当时壮族地区的常见病和多发病。《后汉书·马援传》载，"出征交趾，士多瘴气""军吏经瘴疫死者十四五"，可见瘴气危害之甚。壮族先民总结了具有民族特色的祛瘴法。每年春、夏季将自采的草药扎成药把挂于门外或放置房中，以辟秽祛瘴。常用的药物有菖蒲叶、佩兰叶、艾叶、青蒿叶等。家中若有未成年孩童，则令其佩戴各种香药制成的药囊，意在扶正祛瘴。常用的药物有檀香、苍术、木香等。在瘴疠流行季节，村寨里无论男女老幼，都佩戴药囊，以避邪防瘴，预防或减少瘴疫的发生。这些防瘴习俗一直沿用至今。

（2）鼻饮。在壮族地区，流传着一种洗鼻及雾化吸入以防病的方法，即煎取某些草药液令患者吸入洗鼻，或蒸煮草药化为气雾，令患者吸入，以预防一些时疫疾病。这种方法在古代称为"鼻饮"。鼻饮在古越族中流传，史书、志书多有记载，最早见于汉代的《异物志》，"乌浒，南蛮之别名，巢居鼻饮"。宋代周去非的《岭外代答》对鼻饮的方法做了比较详细的描述："邕州溪峒及钦州村落，俗多鼻饮。鼻饮之法，以瓢盛少水，置盐及山姜汁数滴于水中。瓢则有窍，施小管如瓶嘴，插诸鼻中，导水升脑，循脑而下入喉……饮时必口噍鱼鲊一片，然后才安流入鼻，不与气相激。既饮必噫气，以为凉脑快膈，莫若此也。"这种奇特的卫生民俗包含着物理降温和黏膜给药等科学知识，对鼻病、喉病、呼吸系统病证都有一定的疗效。

（3）嚼槟榔。在广西龙州、防城港、上思和宁明等地的壮族村庄里，盛行着"客至不设茶，唯以槟榔为礼"的习俗。《平乐县志》说："气多痞瘴，槟榔之嚼，甘如饔飧。"从药用价值来看，槟榔能辟秽除瘴，行气利水，杀虫消积。可以说，壮族人民嚼食槟榔的一个重要原因是用槟榔来防治瘴气。

5. 饮食养生习俗

（1）岁时饮食。壮族地区自古以来就有注重岁时饮食养生的习俗，如农历正月底采白头翁、艾叶和米为粽，白头翁、艾叶均为壮医常用药物；农历三月初三，人们多采金银花、青艾等制成糯米糍粑，传说吃此糍粑能祛病，令身体健康；农历四月初八为浴佛节，壮族习俗是炊乌米饭，食之以辟疫；农历五月初五，老少饮菖蒲酒、雄黄酒以辟疠疫。壮族岁时饮食养生的习俗，既讲究食物的调养，又讲究药物的作用，符合壮医养生保健的精神，深受群众的欢迎。

（2）壮族药膳。壮族人民在长期的生活实践中总结出不少由食物、药物和调料组成的具有防病治病、强身益寿功效的药膳，如龙虎（蛇、猫）斗、龙凤（蛇、鸡）会、三蛇（眼镜蛇、金环蛇、灰鼠蛇）酒，又如流行于右江一带的"果粑"（牛奶果、糯米）、"花团"（糯米、南瓜花、花生、芝麻、猪排骨）。由于壮族地区新鲜草药和动物药十分丰富，因此壮族人民常用鲜草药和血肉有情之品治疗疾病。例如，以山羊肉、麻雀肉、鲜嫩的益母草、黑豆相互配合作饮食治疗，可以防治妇女不孕；各种蛇肉汤或乌猿酒，可以防治骨关节疾患，治疗历年不愈者；猪肉或老母鸭、水鸭、鹧鸪肉煲莲藕，可以防治阴伤干咳。

五、明显的壮汉文化交流印记

壮族作为中华民族大家庭的一员，其文化深受中华汉文化的影响。从出土的文物来看，先秦时期汉文化早已浸润岭南。广西武鸣勉岭出土了具有中原商代风格的青铜器皿，桂林兴安出土了商代兽面纹铜卣，钦州大寺镇出土了商代中原风格石磬，说明商代中原文化已影响到广西南部，表明壮汉文化的交流始于先秦时期。随着汉字的传入、学校的建立、儒家和道家等思想的传播，壮族文化吸收了汉文化的适用部分，经过长期的社会历史发展，形成了壮族文化在表面上与汉文化无异，而在思想观念等深层结构方面仍保留着壮族文化的特点。

壮汉文化交流对壮医药文化的形成和发展产生了不可忽视的影响。先秦时期的一些古籍记载了壮族先民早期的医疗实践活动。从目前已有的资料来看，壮医药的记载始于汉代，然后历代有所增加。据文献记载，晋代的葛洪等医药学家、唐代的柳宗元等文人流官，都曾把中医药传播到壮族地区。宋代咸平初年，广南西路转运使陈尧叟"集验方刻石桂州驿"，邕州知府范旻"下令禁淫祀""市药以施治""并刻疗病方书，置诸厅壁"。明代李时珍的《本草纲目》是一部内容丰富、收载广泛的医药学巨著，收载了不少岭南地区的壮族草药，最突出的是壮族人民对名贵壮药——田七的开发和应用。在与汉族的长期交往和壮汉文化的交流中，有大量关于壮医药的真实资料以汉文形式记载于各种文献之中，有的则以文物的形式展现出来。

壮族聚居和分布地区处于亚热带，虽然平均气温较高，但是四季仍较分明。日月穿梭，昼夜更替，寒暑消长，冬去春来，使壮族先民很早就产生了阴阳的概念，加上与中原汉族文化的交流及受其影响，阴阳概念在生产、生活中的应用就更为广泛了。阴阳概念也被运用到壮医学上，形成了"阴阳为本"的基本理念，该理念作为解释大自然和人体生理病理之间种种复杂关系的说理工具。

第二节　壮医药文化的表现形态

作为壮医药与壮族传统文化交融、结合、渗透形成的产物，壮医药文化的表现形式是多种多样的。有的以相对独立的物质或非物质的形式表现出来，如药线、骨弓、药锤等一些治疗器具；大部分则隐含在其他文化丛的表现形式当中，如以神话、习俗、山歌、药市等形式表现出来。具体而言，壮医药文化可以分为物态文化、神话文化、巫医文化、符号文化、口碑文化、习俗文化、歌谣文化、药食文化、生殖文化、体育文化等。

一、物态文化

物态文化是人类在长期改造客观世界的活动中所形成的一切物质生产活动及其产品的总和，是文化中可以具体感知的、摸得着、看得见的东西，是具有物质形态的文化事物。壮医药在漫长的发展过程中，逐步形成了各种治疗工具和治疗方法，从原始社会时期的石片、骨器、骨针、陶器，到先秦两汉时期的青铜针、银针，直至今天广泛使用的各种针具、药线、牛角、竹罐、药锤等壮医医疗工具以及药物熏蒸、药物熏洗、药物敷贴、药佩、药刮、滚蛋等治疗方法，都是具有物质实体的文化事物。北宋时期的《欧希范五脏图》所绘内容主要为人体内脏图谱，这是我国医学史上第一张有记载的实绘人体解剖图，也是壮医药发展史上具有标志性意义的实物图谱。壮族地区地处岭南亚热带，药物资源十分丰富，不少壮药较早地得到开发利用，有些还成为著名的中药材，在《神农本草经》收载的365种药物中，就有壮族地区盛产的菌桂、牡桂、薏苡仁、丹砂、钟乳石等。田七、肉桂、八角茴香、薏苡仁、罗汉果、珍珠、蛤蚧等均为主产于壮族地区的名贵药材。特别值得一提的是田七，其主产于壮族聚居的广西百色市田阳、田东、那坡、德保、靖西一带，是一味著名的壮药，是壮族对我国传统医药乃至世界传统医药的重要贡献。以上这些医疗工具、治疗方法、药材均具有实物的属性，属于壮医药物质文化的主要形式。

二、神话文化

神话是古代人们对世界起源、自然现象和社会状况的主观想象和幻想，是各民族文化长河中的瑰宝。神话传说深刻地体现着一个民族的早期文化，并在以后的历史进程中积淀在民族精神的底层，转变为一种集体的无意识，深刻地影响文化整体的发展。在壮族地区流行有神医三界公的传说，这是壮民族与医药相关的神话文化的代表。传说中的三界公乃仙童转世，曾于山中遇仙，仙授以五彩带、仙棒、仙桃和金字书法宝，三界公吃下仙桃后变成神医，专为贫苦乡人治病。治病时在病人患处缠上五彩带，以仙棒轻轻敲三下，则骨折脚跛的人就能奔走，浮肿病人就能恢复健康，多年的瞎子就能重见光明。在瘟疫盛行期间，三界公广发"驱瘟灵"，使患者药到病除，起死回生，且分文不取，深受乡人的爱戴。为了纪念这位神医，祈求保佑，消灾祛病，壮族地区多处修建有"三界庙"，至今广西忻城县土司衙门旧址附近仍保存有一座清代修建的"三界庙"，此庙常年香火不断。神医三界公的传说生动地反映了壮族人民对真、善、美的追求，成为承载壮族人民防病治病思想的重要载体和表达方式。

三、巫医文化

在人类文化中，最早试图征服自然界的手段是巫术。巫医现象从远古时期就已产生，是人类文化的一个组成部分，它曾对传统医学的形成起到孕育与催生的作用。巫医与神职医生是世界上几乎所有民族在早期都出现过的职业。壮族地区巫医文化古已有之，壮族先民对于自然界的种种现象无法理解，于是他们就想象在这些自然现象的背后，一定有某种威力无比的神秘的神灵在起作用，从这种"万物有灵"的认识，推想人自身及行为与自然界之间存在着各种神秘的关系。壮族先民重巫，文献不乏记载。汉代越巫之风，亦曾轰动京师。明代邝露的《赤雅》记载："汉元封二年（公元前 109 年）平越，得越巫，适有祠祷之事，令祠上帝，祭百鬼，用鸡卜。斯时方士如云，儒臣如雨，天子有事，不昆命于元龟，降用夷礼，廷臣莫敢致诤，意其术大有可观者矣。"可见壮族巫文化影响之深广。清代，南方壮族地区仍盛行巫风。直到现代，壮族地区仍见巫之遗风。至今，在广西部分城乡还可见到一种治小儿夜啼的符咒法，把写有"天皇皇，地皇皇，我家有个小哭王，路人行过念一念，一觉睡到大天光"的符咒丢在路口或贴在路边的树干、电线杆、墙壁上，路人走过念一念，小孩的夜啼病就好了，这是巫医文化的一个例证。刘锡蕃在《岭表纪蛮·杂述》中对巫医治病的过程有较为详细的记载："蛮人以草药医治跌打损伤及痈疮毒外科一切杂疾，每有奇效，然亦以迷信出之。"并有目睹为证："予尝见一患痈者，延僮老治疾。其人至，病家以雄鸡、毫银、水、米、诸事陈于堂。术者先取银纳袋中。脱草履于地，取水念咒。喷患处，操刀割之，脓血迸流，而病者毫无痛苦。脓尽，敷以药即愈。"壮医与巫术的关系是十分密切的，医巫同源、医巫并存是壮族医学发展过程中的一大特点。以巫术驱邪或治病，曾是壮族社会历史上一种十分普遍的现象。从医学发展的观点来看，巫医的存在确实阻碍了壮医的发展，但如果用历史唯物主义和辩证唯物主义的观点去看问题，巫医的产生和发展又是壮医产生和发展过程中一个不可替代的历史。

四、符号文化

符号是指具有某种代表意义或性质的标识。德国哲学家卡西尔在《人论》中说"人是符号的动物"。符号是人类约定俗成的对象指称，也是人类表达思想的工具。符号的创造总是与一定的文化意义相联系的，生活中人们可以通过相互交流，体认或传播符号所蕴含的信息、情感或态度。亦即，符号能够反映一定时间与空间中，某一族群社会相对稳定的思维方式、价值取向与情感诉求。作为工具性存在的符号，每一种符号体系都有特殊的意义，符号创造在某种程度上意味着种种文化创造。在广西左江流域一带，共发现了大量笔触粗犷、风格浑朴的巨型壁画，其中宁明县花山崖壁画的规模在我国已发现的崖壁画中首屈一指，在国外亦属罕见。经考证，这些崖壁画为先秦时期瓯骆先民所作。关于崖壁画的文化内涵，其中一个观点认为它是壮医为防病强身绘制的功夫动作图。利用舞蹈导引气功等方法防治疾病，是古代壮医的一大特色。有学者将之与春秋战国时期带气功铭文的玉佩和长沙马王堆汉墓的导引图帛画并列为中国三大气功文物。花山崖壁画是古代壮族人民与疾病做斗争的方式方法的形象化表述，显示了壮医药文化的独特风貌与内涵。

五、口碑文化

"口碑"一词，《古汉语大词典》《辞源》《汉语大词典》等工具书均有注解。比较集中的解释是，比喻群众口头上的称颂。另外，"口碑"还泛指众人的议论、群众的口头传说、社会上流传的口头热语。广西壮医医院的谢爱泽认为，"口碑"是指"口耳相传（包括家传、师承），没有文化记载，代代相传（者）"，壮医药口碑资料是以民族语言为载体的，通过口耳相传流传下来的壮医知识。壮族民间医药经验能历经千年流传至今，最主要的原因是民间存在着丰富的口碑资料。口碑资料中有的是医者亲身经历的记录，有的仅仅由口头转述。例如，罗勒、佛手、九里香治疗腹痛和肚胀；小茴香和水田七，胃痛服了真有益；花椒和干姜，胃寒是良方；茉莉花根和香附子，跌打扭伤痛即除。一些壮医的口碑资料并不只是局限于壮医之间流传，还被作为一种生活常识在民间普通百姓中世代相传。例如，壮族地区群众普遍懂得药物"斑鸠站"可以治疗疟疾，田基黄、鸡骨草、黄花倒水莲、无娘藤、不出林等是治疗肝炎的要药。历经千百年的发展，壮族人民运用口碑形式传承壮医药已经在不知不觉中形成了一种文化氛围。这种口碑形式传承医药涉及的范围非常广泛，已经深入到民间，形式多种多样，在很大程度上充实并延续了壮医药知识库，并且为壮医药理论的形成创造了条件。

六、习俗文化

习俗，顾名思义，是习惯风俗的意思。习俗文化是与生活紧密相连的文化现象，是一个民族经过长时间积累、吸取和改造后，在物质生活和文化生活方面广泛流行的共同的喜好、风尚、习气、禁忌和信仰。医药习俗文化是各民族人民在长期的生产、生活实践中形成的，被本民族或社会所认同并世代相传的，关于治病、防病、保健的相关知识文化的总称。壮族在漫长的历史发展过程中，形成了包括生活卫生、崇巫尊祖、防病保健、防疫防毒等丰富多彩的医药习俗文化（具体内容见第二章第一节）。壮医药习俗文化是在壮族地区特有的自然环境、地理环境、社会环境和民族文化背景下，壮族人民在长期的生产生活实践中，因地制宜，用不同的方式积累起来的关于治病、防病、保健的智慧结晶，具有多样的文化载体和文化表现形式，内

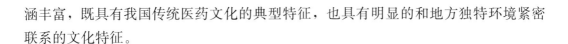

涵丰富，既具有我国传统医药文化的典型特征，也具有明显的和地方独特环境紧密联系的文化特征。

七、歌谣文化

歌谣是民歌、民谣的统称。壮族是一个能歌善舞的民族，壮族歌谣题材广泛、内容丰富，涵盖了壮族人民生活的一切领域。除了男女之间的感情交流，壮族的生活习惯、农耕工艺、民情世俗、社会形态乃至医药等均在歌谣中大量出现。壮族歌谣中包含大量的医事保健（如季节气候与疾病、婚姻生育、居住环境、房屋建设、情志）、医药理论、疾病症状、治疗技法、方剂及药物功效等方面的内容，在壮医药传承过程中发挥了重要的作用。"春分有雨病人稀，初一翻风又落雨，沿村病疫定然凶；立夏东风吹发发，沿村没有病人魔；季秋初一莫逢霜，人民疾病少提防；重阳无雨三冬旱，月中亢旱病人忙；凑巧遇逢壬子日，灾伤疾病损人民；初一西风盗贼多，更兼大雪有灾魔"，这首民歌讲述了气候变化与疾病的关系，教导人们在气候变化时要注意防病。"寒手热背肿在梅，瘰肌痛沿麻络央，唯有痒疾抓长子，各疾施治不离乡"是壮医药线点灸疗法取穴规律的总结。民歌中对药物功效记载的内容大致可分为两种：一种是概括药物功效的共性，如"每棵都成药，有苦也有辣，辣的能治瘀，苦的能清热；有酸也有甜，酸的能吸汗，甜的能补气"；另一种是阐述单味药物的功效，如"瘀证常用南蛇簕，医治跌打和骨折，含咽根本除骨鲠，瘰疬功效也不劣"。可以说壮族歌谣是一部壮民族古代原生态的百科全书。

八、药食文化

药食文化是人类医药文化中普遍经历过的阶段和重要特征。我国自古有"神农尝百草，一日而遇七十毒"识别药物的传说。在人类社会的早期，由于医疗经验的缺乏，先民总是在可食之物范围内，认识到某一食品除具有填腹充饥的作用外，尚有治疗疾病的效果，由此逐步积累了一些药食的初步经验。因此，食为药之先，对药用的认识是对食用认识深化的结果，而药物与食品之间又具有互补作用，从而形成了具有民族特色的药食文化。壮族是最早的稻作民族之一。稻类不仅是古代壮族人民充饥之食，而且还被作为健脾胃、益肾气、延年益寿的食疗壮药，加工成药粥、药酒、药饭、药糕等药膳食用。如贺州市的黑糯米酿酒"沽于市有名色"，桂平市黑糯米酿成的甜酒具有"补中益气而及肾"的功效。除粮食作物被壮族先民发现有良好的食疗保健作用外，水果、蔬菜、动物、调料等能补充营养的大部分食品也有特定的食疗功效。橙能解鱼蟹毒；核炒研末冲酒服，可治闪挫腰痛；紫苏"食之不饥，可以释劳"；枸杞菜"味甘平，食之能清心明目"……壮族民间历来流传着生饮蛇血治风湿，老鼠滋补之功"一鼠当三鸡"，蚂蚁治风湿，蛤蚧、麻雀、公鸡蛋（公鸡睾丸）滋补壮阳等用药经验。由于特殊的气候和地理环境，壮族地区药食两用的动植物资源丰富、品种繁多，为药食文化的形成和发展提供了得天独厚的条件。

九、生殖文化

生殖是人类生存至今的一个古老而又永恒的话题。可以这样说，人类在地球上有多长的生存历史，生殖就有多长的历史。恩格斯在第一版《家庭、私有制和国家的起源》的序言中指出，生产本身有两种："一方面是生活资料即食物、衣服、住房以及为此所必需的工具的生产；另一方面是人类自身的生产，即种的繁衍。"在远古人类的洪荒初辟时代，人类自身的繁殖是社会发展的决定因素，远比物质资料的生产更为重要，"生育是种族的绝对义务，就像死亡是个人不可抗拒的命运一样"。生殖崇拜也就成为一种遍及世界的历史现象。壮族是一个历史悠久的古老民族，壮族民间对人类的生殖繁衍也有自己的理解。壮族民间信奉花婆神，她是专管生育儿女的女神，又称"花王圣母"。壮族民间认为儿女是花婆庭院里的花朵，枯荣全凭花婆主宰。婴儿出生，即在床头铺上纸花，逢年过节由母亲领孩子祭花婆。孩子生病，也要祭请花婆保佑。壮族先民对于生殖的崇拜，在一些动物身上得到了体现。在壮族地区，一直流传着许多关于青蛙的传说，一方面，青蛙由于自身的体形以及强盛的生殖力，被先民视为女性或男性的化身；另一方面，人们又将其与壮族地区的生育神——雷神相联系，借此增强青蛙的生殖力，青蛙在壮族生殖崇拜文化中具有独特的地位。在骆越文化考古考察工作中，专家在环大明山地区发现男根形态的大型石祖一直被当地村民所供奉。另外，在宁明县花山崖壁画上，能清晰地看到数千年前壮族祖先描绘的两幅人交媾图，这些都体现了壮族人民历来对人类的生殖有着非同寻常的崇拜。

十、体育文化

壮族先民很早就意识到通过体育锻炼可以增强体质，预防疾病。宁明县花山崖壁画所绘的人像，正面的多为两手上举，肘部弯曲成 $90°\sim110°$，两膝关节弯曲成 $90°\sim110°$，呈半蹲状；侧身的人像多排列成行，两腿向后弯曲，两手向上伸张。专家研究认为，不管是正面的人像还是侧面的人像，都是一种典型的舞蹈动作或功夫动作形象。舞蹈在早期医疗实践中的地位，从马王堆汉墓出土的导引图、华佗的五禽戏中可以得到证实。壮族地区由于特殊的自然地理环境，常年阴湿多雨，脚气、风湿、身重等为常见多发之病证，严重影响了人们的生产和生活。因此，壮族先民创造了这些具有宣导滞着、疏利关节作用的舞蹈动作，并作为永世流传的防治疾病的方法绘制下来。至今，壮乡人民仍喜爱体育活动及歌舞，常在节日里开展抛绣球、赛龙舟、踩高跷、舞龙、舞狮、拾天灯等传统健身活动，这与壮医十分强调"未病先防"的预防保健观念是密不可分的。

参考文献：

[1] 黄汉儒. 中国壮医学 [M]. 南宁：广西民族出版社，2000.

[2] 蓝日春，刘智生，覃文波. 浅谈骆越文化与壮医药文化的关系 [J]. 中国民族医药杂志，2008 (12)：1-6.

[3] 庞宇舟. 壮族医药卫生习俗述略 [J]. 中国民族民间医药，2008 (3)：3-5.

[4] 何新. 艺术现象的符号——文化学阐释 [M]. 北京：人民文学出版社，1987.

[5] 林辰. 浅析壮族巫文化对壮医药发展的影响 [C]. 第一届中泰传统医药和天然药物研究学术研讨会论文集，2006.

[6] 刘珂珂，张梅. 人·符号·文化 [J]. 江苏社会科学，2012 (5)：28-31.

[7] 谢爱泽. 壮族医药口碑资料研究 [C]. 2005 全国首届壮医药学术会议暨全国民族医药经验交流会论文汇编，2005.

[8] 莫清莲，黄萍，黄海波. 略论壮族民歌在壮医传承中的作用 [J]. 中国民族民间医药，2019 (21)：25-27.

[9] 马克思，恩格斯. 马克思恩格斯选集：第 4 卷 [M]. 北京：人民出版社，1972.

[10] O. A. 魏勒. 性崇拜 [M]. 史频，译. 北京：中国文联出版公司，1988.

[11] 廖明君. 动物崇拜与生殖崇拜 [J]. 广西民族学院学报：哲学社会科学版，1995 (3)：23-28.

[12] 庞宇舟. 花山岩画壮医学内涵探析 [J]. 光明中医，2008，23 (12)：1871-1873.

第三章 壮医药与壮族哲学、宗教信仰文化

第一节 壮医药与壮族哲学

远古时期的广西地区，气候温暖，雨水丰沛，河流纵横，森林茂密，动物繁多，岩洞遍布，是原始人类理想的生息繁衍之地。壮族人民自古以来就生息繁衍在岭南这块广阔而肥沃的土地上，他们披荆斩棘，辛勤劳动，建设美好的家园。近代以来的考古发掘研究成果及壮族民间有关远古时代的神话传说，从不同方面向我们展示了壮族先民探索、征服大自然的艰苦历程。壮族先民在征服大自然的伟大斗争中，既创造了物质文化，也产生了一些淳朴、自然的观念，对宇宙的起源、人类万物的来源有了粗浅的看法。随着壮族社会的发展，人们实践的深入，壮族先民视野不断扩大，认识也逐渐加深，对自然和社会的种种现象有了自己的看法，即有了自己的世界观。当然，这种对世界的看法，还是带有朴素性的直观认识。壮族的哲学思想，也是中华民族哲学思想的一个重要组成部分。

壮医药的形成和发展，经历了漫长的历史时期。壮医药的形成，是以壮族先民千百年的生产生活及临床实践为基础的。壮族先民为了顺应自然，适应自然，就不得不探索大自然的奥秘，形成对可感的外部环境的认识，产生了与生息繁衍密切相关的各种意识形态，其中包括关于自身同自然界的关系，或者是关于人与人之间的关系，或者是关于自身的肉体组织的观念。

一、壮族哲学思想

黑格尔说："一个民族进入一个时代，在这时精神指向着普遍的对象，用普遍的理智概念去解释自然事物，比如说，要求去认识事物的原因。于是我们可以说，这个民族开始作哲学思考了。"在探索大自然的奥秘时，壮族先民最初的疑问来自于天地的形成和人类自身的起源，也是从天与人的思考中诞生了具有本民族特色的朴素的原始哲学思想。这种原始哲学思想以民间神话传说为载体，流传至今。

1. 关于宇宙的起源说

壮族民间流传的神话传说有很多，大多数以长篇叙事诗歌的形式流传，其中流传较广的有《开天辟地歌》《人神分家》《姆洛甲》《布洛陀》《妈勒访天边》《特康射太阳》《布伯的故事》《铜鼓的传说》等。

《布洛陀》这个古老的神话故事的梗概：很早很早以前，天地没有分家，先是宇宙间旋转着一团大气，那大气团渐渐地越转越急，转着转着，转成了一个大圆蛋。大圆蛋有三个蛋黄，后来大圆蛋爆炸开来，三个蛋黄分为三片，向三个方向飞出去，一片飞到上边，成了天空；一片降到下面，成了海洋；一片落在中间，成了大地。天地分成三界，天空是上界，地上是中界，地下是下界。上界由雷王管理，中界由布洛陀管理，下界由龙王管理。那时，天矮地薄，人们砍柴时斧头常常碰着天，打桩纺织也常常凿穿地皮，弄得上界、下界的人不得安宁，日夜埋怨。于是，布洛陀就叫上界的人把天升高，高到"三十三条楠竹那么高，三十三巉头发吊不到"；叫下界的人把地加厚，厚到"三十三座石山那么厚，三十三巉黄藤穿不透"……这就是古代壮族先民的天地生成说，它有着浓厚的神话色彩，但在神话的外衣下，却也显现出唯物主义的曙光、哲学思想的萌芽。这种唯物主义的曙光，表现为壮族先民已认识到大气存在于天地形成以前，大气旋转而形成一个圆的像蛋的东西，它炸开后成为三片，这三片分别成了天、地、海洋，这不得不说是对天地生成的唯物的解释，蕴含着朴素的唯物自然观。壮族的"气本原说"不仅有朴素唯物论的思想萌芽，而且还有朴素辩证法的思想萌芽。壮族先民意象中作为宇宙本原的"大气"不是僵化不动的，而是交互运动且旋转（运动变化）得越来越急（事物内部矛盾运动越来越激烈）的，由此转成了一个大圆蛋（体积小、密度大）。大圆蛋在爆炸（质变）中产生天、地、海洋。壮族先民以直观具象的思维，用旋转、爆炸来描述物质的运动、发展和变化，并且把世界的形成归结于事物内部的矛盾运动。这种旋转、爆炸产生宇宙的观点，在某种程度上类似于当代关于宇宙起源假说中的"星云说"和大爆炸理论。这样的相似源自于人们对宇宙生成的思考都含有唯物辩证法因素，只不过壮族先民的辩证法思想是朴素辩证法的自然流露。

2. 关于人类的起源说

壮族先民在极其落后的生产方式之下，以直观、朴素的思维"取物观象"，对这个"宇宙之谜"做出了种种夸张的构想，在神话的光环之下亦有哲学思想的闪光。壮族先民对人类起源的描述可分为原生人类和再生人类。

一是花婆姆六甲"抟土造人"，产生原生人类。壮族神话《布洛陀和姆六甲》中说：古时候，宇宙中有一个在旋转着的蛋，后来爆开分为三片，成为天、地、海洋三界。中界的大地上长出一朵花，花中间长出一个女人，这个女人是世界上第一个人。她披头散发，满身长毛，很聪明。她尿湿了大地，然后用湿土捏出了人形，并用辣椒与杨桃分出了男女。

二是"兄妹婚配，再生人类"。主管上界的雷王因恼怒放下大水，淹没了人类，只有一对兄妹躲进葫芦得以生存。为了再生人类，兄妹俩顺从天意，结为夫妻，婚后生下一个肉团，他们把它砍成肉片，撒到野外，结果落在江河里的变成了鱼虾，落在平地上的变成了人类。人们互相婚配，人类就繁衍下来了。

这两种起源说相互联系，都是不同历史发展阶段的产物。姆六甲"抟土造人"之说是壮族先民还不明白男女交合的生殖作用时，根据开花结果的采集经验认为花是人类的起源，现今壮族依然保留着对花的图腾崇拜。"兄妹婚配，再生人类"之说是原始群婚阶段的反映。这样，在壮族神话传说体系中勾勒出人类的演化史：气—天、地、海洋三界—花婆姆六甲—原始人类—再生人类。

3. 关于人与自然之间的关系

在长期的劳动和生活实践中，壮族先民认识到了人与客观世界的辩证统一。人首先要适应自然环境，尊重客观规律，这种尊重主要表现为对神灵的敬畏而产生一系列祈福避凶的膜拜仪式，这是唯心主义的表现。但从另一个角度来看，人类也有了自我觉醒的意识，不断地改造客观世界，使人类适应自然环境而发展。在壮族的神话传说中涌现出许多战天斗地、领导人们同自然抗争的英雄。如英雄人物布洛陀在天地形成后为了改善恶劣的生活环境，带领人们治理天地，找老铁树顶天压地，用计轰雷公上天，赶蛟龙进海，撵老虎入林，教导人们编衣、种植、取火，让人们在大地上安居乐业。《布伯的故事》中有这样的情节：雷王不下雨，布伯上天找雷王算账，他抓住雷王的臂膀，把剑架在雷王的鼻梁上。在《雷鼓的传说》中表现的是人们勇敢抗涝的故事，特依三兄弟造鼓以斗雷王："雷王的威风全靠鼓，我们也做几面鼓，我们的鼓声压住雷王的鼓声，他自然就输了，不敢逞威风。"《特康射太阳》中的特康是类似于汉族后羿的英雄。布洛陀、布伯、特依三兄弟、特康等英雄的事迹实际上是广大劳动人民与大自然抗争的缩影，虽然看起来离奇幼稚，但是都间接地反映出人类的进取精神，同时也歌颂了人们与大自然抗争的勇气。人们对自然由无限信仰到蔑视（代表自然力的）神灵并与其抗争，也是朴素唯物主义思想升华的过程。

二、壮族哲学文化的基本特点

1. 古朴的自然观念和对自然的崇拜

远古时代，由于社会生产力水平十分低下，科学知识极端贫乏，因此壮族先民对于各种自然现象，如打雷、闪电、刮风、洪水、干旱、山崩、地裂以及日月轮转等无法理解，于是他们就想象在这些自然力的背后，一定有一种威力无比的神秘的东西在支配着。他们认为打雷有雷公，闪电有电母，刮风有风婆，下雨有雷王，海有龙王，山有山神，地有地神，日月也有神，等等。壮族先民还认为草木、飞禽、走兽也有神灵，把这些自然界及自然现象人格化、神化，从而产生了自然崇拜的观念。

2. 人能胜天地的思想

人能胜天地的思想，是壮族先民在长期与自然界的斗争中，不断总结经验而形成的。随着壮族社会生产力水平的提高，人们对自然界认识的加深，壮族先民在战天斗地中逐渐认识到自己的力量，初步产生了人类能够战胜天地的思想。壮族先民的这种思想，不是从他们的生产、生活中直接反映出来的，而是通过许多故事传说间接地表现出来的。通过把现实社会中的人、物理想化，塑造出一些英雄人物和神化了的人物，与天斗、与地斗，获得胜利而表现出来的，反映出壮族先民朴素的人能战胜天地的思想。

壮族先民在与大自然的斗争中不仅有了人能战胜天地的思想，而且还能认识到人能够改变环境，战胜洪水猛兽。在叙事诗歌《岑逊王》中就记载了壮族先民战胜洪水猛兽的故事。故事说，古时江岩（今广西田阳县田州镇）有个人叫岑逊，他看见洪水时常泛滥，淹死无数生灵，人们不得不搬到山上去住，但在那里又遭受毒蛇猛兽之害。于是，他发誓要治服洪水，消灭毒蛇猛兽。为了治理水害，他跋山涉水，走遍了壮乡村寨，观流泉，看山势，还向人们讲授洪水猛兽之害，克服了数不尽的困难，走了 720 天，和毒蛇猛兽搏斗了 1044 次，终于胜利地回到了家乡。回家后，他开始挖山劈岭，疏通河道，治平了山洪，也消灭了猛兽。从此，人们安居乐业，过着太平的生活。这个故事道出了人们要战胜洪水、消灭野兽，首先就得了解水流山势、野兽出没的实情。而要了解这些情况，就得跋山涉水，察地形，观流泉，看洪水奔流的去路。从这一点来说，那时人们已朦胧地认识到要了解情况，就要深入实际的道理，初步懂得了要战胜洪水，首先要认识水流的性质和特点。虽然这种认识还是属于经验性的，但是距今几千年的壮族先民能有这种认识思想，无疑是十分宝贵的。当然这种认识不是一朝一夕就能形成的，而是壮族人民世世代代在生产斗争中长期积累经验的结果。总之，这个故事虽然含有浓厚的神话色彩，但是也反映了壮族先民已认识到自己的力量，有了人能胜天地的思想萌芽。

3. 巫文化在壮族哲学文化中占有重要地位

生产力水平十分低下的壮族原始先民，对自然界的各种现象，如地震、洪水、火山爆发等，甚至对日常生活中的日出、日落、刮风、下雨、雷鸣、闪电等无穷变化的大自然奥秘都无法解释，特别是对人在夜间做梦和生老病死更是感到神秘莫测。因此，他们开始无边无际的幻想，最终臆断世界之外一定存在着某种超自然的力量和神秘的境界主宰自然和社会。在他们看来，风调雨顺能使万物顺利生长等有利于他们采集、生活的事是主宰自然的神秘力量对人类及大自然发善的表现；而洪水、地震等给人类造成的灾难，是主宰自然的神秘力量凶狠、愤怒的发泄。于是，他们便幻想着去寻找一种超自然的神力，通过它来消灾除祸，驱瘟防病，排除饥饿，并能让气候、动物、庄稼、健康、寿命等遵从他们的意愿，使他们在心灵上得到安慰，在精神上有所寄托，这样就产生了巫文化。

巫文化的产生与当时生产力的发展水平低下，反映于意识形态上的自然崇拜中万物有灵的宗教观念未根除有关系。壮族先民把一切自然现象人格化、神灵化，认为万物都有灵魂，尤其是与生产相关的自然力，如山、川、日、月、雷、电、风、雨、水、火、土等，都有"神灵"。人们企图以祭祀的方式，去取得自然力的欢心，博得自然的恩赐，山有山神，水有水鬼，地有地母，都需要祭祀。这些原始信仰，往往是巫术与宗教不分，占卜、祭祀、超度亡灵都夹杂有巫术。

巫文化即巫术文化。巫文化的核心是信仰鬼神，其在壮族哲学文化中占有重要的地位，它不仅影响壮族的民间宗教文化、文学艺术，而且影响民俗、医药、饮食、器皿、经济生活、天文历法、教育、音乐、舞蹈、美术、工艺、功法等各个方面。

三、壮族哲学对壮医药的影响

壮族是中华民族的重要组成部分。由于壮族聚居地区特殊的地理环境和政治、经济、文化等因素，壮族的社会历史发展具有一些明显的特点，这些特点对壮族医药的存在和发展有着重大的影响。壮族医药具有明显的民族性和区域性，其形成及发展除了与壮族地区特定的社会历史有密切关系，还与其自然地理环境、气候特点、经济、文化、民俗等有密切关系。

不同的哲学文化都可能发展出其独特的哲学思维方式，壮族哲学对自然的认识、对人体的认识都深深地影响和渗透到壮医药当中，诸如壮族哲学中对于人与自然之间的关系——天、地、人三气同步的认识，人禀天地之气而生，为万物之灵的观点，人类在掌握自然规律的基础上可以改变自然的"人能胜天地"的认识。这些内容既是哲学领域研究的问题，也是壮医药学所探讨的内容，在壮族许多的口头叙事诗歌中都有所反映。

第二节　壮医药与壮族宗教信仰文化

一、道教、佛教与壮族宗教文化

秦汉时期之后，随着中央集权封建王朝对壮族地区统治的不断加强，壮族与汉族在政治、经济、文化方面交流的不断加强，汉族道教和一些外来宗教先后传入壮族地区，与壮族地区原有的文化相结合，壮族文化和宗教互相影响，巫、师、道、佛互相混杂，形成了壮族民间宗教文化的复杂性与多元性。

1. 道教与壮族宗教文化

道教是最早传入壮族地区的外来宗教。道教产生于中原地区，东汉时期开始传入广西。据广西宗教研究学者考证，东汉时期，刘根、华子期、廖平、廖冲、廖扶等人都曾在今容县都峤山修道。清代嘉庆年间的《广西通志》卷二百四十《记博白县事》说："紫阳观，在城西南六十里。在紫阳岩南，汉刘宗远建。"由此可知，汉代广西已经有了道教传播。东晋时期，葛洪听说交趾（泛指南方，当时辖两广及越南等地）产丹砂，求为勾漏（今广西北流）令，入岭南著书传道，促进了道教在岭南的传播。隋唐时期，道教主要是在桂东南一带传播；到了宋代，道教逐渐从桂东南向左江、右江流域和桂西北传播，并逐渐与壮族原始宗教文化融合。道教传入壮族地区后，很快就和壮族民间信鬼神、好淫祀、病鲜求医、专事巫觋的原始信仰习俗联系起来，满足了壮族社会的需要，从而促进了壮族原始习俗、文化和道教的相互影响、相互渗透，促进了道教在壮族地区的传播及壮族哲学文化的发展。

道教在传入壮族地区后，也发生了很大的变化。道教为了满足壮族群众迷信鬼神的心理需要，先后吸收了壮族原始信仰和佛教的一些成分，任意发展道教内容，自由地改变道教的形式，既尊奉太上老君，同时又融入壮族原始宗教和佛教的一些内容，把道、师、佛等内容杂糅起来，使道教更能为封建统治阶级和壮族社会所接受。道教的道公，壮族称之为"公道"，为道者不出家，可以婚娶成家立业，不吃素，只忌食牛肉、狗肉，禁杀牲；其活动主要是为人设斋打醮、操办丧事、超度亡灵、作会诵经、堪舆择日、免劫除灾等。其经文用汉字书写，诵时亦用汉语。因其专事念诵经符咒而少解经文，加之读音不准，念时装模作样喃喃谟谟，故民间又称其为"喃谟"。

2. 佛教与壮族宗教文化

佛教是外来宗教。学术界认为，佛教自印度传入中国：一是从印度西北经波斯越葱岭入新疆，进入甘肃、陕西、河南、河北等地；二是从印度东北经缅甸入云南、四川，再沿长江、汉水而下，传播于长江流域；三是从印度恒河越印度海域进入中国广州或越南再入中国两广地区；四是由印度沿海经马来半岛、南海群岛入中国东南沿海各省区。广西宗教界学者对大量出土的文物进行考证后认为，汉代末年，佛教便由海上经扶南（今柬埔寨）传入交趾郡合浦港，再从合浦港沿交广通道在广西内地传播。佛教传入壮族地区后，在壮族原始信仰和文化的影响下，迅速走向世俗化、巫教化。宋代之后，壮族地区最流行的佛教是禅宗和净土宗，前者见性成佛，后者持名念佛，将佛教从烦琐的经书中解脱出来，走向民间和世俗。明代以后，佛教进一步禅、净合一，儒、道、释合一，佛经简化为通俗易懂的劝善书，佛像多塑接近民众的观音、弥勒，修持简化为行善修德，普度众生。因此，壮族地区的佛教僧侣不一定是"和尚"，而是"花僧"，即可结婚成家立业，可吃荤，每月只选几天吃素。故《百粤风土记》说，广西"僧多留发，娶妻生子，谓之在家僧"。《投荒杂录》也记载："南人率不信释氏，虽有一二佛寺，吏课其为僧，以督责释之土田及施财。间有一二僧，喜拥妇食肉，但居其家，不能少解佛事。土人以女配僧，呼之为师郎。或有疾，以纸为圆钱，置佛像旁，或请僧设食。翌日，宰羊豕以啖之，目曰出斋。"其活动主要是为人受戒、超度亡灵、卜卦算命、做斋赶鬼、安祖葬坟。有的壮族地区做道场时，和尚、道公、巫师混在一起，文昌庙、观音庙、真武庙、关公庙、土地庙并列或置于同一神坛之上，与汉族地区正统的佛教大不一样。

从佛教和道教在壮族地区的传播来看，佛教的影响不如道教的大。道教是中国本土宗教，它的基本理论与中国古代原始信仰中的神秘思想及巫术是一脉相通的，原始宗教中的自然崇拜对象基本上都被道教全部包容，加上道教传入壮族地区后能较全面地介入壮族社会的生产、生活，把壮族古老的原始宗教中的神灵和信仰及后来新产生的神灵与信仰全部融入道教信仰中，因此道教传入壮族地区后能较快地与壮族原始信仰融合——道教吸纳壮族原始信仰中的各种神祇为自己的崇拜对象，壮族原始宗教则借助道教的宗教仪式来完成信仰实践的过程。佛教在壮族地区影响不大，原因是多方面的。《广西通志·宗教志》认为："广西佛教虽从海路传入较早，但通道旁区域经济不发达，文化较闭塞，广大地区尚属土著民族势力。原始巫教呈压倒优势，外来佛教影响甚微。"佛教作为一种外来宗教，它和壮族的多神崇拜观念有一定的差异。虽然佛教在传入壮族地区的过程中也尽量吸纳壮族民间神祇，注意从壮族民间信仰文化体系中吸取养料，但是佛教和壮族传统文化的交流、融合还是不够的。虽然佛教早在汉代就传入广西，但是其寺院多分布在桂东南和桂北等汉族聚居区，壮族聚居区的佛教寺院较少。因此，佛教在壮族地区的传播面并不广，其信徒数量并不多。这不是说佛教在壮族地区的世俗化不成功，而是佛教和壮族的传统文化融合不够，不能全面地介入壮族的社会生产、生活。它对现实和未来世界的看法、解决问题的手段，都不能满足壮族民众的精神需求。壮族先民对待人生抱着积极的态度，他们热爱生活，在生产斗争中遇到种种无法解决的困难时，也会乞求神灵的帮助，如上山狩猎希望能猎获野兽且不被伤害，春种缺水希望雷王降雨。人们崇拜神灵的目的是为了解决现实生活中的实际困难，如果崇拜的神灵不灵，人们就会对它加以惩罚，迫使它为自己的现实需求服务。如久旱要求雷王降雨，若总是不降雨，人们便将庙中的神像捆绑倒吊，抬去游村，给人鞭打、泼水，令其上天通报雷王，限期降雨。这种以实用为主的信仰观念与佛教的因果报应观念是完全背道而驰的。反之，壮族原始信仰在与道教、佛教交流的过程中，广泛地吸收了道教、佛教的信仰资源，成为新的民间宗教信仰。壮族民众在参加宗教祭祀活动时，并不在意它属于哪一个宗教，而是在意它是否与地方及民族传统文化有关。壮族民众真正崇拜的是混杂了来源不同的信仰和仪式的民间宗教。

因此，佛教传入壮族地区后，其原有的宗教理论因不能适应壮族社会的生产、生活需要而没有得到很好的发展。因此，佛教的影响不大就不足为奇了。

二、道教、佛教对壮医药的影响

1. 道教对壮医药的影响

随着道教传入壮族地区，道家的代表人物老子和庄子等人的思想也逐渐在壮族民间为人熟知，壮医药根植于壮族民间传统文化的土壤，我们可以从壮医药的部分理论中看到道家思想对壮医药的影响。

（1）道家的宇宙观与整体观对壮医药的影响

道教的教理教义都是围绕生命展开的，生命问题是道教思想的枢纽。道教认为，人类只有顺应自然界的变化，才能达到颐养天年的最终目的。这与壮医药理论中的"天、地、人三气同步学说"较为相似，"天、地、人三气同步"是根据壮语"人不得逆天地"或"人必须顺天地"意译过来的，其主要内涵如下：①人禀天地之气而生，为万物之灵。②人的生、长、壮、老、死生命周期，受天地之气涵养和制约，人气与天地之气息息相通。③天地之气为人体造就了生存和健康的一定"常度"，但天地之气在不断地变化。日夜小变化，四季大变化，是为正常变化；而地震、火山、台风、洪水、陨石雨等爆发则是异常变化，是为灾变。人作为万物之灵，对天地之气的变化有一定的主动适应能力，如天黑了会引火照明，天热了会出汗，天冷了会加衣被，洪水来临会登高躲避，等等。甚至妇女月事也与月亮的盈亏周期有关。对于天地之气的这些变化，人如能主动适应，就可维持生存和健康的"常度"；如不能适应，就会受到伤害并导致疾病的发生。④人体也是一个小天地，是一个有限的小宇宙单元。壮医认为，整个人体可分为三部：上部天（壮语称为"巧"），包括外延；下部地（壮语称为"胴"），包括内景；中部为人（壮语称为"廊"）。人体内三部之气只有同步运行，制约化生，才能生生不息。形体与功能相一致，大体上天气主降，地气主升，人气主和。升降适宜，中和涵养，则气血调和，阴阳平衡，脏腑自安，并能适应大宇宙的变化。⑤人体的结构与功能，先天之气与后天之气，共同形成了人体的适应能力与防卫能力，从而达到天、地、人三气同步的健康境界。

可见道教的"道法自然""天人合一"的哲学思想与壮医"天、地、人三气同步学说"有异曲同工之妙。

（2）道教"祝由符咒"对壮医药的影响

除了理论方面，道教的"祝由符咒"对壮医药也有一定的影响。"祝由符咒"是古时道家用来祈祷、祭祀，以祈求先祖庇佑、鬼神宽恕的法术，也被巫医和道医用作一种治病手段，他们认为通过"祝由符咒"可将蛊毒驱除体外。道教的"祝由符咒"除用以祈福禳灾外，主要用来为人治病。此法可使病人排除焦虑、紧张、忧郁等不良情绪，从而使气机调畅。

壮族传统信仰观念认为，灵魂能支配人的精神，并对生物体的生命起着庇佑的作用，是一种超自然的力量。如果一个人丧失了灵魂，其躯体就会丧失活动和生长能力，呼吸也就随之停止而死亡，因此魂能保命和保身体健康。"丢了魂"就会生病，而举行招魂仪式就能治病。壮族民间至今仍然流行着多种以"禳鬼降神"为主要内容，以祈求"神灵"庇佑、"病去人安"为目的的不同形式的巫医活动。

（3）道教"服气导引"对壮医药的影响

"服气"是一种以气息吐纳为主，以导引、按摩为辅的养生技法；"导引"是用意念以自力引导肢体运动，以使气血平和。壮医也强调"未病先防"在养生保健中的重要作用。壮医通过一些传统的舞蹈动作来缓解和治疗部分疾病。根据宁明花山崖壁画及壮乡铜鼓上的舞蹈造型、气功图谱及沿袭至今的在农闲、节日里开展的一些传统健身活动，可知壮族人民崇尚气功，这与道教的"服气导引"是分不开的。

2. 佛教对壮医药的影响

虽然佛教早在汉代就已传入广西，但是壮族聚居区的佛教寺院并不多。在历史上，佛教在壮族地区的传播面并不广，其信徒数量并不多，对壮族文化的影响不如道教。佛教对现实和未来世界的看法、解决问题的手段，都不能满足壮族民众的精神需要。但这并不能说佛教对壮医药没有影响，在佛教传播的过程中，佛教的部分教义和思想与壮医药的思想也有相似之处。

"四大"是佛教用语，指地、水、火、风四种物质，佛教认为这四种物质是构成世界的基本元素，一切物质为"四大"所生，人身也是由"四大"构成，"四大"平衡则人体健康，"四大"失衡则发病。这种"四大"理论与壮医药的"三气"同步理论有相似之处。壮医"三气"同步主要是通过人体内的谷道、水道和气道及其相关的枢纽脏腑的制化协调作用来实现的。谷道（壮语称为"条根埃"）主要是指食管和胃肠，其化生的枢纽脏腑在肝、胆、胰。水道的调节枢纽为肾与膀胱。水为生命之源，人体由水道进水、出水，与大自然发生最直接、最密切的联系。水道与谷道同源而分流，在吸取水谷精微营养物质后，由谷道排出粪便，水道则主要排出汗、尿。气道是人体与大自然之气相互交换的通道，进出于口、鼻，其交换枢纽脏腑为肺。"三道"畅通，调节有度，人体之气就能与天地之气保持同步协调平衡，即健康状态；"三道"阻塞或调节失度，则"三气"不能同步而致疾病丛生。

可见佛教"四大"的病因学说与壮医的"三气"同步理论异曲同工，除此之外，佛教普度众生的慈悲思想和救死扶伤的医学道德观对壮医的医德医风也有积极的影响。

三、壮族巫术文化与壮医药

1. 壮族巫术文化

一方面，壮族先民由于信仰鬼神而产生了巫文化，在原始社会图腾崇拜的基础上，壮族先民有关巫的思想观念根深蒂固，至今仍可见其遗风。另一方面，从流传至今的壮族民间叙事歌谣、传说和民间故事等口头文学中，可以窥见壮族先民怎样处理自然、社会、人体以及它们相互之间的关系。

据研究，左江崖壁画体现了壮族先民对日、月、星辰的崇拜，对此古籍不乏记载，直到近现代，壮族地区的巫风仍有所遗存。巫文化对壮医药的影响，先是"巫""医"合一，后是"医""巫"并存，最后"医"盛于"巫"。古时壮巫分巫婆和魔公，主家有病痛或灾难时，请巫婆和神对话，问明病灾的缘由，再择吉日请魔公行法事，杀畜禽敬祭，劝离神仙，禳解厄难，舞刀剑，烧油锅，镇妖赶鬼。壮族民间传说三界公能驱邪除魔，保境安民，人们奉其为医神而立庙祭祀，旧时壮族地区较大的村寨都立有药王庙，每年定期祭祀，这就是巫文化的反映。从考古发掘资料来看，春秋战国时期之后，广西壮族地区就已出现巫觋。据我国考古学家研究，广西左江流域崖壁画中的舞蹈人群图像应是宗教祭祀图像，画面中心装束特殊、气宇轩昂的高大正身人像应是祭典的主持者，是主持祭典的巫觋和领舞人。据考证，该崖壁画是壮族先民在战国至两汉时期创作绘制的，至今已有 2000 多年的历史。壮族先民重巫，文献中不乏记载，汉代越巫风曾在中原地区广为传播。《史记》卷十二《孝武本纪》中记载："是时既灭南越，越人勇之乃言'越人俗信鬼，而其祠皆见鬼，数有效……，乃令越巫立越祝祠，安台无坛，亦祠天神上帝百鬼，而以鸡卜。"可见壮族巫文化影响之深广。清代，壮族地区仍盛行巫风。直到现代，壮族地区仍见巫之遗风。

2. 壮医药与壮族巫文化的关系

医巫同源、医巫并存是壮族地区文化发展的特点，对壮医药产生了重大的影响。壮族医药中医巫并存的情况长期存在，壮医药对某些疾病确实有较好的疗效，往往以巫医的形式出现，这在新中国成立以前，特别是边远山区的壮族民间更是如此。宁明花山崖壁画的人物形象，除了舞蹈动作，还有些可能是诊疗图，既有施术者和持器（具）者，又有受术者。结合崖壁画的祭祀场面，联系壮族先民的巫文化特点，我们可以说崖壁画有巫医治病的内容。刘锡蕃的《岭表纪蛮·杂述》对此有明确的记载："蛮人以草药医治跌打损伤及痈疽疮毒外科一切杂疾，每有奇效，然亦以迷信出之。"并有目睹为证："予尝见一患痛者，延僮老治疾，其人至，病家以雄鸡、毫银、水、米、诸事陈于堂。术者先取银纳袋中，脱草履于地，取水念咒，喷患处，操刀割之，脓血迸流，而病者毫无痛苦。脓尽，敷以药即愈。"这确实是对历史上壮医治病的比较客观的记载，直到现代，壮医仍然在某种程度上保留着这种独特的治疗形式，不同的是，念咒的角色由患者的亲属来担任。如果把这种治疗形式视为纯粹的迷信加以摒弃，无疑会连同其中合理的医学内容一起丢掉。念咒语、喷符水并不妨碍壮医的施术和用药，也不能否定壮医的确切疗效，有些历史记载说壮族"病不服药，惟事祭寨"是片面的，至少是夸大了巫的作用。

参考文献：

[1] 黄庆印. 论壮族哲学思想特点及其研究意义 [J]. 广西民族学院学报：哲学社会科学版，1995（1）：36－39.

[2] 马克思，恩格斯. 马克思恩格斯选集·德意志意识形态节选：第 1 卷 [M]. 北京：人民出版社，1995.

[3] 黑格尔. 哲学史讲演录：第 1 卷 [M]. 北京：商务印书馆，1983.

[4] 民族院校公共哲学课教材编写组. 中国少数民族哲学和社会思想资料选编 [M]. 天津：天津教育出版社，1988.

[5] 李富强. 人类学视野中的壮族传统文化 [M]. 南宁：广西人民出版社，1999.

[6] 朱名遂，谢春明. 广西通志·宗教志 [M]. 南宁：广西人民出版社，1995.

第四章　壮医药与壮族稻作文化

中央民族大学梁庭望教授在《水稻人工栽培的发明与稻作文化》一文中提出："中国是世界上最早发明水稻人工栽培的国家；最早发明水稻人工栽培的是江南越人的先民，江南越人是当今江南汉族和华南、西南壮侗语诸族（壮族、侗族、布依族、傣族、黎族、仡佬族、水族、仫佬族、毛南族）的祖先，壮侗语诸族的先民对中国最早发明水稻人工栽培做出了重大贡献。"中国是世界上最早进行水稻人工栽培的国家，稻作文化是中华文明和世界文明的重要文化遗产。稻作文化是骆越文化的重要标志，出土文物及研究表明，古骆越地区有广泛的野生稻存在，骆越人较早认识野生稻，并和苍梧人、西瓯人一起，最先发明了水稻人工栽培法，为中华民族和全人类做出了巨大的贡献。

第一节　壮族稻作文化及其特征

壮族先民把野生稻驯化为栽培稻，是我国最早创造稻作文明的民族之一。生产方式决定文明类型。壮族是稻作民族，他们称水田为"那"，冠以"那"字的地名遍布我国珠江流域及整个东南亚地区。文化生态学视野中的壮族文化，不仅表现为一种稻作文明类型，而且以其整体性显示出区域文化的个性特质。"那"字地名蕴藏的稻作文化和民族文化的丰富内涵，成为生息于这一地区的人们共同的鲜明标志和历史印记，故我们称之为"那文化"。

壮族先民居住的珠江流域属亚热带地区，地理气候环境适宜水稻生长。这一地区自古以来就是我国典型的稻作文化区，野生稻分布广泛，是稻作农业的起源地之一。壮族先民在长期采集野生稻谷的过程中，逐渐认识和掌握了水稻的生长规律，"从潮水上下"，垦殖"雒田"，栽培水稻。湖南省南部道县玉蟾岩遗址和广东省英德市牛栏洞遗址发现距今约 1 万年的稻谷遗存。根据历史文献记载、考古发现和体质人类学研究，这一地区的原始人类就是壮侗语诸族先民，汉族、瑶族、苗族等民族是在秦汉以后才陆续进入这一地区的，因此壮族先民是这一地区稻作文明的创造者。史书记载的"雒田"，实为越语的"麓那"，即山岭谷间的一片田的半音半义的译称。至今，在广西、广东等古越人居住的珠江流域广大地区，仍保留着大量的含"麓"（雒、六、禄、渌、绿、鹿、罗）的地名。含"那"（意为水田）字的地名则更是不计其数。此外，汉语古籍如《山海经》《诗经》《说文解字》中的"耗""膏"

"粳"等字，是壮语中野生稻、稻、稻谷、稻米、稻米饭的汉字记音。遍布壮族各地的冠以"那"字的地名，大者有县名、乡（镇）名，小者有圩场、村庄、田峒、田块名，形成了特有的地域性地名文化景观，构成了珠江流域特有的一种文化形态。而华南到东南亚地区"那"地名分布的广大地域，则形成了"那文化圈"，其具有深厚的文化内涵。壮族及其先民在长期的历史发展过程中，形成了一个据"那"而作、依"那"而居、赖"那"而食、靠"那"而穿、因"那"而乐、为"那"而用、因"那"而涵化的以"那"为本的生产生活模式及"那文化"体系。

一、据"那"而作的生产文化

其主要表现为双肩石斧和大石铲文化。双肩石斧等新石器工具的出现，产生了原始农业，野生稻被驯化为栽培稻。为适应稻作农业的发展，壮族先民不断创造由简单到复杂、由低级到高级的生产工具。新石器晚期出现的大石铲文化，就是壮族先民稻作生产方式及其功利目的的产物。20世纪50年代以来，在邕江及其上游流域发现60多处距今约5000年的颇具规模的大石铲遗址。大石铲通体磨光，棱角分明，曲线柔和，美观精致，特别是形体硕大、造型优美、磨制精致的石铲，成为艺术珍品，令人惊叹不已。大石铲是从双肩石斧演变而来的，是适应沼泽地和水田劳作的工具，随后演化为一种祭祀神器，它注入了古壮族先民对大石铲的崇敬，对丰稔的虔诚祈求，对劳动的热情。大石铲的产生，标志着新石器时代壮族先民生产力的巨大进步，标志着稻作农业发展已具有一定的规模和水平，标志着壮族先民源于稻作生活的祀神意识、审美观念和艺术创造达到了一定的高度。

二、依"那"而居的居住文化

其主要表现为干栏文化。壮语称房屋为"栏"，把在底架上建造的房屋称为"干栏"，或称"更栏"，意为架设在上方的房子。壮族的聚落主要分布在水源丰富的田峒周围，其干栏则沿着田峒周围的山岭，依山势而建，其建筑形式是用木柱穿斗架檩，构成离地面一定高度的底架，再在底架上建造房屋，楼上住人，楼下圈养牲畜和贮存物件。这种建筑形式为适应南方山区潮湿多雨、地势不平的环境而建造，具有防潮、防兽害、防盗、利于通风采光和节约用地的特点。《魏书·僚传》记载，最初是"依树积木以居其上，名曰干阑。干阑大小，随其家口数"。经过长期的历史发展，干栏从建筑过程到其整体和局部的结构及功能特征，都具有丰富的文化内涵。干栏建筑反映了壮族先民对自然环境的适应能力，是我国古代建筑遗产的重要组成部分，如今这种建筑形式在我国南方山区的乡村中仍然存在。

三、赖"那"而食的饮食文化

20世纪60年代起，考古工作者就在邕宁、武鸣、横县、扶绥等县（区）沿邕江及其上游的左江、右江两岸新石器时代早期的贝丘遗址中发现了石杵、石磨棒、石磨盘、石锤等加工谷物的工具，在桂林市甑皮岩遗址出土了距今9000多年的新石器时代早期的陶片。根据遗传学资料，当时这一地区加工的谷物主要是稻谷，麦、粟等是后来传入这一地区的，而根据民族考古学，陶器是适应食用谷物的需要而出现的。这些表明早在距今9000多年的新石器时代早期壮族地区便开始食用稻米，并发明了与食用稻米有关的杵、磨、锤、陶罐等加工工具和炊煮工具。成书于公元前1100多年的《诗经》中的《大雅·公刘》有"乃积乃仓，乃裹餱粮"，其中的"餱粮"（又写作"糇粮"），源于古越族语言，与北方的"粮"同义，至今壮族人民仍称稻、稻谷、稻米、稻米饭为"糇"或"膏"。这就说明，壮族先民在远古时代就学会将稻米煮熟食用，而且随着稻的传播，其传入我国中原地区，并被记录于《诗经》之中。壮族和傣族民间都有"水里有鱼类，田里有稻米"的俗语，这就是壮族先民"饭稻羹鱼"，赖"那"而食，以"那"为中心的饮食文化的生动反映。壮族先民适应自然环境，反复地筛选、培育糯稻，并广泛种植，使之成为生活中的重要食物，形成了以糯米为主食的粮食加工制品。除以糯米作为主食外，糯米还被壮族先民做成五色糯米饭、糍粑、粽子等，形成了喜食糯米的一系列民间饮食文化。

四、靠"那"而穿的服饰文化

壮族先民稻作农业的发展，带动了棉、麻纺织业及服饰加工业的发展。壮族地区富含细长纤维的麻类资源丰富，不仅有野生麻，而且还有人工种植的麻，因此麻纺织业有着十分悠久的历史。壮族地区新石器时代文化遗址中就出土了石制和陶制的纺轮，是用于麻纤维旋转加捻的工具。《汉书·地理志》记载："粤地……处近海，多犀、象、玳瑁、珠玑、银、铜、果、布之凑。"颜师古注："布谓诸杂细布皆是也。"我国古时称布的主要是麻、苎、葛等植物纤维织品，《小尔雅》记载"麻（苎）葛曰布"，说明壮族先民很早以前就会用麻类纤维织布了。广西平乐县银山岭战国墓出土的遗物中，男墓有兵器而无陶纺轮，女墓有陶纺轮而无兵器，反映了当时壮族先民男女自然分工，女子主要从事纺织的社会现象，说明当时麻纺织业已有了较大的发展。《尚书·禹贡》说扬州"岛夷卉服，厥篚织贝"，这里的扬州是指淮河以南至南海的广大地区，贝就是吉贝、劫贝、古贝的简称，古贝当其音译。织贝即用棉花制成的织品，壮侗语族的壮语、布依语、临高语、傣语、黎语，以及越南的侬语、岱语，老挝的老语，泰国的泰语等称棉、棉花等，是同源词，并与吉贝、劫贝、古贝的"贝"有关，说明这些民族在迁居各地之前，种植和使用棉花已经是他们共同生活中的一部分。因此，可以说壮族先民是最早种植和使用棉花的民族之一。

五、因"那"而乐的节日文化

节日文化体现整个民族文化的全民性、认同性。壮族节日文化和稻作农耕生活密切相关，是物质文化、行为文化和观念文化综合的表现形态，是稻作文明类型和壮族文化群体的象征。围绕着稻作农耕，在壮族先民的观念中形成了一系列的崇拜对象，并形成了以祭祀这些崇拜对象为中心的节日活动。例如，红水河一带从农历正月初一到十五过蛙婆节，举行祭祀蛙神活动；新年祭祀牛栏；春节过后举行开耕仪式；农历三四月插秧时举行祭祀秧田活动；农历五月、六月秧苗返青时过禾魂节和牛魂节，举行祭祀禾苗和祭祀牛魂仪式；农历七月稻谷结实泛黄时过尝新节；农历十月霜降收获以后过糍粑节。每个节日都举行一定的仪式并有相应的壮族歌谣，不少地方在插秧、收割时都举行隆重的峒场歌会，通过这些活动以满足他们对物质生活和精神生活的追求。

六、为"那"而用的宗教文化

壮族的宗教有三个层次：①原始宗教；②原生性民间宗教，即麽教和师教；③人为宗教，即道教和佛教。原始宗教的自然崇拜、鬼神崇拜、图腾崇拜和生殖崇拜大抵只是残余形态，他们受到渔猎文化的涵化，也受到稻作文化的涵化。唯有祖先崇拜比较"顽强"，并且被纳入稻作文化系统之中。祭祖先的目的在于祈求人丁兴旺、老少平安、五谷丰登、禽畜繁衍，也同样用稻米制品及其转化物去祈求这两种生产的繁荣。至于原生性民间宗教和人为宗教，其教义和仪式的中心也都是祈求人丁兴旺、老少平安、五谷丰登、禽畜繁衍，也同样用稻米制品及其转化物去祈求这两种生产的繁荣。从总体上来看，这三个层次都纳入稻作文化系统之中。《壮族麽经布洛陀影印译注》收入的 29 种经书中，物的生产部分是以水稻为中心的，各部在造天地之后，便造田、菜园、干栏、牛、泉水、水车、谷仓，接着先招稻魂，然后招牛马魂、猪魂、鸡鸭鹅魂，最后招鱼魂，可见水稻的中心地位明显。

七、因"那"而涵化的艺术文化

壮族的文学艺术充满浓厚的稻作文化氛围，如神话。古越人崇拜蛙，尤其是壮族，蛙是全民族最尊崇的图腾。神话说，壮族三大神是三兄妹，大哥雷公是天神，二哥布洛陀是地神，三妹图额是水神（鳄鱼、犀牛、河马的合体），大哥与三妹私通，生了个怪胎蛙神。它本与父亲住在天上，后来被派到人间做天使，田间有虫它去捉，田间缺水它叫父亲放水。后来被尊为"祖先"，壮话称它为"龚叟"，意思是"你们的祖爷"。三兄妹显然是渔猎文化的代码，蛙则是稻作文化的代码，这里用神话来演绎壮族从渔猎时代到稻作农耕的演变。壮族稻种来源的神话叫作《狗偷稻种》，说稻种是狗到天上偷来的，因此从前广西西北部壮族人民新谷登场的第一顿米饭得先打一碗喂狗，感谢它偷来稻种。由于壮族先民带狗打猎中发现狗身上粘着野生稻粒，引起人们的注意而发现稻种。在壮族的洪水神话《布伯的故事》里，起因

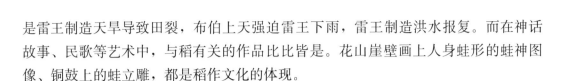

是雷王制造天旱导致田裂，布伯上天强迫雷王下雨，雷王制造洪水报复。而在神话故事、民歌等艺术中，与稻有关的作品比比皆是。花山崖壁画上人身蛙形的蛙神图像、铜鼓上的蛙立雕，都是稻作文化的体现。

第二节 壮医药与稻作文化

大量的考古资料均证明，壮族是一个典型的稻作民族。据专家考证，广西的左江、右江地区及邕江流域是壮族先民——西瓯、骆越民族的原始家园和稻作农业的起源中心之一。稻作文化是西瓯、骆越民族的基本或者说主要的文化特征。

一、稻作文化与壮医药起源

据考证，早在距今 9000 多年的新石器时代早期，广西壮族地区就出现了最初的稻作农业，其后壮族稻作文化历代均有发展。直至今天，稻作文化对壮族社会生活方方面面的影响仍然根深蒂固。医药的起源，与原始农业及畜牧业的发展有着十分密切的关系。关于医药起源的传说很多，《帝王世纪》记载："伏羲氏……乃尝味百药而制九针，以拯夭枉焉。"《史记纲鉴》记载："神农尝百草，始有医药。"《史记·补三皇本纪》记载："神农氏以赭鞭鞭草木，始尝百草，始有医药。"在关于医药起源的传说中，较多的是关于伏羲氏和神农氏的传说。后世多数人认为，神农氏可视为原始农业的代表，而伏羲氏则为早期畜牧业的代表，表明医药的起源与原始农业和原始畜牧业有密切的关系。这些有关医药起源的传说，不仅是我国传统中医药起源的写照，而且也是壮医药起源的真实写照。

在氏族社会的末期，壮族地区的工具制作技术已有所进步，原始农业和渔猎经济都有了较显著的发展。壮族地区原始农业的发展，使壮族先民在农作物栽培的过程中，有条件对更多的植物进行长期细致地观察和进一步的尝试，使部分野生植物药由野生变为人工栽培，从而认识更多的植物药。而渔猎经济的兴起，又为壮族先民提供了较多的鱼肉类食物，在实践中，壮族先民又认识了一些动物药。经过反复的实践与观察，并对这些原始朴素的经验加以总结，逐渐有了壮族药物的起源。

二、稻作文化与壮族养生防病

通过长期的生产、生活实践，壮族人民用自己非凡的智慧，不仅创造了悠久灿烂的壮族文化，而且还创造了与稻作文化密切相关的、人们喜闻乐见的、具有民族内涵的壮族传统体育文化，产生了打铜鼓、打扁担、踩风车、蚂蚜舞、抛绣球等风格独特的壮族传统体育项目。这些壮族传统体育项目非常接近自然，或是劳动的再现，或是技术动作的升华，大多反映了稻作过程中的农耕、祭祀、民俗等活动。因此，壮族传统体育项目成为壮族人民生活中重要的组成部分而世代相传。

打铜鼓源于2000多年前的西瓯、骆越民族举行祭祀和召集战斗的活动。战国时代绘制的广西左江流域花山崖壁画群中，展现打铜鼓的场面比比皆是。秦汉时期以后，封建王朝对岭南的统治不断加强，政治逐渐稳定，社会经济不断发展，各民族之间广泛开展经济、文化交流，打铜鼓活动也在各民族间广泛开展。众多研究已证明，铜鼓文化是源于稻作农业的一种文化。铜鼓纹饰中太阳、雷纹、水波纹以及蛙纹等都与稻作文化有关。壮族民间收藏铜鼓时，有用稻草绳拴其耳，或将铜鼓倒置盛满稻谷的习俗，谓之"养鼓"。铜鼓的功能主要是在家中用稻谷养铜鼓以增加其灵性，或者与神灵沟通，或者传递信息。壮族先民创制的铜鼓，最初是作为炊具之用，后来逐渐扩展到以鼓娱神，以鼓祈雨，以鼓聚众，以鼓号令军阵，以鼓歌舞，以鼓作为权力与财富的象征，等等。稻作文化与铜鼓文化的形成与发展，是一个相互影响、相互促进的过程。壮族民间有一句俗语："铜鼓不响，庄稼不长。"由铜鼓而形成的打铜鼓活动，可以说与稻作农业有很大的关系。打铜鼓现已成为壮族人民喜闻乐见的一项民族传统体育活动。如今红水河流域的东兰、天峨、巴马、凤山等地，壮族聚居区每年举行的蚂蚜节依然盛行打铜鼓。击打时，铜鼓后面还有一个人持木桶套于鼓后，这样一敲一拉，发出"咚呼""咚呼"的音响节奏。鼓声协调悦耳，击鼓者伴着旋律边鼓边舞。他们充分施展自己的拿手技艺，时而左旋，时而右转，动作刚劲敏捷，快慢相间，鼓声此起彼伏，节奏分明；鼓阵庄严雄浑，动人心魄。打铜鼓的动作粗犷古朴，情调高昂，体现出壮族人民淳朴、刚毅和勇敢顽强的民族精神。打铜鼓活动不但可以增强人们的力量、灵敏性和耐久力，而且可以培养人们坚毅、果敢、勇于进取和积极向上的优秀品质。

扁担是人类最早使用、也是保持时间最久的运输工具之一。由谷物加工劳动形成的打扁担是深受壮族民间喜爱的一项体育活动，是一种由壮族稻作生产劳动发展演变而来的体育活动，因使用扁担器具，故名"打扁担"。打扁担起源于"打春堂"，壮话叫"特榔"，也称"谷榔""谷鲁榔"，壮族人民又称打扁担为"虏烈""打虏烈"。打扁担的场地可大可小，人数为四人、六人、八人、十人不等，以双数为宜。打扁担时，大家围在长凳两边每人拿着扁担，双手握扁担中部，按传统节奏用扁担两端敲打长凳，打法变化多端。打扁担活动的传统套路是根据壮族人民的劳动过程来设计的，有"打春堂""全家乐""大团圆""插秧""车水""打谷""庆丰收"等。动作有上下对撑，站立和下蹲，原地和行进，以及转身和跳跃，加之伴以锣鼓和不时发出的"咳咳"呼声，表现出强烈的节奏感。节日的打扁担活动是模拟农事活动中的耙田、插秧、戽水、收割、打谷、舂米等姿势动作，既是对稻作生产过程的模拟再现，也是对全年生产活动的总结，更是希望通过轰轰烈烈、喜庆热闹的类同性表演庇佑来年丰硕的稻作生产。

水稻种植需要耐心、细心、恒心。长期的稻作农耕，磨砺了壮族人民的性格，使他们形成了温和内向、吃苦耐劳、耐心容忍、互助礼让、外柔内刚的民族性格。水稻是一种比较娇气的农作物，种植需要经过整秧田、浸种、育秧、耙田、插秧、返青、分蘖、幼穗分化、孕穗、抽穗、乳熟、黄熟、完熟等 10 多个大小阶段和程序。从秧苗如针开始到稻谷成熟的几个月里，人们必须像抚育婴儿那样精心护理，随时注意气温、排灌、催肥、除草、防虫、防病、防倒伏。收割期还要防禽畜祸害和梅雨天气，耐心细致，急躁不得。水田和旱地不同，前者要选择阳光充足、地面较平、靠近水源、不旱不涝的地方，不是随便找一块地就可以耕田的，因而要求人们的居住地相对稳定，尽量减少流动。这就形成了壮族人民温和内向、不喜流动、不爱张扬、耐心容忍的性格。现在人们看到的桂林山水、八宝风光，殊不知古代这些地方森林环绕，数百里无日色，炎热多雨，瘴气弥漫，虫蛇怪兽遍地横行，并非人类理想的生存之地。直到宋代，广西仍被称为"大法场"（宋代周去非的《岭外代答》），唐代、宋代、元代、明代时期广西是贬谪犯人的地方。唐代诗人沈佺期被流放路过广西北流时写道："昔传瘴江路，今到鬼门关。此地无人老，迁流几客还。"在这样的条件下，壮族人民要顶着酷热瘴气泡在水田里，其辛苦可想而知。天长日久，壮族人民磨炼出吃苦耐劳的品格，表面温和，内心坚强；没有攻击性，但在维护自己的劳动成果时十分勇敢。因此，《赤雅》曰："假兵鸷悍天下称最。"这就是壮族人民外柔内刚的直接体现。汉族是农业民族，壮族也是农业民族，在文化上容易相通，而壮族人民学到了儒家的温良恭谦，甚至把二十四孝改编为 24 首长诗，这在中原地区是没有的。

从河姆渡文化的发掘中得知，在七八千年前，百越民族的祖先已有种植水稻的历史。到骆越时代，壮族先民不仅会种植水稻，而且大量种植棉花和纺纱织布，把稻作文明推向更高的程度。谷以养命，布以御寒，谷从土生，故壮族人民也被称为"土人"。古人称水田为"那"，意为山岭谷地间的一片田，"那"字蕴藏着壮族先民稻作文化的丰富内涵。由"那文化"产生的陶器文化和大石铲文化，对烧煮食物、饮食卫生的发展起到了促进作用，尤其是壮族先民发明陶器后，渔猎熟食进步了，更有利于人体各组织器官，特别是大脑的发育成长，预防和减少了肠胃病的发生，体现了壮族先民养生防病观念的初步形成。值得一提的是，壮族先民奇特的"防治未病"的卫生习俗——鼻饮。《汉书·贾捐之传》云："骆越之人，父子同川而浴，相习以鼻饮。"《魏书·僚传》亦云："僚者，盖南蛮之别种……其口中嚼时并鼻饮。"宋代范成大著的《桂海虞衡志》云："南人习鼻饮，有陶器如杯碗，旁植一小管若瓶嘴，以鼻就管吸酒浆。暑月以饮水，云水自鼻入咽，快不可言，邕州人已如此。"宋代周去非著的《岭外代答》云："鼻饮之法，以瓢盛少水，置盐及山姜汁数滴于水中，瓢则有窍，施小管如瓶嘴，插诸鼻中，导水升脑，循脑而下入喉。富者以银为之，次以锡，次陶器，次瓢。饮时……然后水安流入鼻，不与气相激。既饮必噫气，以为凉脑快膈，莫若此也。"鼻饮具有"凉脑快膈"的功效，这是壮族先民为了抵御南方湿热地气和动植物腐臭之气混合而成的瘴毒及防暑降温而创造的一种保健习俗。至今，壮医使用的洗鼻雾化疗法，对鼻病、喉病、呼吸系统病证均有一定的防治效果。

第三节　壮医理论与稻作文化

一、稻作文化孕育了壮医"三道"理论

稻作文化是骆越文化的重要标志，是中华文明和世界文明的重要文化遗产。出土文物及研究表明，古骆越地区有广泛的野生稻存在，骆越人较早认识野生稻，与苍梧人、西瓯人一起，最先发明了水稻人工栽培法，为中华民族和全人类做出了巨大的贡献。南宁市亭子圩遗址出土的原始稻谷脱壳工具，经 ^{14}C 年代测定，年代为距今 11000 年，仅次于湖南省道县壮族苍梧部祖先留下的距今 20000～12000 年的炭化稻粒，比江西省万年县距今 10000 年的稻谷遗址早了至少 2000 年。早在骆田时代，骆越人就已经掌握了整治田畴技术，利用潮水涨退选择田块。《史记·南越王传》索引《广州记》云："交趾有骆田，仰潮水上下，人食其田，名为'骆人'。"广西民族学家覃乃昌先生说："壮族地区早在距今 9000 多年就出现了原始的稻作农业，成为稻作农业的起源地之一。"

水稻在壮族生活中占有举足轻重的地位，对壮族人民心理产生了深刻的影响，形成了对水稻的特殊观念。（1）稻米高贵观念。壮族人民认为稻米来自天上，非人间作物，因而在一切粮食作物中，稻米等级最高，故祭祀、宴请贵客一定要用大米食品。（2）稻魂观念。壮族人民认为，田有田神，禾有禾神，开耕前要祭祀，减收要招禾魂。（3）稻人互渗观念。我国古代普遍有天人感应观念，这种观念体现在《周易》中。壮族人民对水稻就保留了这种观念。古时歌圩，要让男女青年在田间模拟交媾，认为这样禾苗灌浆才饱满。插秧时如果让穿白衣人先下田，不仅失收，而且还要遭到报应。有的地方认为歌圩上唱歌越多，禾苗越高兴，当年稻谷越丰收。有的地方还认为稻草或禾苗可以避邪，挂一把于门外可避百鬼；有的人挂一小把稻草在腰间，可避野鬼，走路时心中有安全感。（4）稻米即生命的观念。壮族人民普遍认为稻米代表人的生命，故以之添寿。壮族老人过生日时，要由子女在师公诵经时往其寿门缸里面添新米，故壮族人民把做寿称为"补粮"，意思是里面的米可以掏出一点熬粥补寿，但绝对不能掏空，否则意味着生命即将终结，不吉利。因此，壮族把人的幸福长寿叫作"稻米命"，苦命叫作"（野）菜命"。这些观念到现在并没有

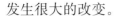

发生很大的改变。

　　壮族稻作文化的兴起，不仅对壮医药的起源起到了积极的促进作用，而且对壮医药后来的发展也有着深刻的影响。壮族是一个典型的稻作民族，稻作文化直接与"食"有关，随着稻作技术的不断进步，壮族人民餐桌之物越来越丰富，并逐渐总结出"食"对养生保健、祛病逐邪的作用。壮医素有"药补不如食补"之说，即与稻作文化及饮食文化有密切的关系。壮族稻作文化还与壮医理论的形成有密切的渊源。据考证，壮族是我国最早种植水稻的民族之一，壮族先民在实践中观察到，水稻察天地之气以生长，赖天地之气以收藏，而人体则赖谷物以养，一日三餐不可或缺，于是将谷物得以进入人体并消化吸收之通道称为"谷道"。壮族先民在实践中还观察到，大自然中水和气对农作物的生长是非常重要的，没有水和气，或者水、气过多或过少，都不利于农作物的生长。同样，水和气对人体也是非常重要的，于是在壮医理论体系中，将人体另外两条极重要的水液交换和气体交换的通道称之为"水道"和"气道"。"谷道""气道""水道"三道理论是壮医理论的核心内容之一，其提出源于壮族先民对人与大自然的朴素认识和实践经验的总结，可以明显地看出这三道理论中壮族稻作文化的痕迹。

二、稻作文化与壮医阴阳理论

　　古代人们认为太阳每天清晨从东方升起（重生），给大自然以光明和温暖，傍晚从西边落下（死亡），给大自然以黑暗与死寂，具有死而复生的能力及给万物以生机的能力；同时先民的农耕生产，特别是稻作生产对阳光的需求和依赖，希望太阳多给人们一些光和热，让人们有吃有穿、身体健康。先民们就自然而然地对"生生之谓易"的太阳产生了敬畏的心理，从而萌发了崇拜太阳的思想，尊之为神，称"太阳神"。古人崇拜太阳，必然要仔细观察太阳，研究太阳的运动。而"阴阳"二字就是对太阳运动（生与死）的形象描述。清晨，太阳升起（生），光芒四射属"阳"字表述的意蕴，自然界呈现一派生机与活力；傍晚，太阳落山（死），光芒被遮，属"阴"字表述的意蕴，自然界呈现一派死气与萧条。于是自然而然地形成了自然界万事万物都是在太阳的阴与阳（即生与死）的变化中而变化着的，自然而然地将太阳上升成为宇宙主宰之神的地位。太阳的光和热不仅是农作物生长的条件，而且太阳的规律运行本身亦为定居的农夫们提供了最基本的行为模式（所谓"日出而作，日入而息"）、基础的空间和时间观念，因此太阳成为人们认识宇宙秩序，给自然万物编码分类的坐标符号。由于人类是借助太阳的升落而确定东西方位和昼夜之别的，因此它实际上是空间意识和时间意识得以建立的最主要的天然尺度。正是有了日神（太阳）信仰，才使本来原始朴素的"阴阳"概念上升成为对中国传统文化影响至为深远的阴阳学说。作为一种系统的方法论，阴阳学说形成于晚周秦汉时期之际，但其基本概念早就孕育在中国上古日神信仰观念的母腹中了。

水稻生长在南方，南方气候炎热，昼白夜黑，阴生阳长，因稻作文化的不断发展，由此延伸出了壮医阴阳理论。明代的《广西通志·卷十七》曰，壮族民间"笃信阴阳"。稻作文化使壮族先民对阴阳有了较早的认识，形成了壮医最初的阴阳概念。阴阳对立，阴阳互根，阴阳消长，阴阳平衡，阴阳转化，揭示了大自然万物变化的规律。壮医以阴阳认识人的生老病死、机体的脏腑功能以及人与自然变化的关系，逐步发展形成了阴阳为本的理论，并成为壮医的基本理论。

参考文献：

[1] 梁启成，钟鸣. 中国壮药学 [M]. 南宁：广西民族出版社，2005.

[2] 罗世敏. 大明山的记忆：骆越古国历史文化研究 [M]. 南宁：广西民族出版社，2006.

[3] 苏秉琦. 中国文明起源新探 [M]. 北京：生活·读书·新知三联书店，2000.

[4] 黄汉儒. 中国壮医学 [M]. 南宁：广西民族出版社，2001.

[5] 梁庭望. 壮族的稻作文化和社会发展探索 [J]. 文山师范高等专科学校学报，2006，19（3）：1-5.

[6] 梁庭望. 中国稻作文化的保护与开发利用 [J]. 河池学院学报，2006，26（4）：63-68.

第五章　壮医药与壮族习俗文化

第一节　壮族习俗文化

一、壮族习俗概述

习俗，即习惯、风俗。著名壮族学者梁庭望教授指出，风俗习惯是人们根据自己的生活内容、生活方式和自然条件，在一定的社会物质生产水平下，自然而然地创造出来的，世代相传，成为约束人们思想和行为的规范。通常我们把民间的各种风俗习惯也称为民俗，它包括生产、生活、礼仪、岁时、社会、信仰、游艺和文艺等方面。

一方水土养一方人。我国地域辽阔，民族众多，56 个民族犹如 56 朵鲜花，竞相争艳，装点着祖国大好河山。由于自然条件与社会环境（生产力及物质文化水平等）的差异，各个民族在长期的历史发展过程中，形成并传承了自己独特的行为习惯和生活方式。《晏子春秋》云"百里而异习，千里而殊俗"，道出了不同地区不同民族习俗的差异性。壮族是祖国大家庭中的一朵奇葩，其习俗文化源远流长，是壮族人民精神生活、物质生活和行为方式的重要表现形式。壮族民俗在服饰、饮食、居住、婚嫁、丧葬、信仰、生产、交通、贸易、社会组织及文化艺术等方面，自然地表露出壮族人民的心理特征、行为方式和语言习惯，是壮民族特征的基本构成要素之一，是将壮族人民联结起来的一条纽带，壮族人民可以从这些民俗中找到认同感。

二、壮族习俗文化的特性

壮族习俗文化具有本民族个性。第一，它与古越人有密切的传承关系。如在语言、文学、生活习俗上可以看到古越人文化的延续。第二，封建性相对较少。如妇女在社会生活中有较大的发言权。第三，地区性的差别较大。某一风俗在壮族各支系各地区中常表现出不同的形态，使壮族风俗具有多样性，这可能与其生活的地理环境有较大的关系。第四，具有内向性和隐蔽性。如壮族人民不会从鲜明的外在形象或者张扬的行为个性等方面给人以强烈的印象。第五，受汉族风俗影响较大。如几乎所有的汉族节日都把壮族人民的节日列入其中。

壮医的形成和发展也离不开壮族文化这块肥沃的土壤。壮医与壮族地区的习俗文化有着密切的关系。如壮族习俗"信鬼神，重淫祀"是壮医与巫医并存的根源，断发、文身、服色尚青黑、鼻饮、喜居干栏、捡骨重葬等习俗，亦与医药有关。学习壮族的习俗文化，不仅可以了解壮族人民丰富多彩的精神世界、物质创造和行为特点，而且还可以窥探壮医形成和发展的根源及其赖以生存的文化基础。

第二节　壮医药与壮族药市习俗

一、药市传说

壮族地区草木繁茂，四季常青，药材资源十分丰富。每年农历五月初五，壮乡各村寨的乡民都去赶药市，将各自采摘的各种药材运到圩镇药市出售，或去买药、看药、闻药。壮族民间认为，端午节的草药根肥叶茂，药力宏大，疗效最好。这天去药市，可以饱吸百药之气，进而可以预防疾病，一年之中少生病或不生病。

壮族药市的形成与壮族民间流传的"爷奇斗瘟神"的故事有关。古时候有一位医术高明的老壮医"爷奇"，带领壮族人民大量采集各种山间草药，跟一个在每年农历五月初五就来肆虐人间的瘟神——"都宜"（壮语意即"千年蛇精"）做斗争。这瘟神"都宜"很厉害，凡是有人居住的村寨，它都要去喷射毒气，散布瘟疫，放蛊害人。一家一户对付不了它，一村一寨也奈何它不得。"爷奇"常年为乡亲们治病，并仔细观察"都宜"的恶行，发现它特别害怕艾叶、菖蒲、雄黄、半边莲、七叶一枝花等草药，于是就教人们采集这些草药，或挂在家门，或置备于家中，以抵抗"都宜"的袭击；在"都宜"到来之前，或以草药煎汤内服，或煮水洗浴，可预防瘟疫流行，即使患了病，也会很快痊愈。因为有的村寨采集的草药较多，有的村寨采集的较少，就出现采集不到齐全的品种，"爷奇"就建议大家在农历五月初五把家里的草药都摆到街上来，这样一来可以向瘟神"都宜"示威，二来可以互通有无，交换草药品种，交流防病治病的经验。"都宜"发现各个村寨的群众居然储备了那么多草药，而且联合起来对付它，气焰就不那么嚣张了，最后只好逃之夭夭。"爷奇"不但教会人们采药，而且教会人们种药，被壮族人民尊为"药王"。后来，赶药市便成了壮乡民俗。如今，壮族聚居的靖西、忻城、隆林、贵港等地都还有药市，其中尤以靖西的端午药市最为著名、规模最大。

二、药市与壮医药

据考证，靖西端午药市始于宋代，盛于明清时期。每到端午，当地和周边的那坡、德保、大新等地以及云南富宁县等地的草医药农，都将各自采摘的各种野生新鲜的草药运到靖西县城交易。附近村寨的壮族人民扶老携幼赶往药市去吸百药之气，或向壮医药农请教医药知识，或买回各自所需的草药。赶药市既是交流药材知识和疾病防治经验的好机会，也是壮族人民崇尚医药的体现。

靖西端午药市的形成和发展得益于良好的群众基础和优越的地理环境。靖西市壮族人口占其总人口的 99.4%，是壮族主要聚居地之一，当地壮族人民一直延续着端午赶药市的习俗，每年参与药市节的群众多达数万人。靖西位于桂西南边陲、云贵高原东南边缘，大部分地区处于北回归线以南，属亚热带季风气候，地势较高，平均海拔 800 米，年平均气温 19.1 ℃，年均降水量 1600 毫米，极为适宜生物的多样性生长。优越的地理气候条件，使得该市中药、壮药资源十分丰富，拥有药材资源 3000 多种，被誉为百草之乡，为当地各族群众采集、利用植物药及其药市文化提供了丰富的资源条件。有学者经过实地调查，发现进入药市交易的药用植物多达 564 种，其中有名贵药材（如田七、蛤蚧），也有大宗药材（如金银花、薏苡仁），还有常用地道壮药（如钻地风、九节风、黄花倒水莲、藤杜仲、鸡血藤、岩黄连等）。靖西端午药市的发展，对当地壮医药的开发利用发挥了重要作用。

第三节　壮医药与壮族生活习俗

一、文身

文身，又叫刺青。在人体皮肤上绘制花纹图案，然后以针刺破皮肤，再用颜料（古代人多用青黛）涂染，待创痕愈合后，即成永久性花纹。壮族先民文身的习俗，见于大量的历史文献记载。《汉书·地理志》曰："（越人）文身断发，以避蛟龙之害。"宋代《太平寰宇记》记载，邕州左江、右江各州"其百姓恶是雕题、凿齿、画面、文身"。古代壮族先民除了狩猎，还有一部分人以渔业为生。在南方的江河湖海，常常有很多蛟龙（即鳄鱼）出没，伤害渔民。渔民出于对蛟龙的敬畏，故在身上画它的图案，打扮成"龙子"，祈求蛟龙视其为同类，不要伤害自己。文身习俗的形成最早是出于氏族、部落的图腾标志或称图腾徽号，目的是为了求得图腾神的保佑，如所谓"以避蛟龙之害"者是也；同时又便于彼此间交际和通婚过程中认同和区别；再后来就像衣服上的花纹和银饰一样，被当作一种美的时尚。文身需用浅刺针具作工具，且文身活动带有宗教性质，在一定的历史时期会激励壮族人民去效仿，故文身对壮医浅刺疗法的形成和发展起到了一定的促进作用。

二、断发

断发是古代壮族先民的风俗，即截短头发之意。《庄子·内篇·逍遥游》载"宋人资章甫而适诸越，越人断发文身，无所用之"，所谓断发者，"剪发使短……而不束发加冠之意也"。根据《汉书·地理志》的记载，从吴越到岭南九郡，所有的越人都有断发的风俗。从广西宁明花山岩画上的人物像来看，壮族先民骆越人的发饰确实有断发情况存在。黄现璠著的《壮族通史》指出："断发文身，这是南方海边、大河的近水居民的风尚，同时也是原始民族图腾崇拜的反映。"可见，壮族先民断发的最初目的与文身相似，追求"以象龙子"，这是古代越人崇拜图腾的一种心态。我们还可以从医疗卫生的角度来看待这一习俗。壮族聚居地区气候属亚热带湿润季风气候，年平均气温在 20 ℃左右，夏季日照时间长，雨量丰沛。壮族先民断发亦可能与天气湿热有关，因断发可以使体温易于散发，常被汗湿的头发更易干爽，同时免于被钩挂而挫伤，符合卫生要求。

三、凿齿

凿齿与断发、文身一样，也是壮族先民的一种毁身为饰的方法。凿齿有两种情况：一种是凿去前齿，再装上假牙。《山海经·海外南经》记载："羿与凿齿战于寿华之野，羿射杀之，在昆仑虚东。"（注："凿齿，亦人也，齿如凿，长五六尺。"）《太平广记·雅州风俗》记载："邛雅之夷僚……长则拔去上齿，加狗牙以为华饰。今有四牙长于诸牙而唇高者，则别是一种，能食人。无长齿者不能食人。"这一类"凿齿人"有吃人的恶习。另一种凿齿情况是成年后拔去前齿，作为成年或已婚的标志。张华的《博物志·异俗》记载："僚子……及长，皆拔去上齿牙各一，以为华饰。"元代李京的《云南志略·诸夷风俗》写道："土（都）僚蛮，叙州南、乌蒙北皆是，男子十四、五，则左右击去两齿，然后婚娶。"《太平广记·贵州风俗》（贵州，今广西贵港市）记载："有俚人，皆乌浒，诸夷率同一姓，男女同川而浴，生首子则食之，云宜弟……既嫁，便缺去前一齿。"《番社采风图考》记载："番俗，男女成婚日牵手……男女各折去上齿相遗……"壮族凿齿习俗，追求的是一种质朴的"残缺美"，反映了壮族先民特殊的审美情趣，也是一场别开生面的"成人礼"。另外，凿齿还有一个目的，就是为了便于服药治病。这一说法在《新唐书·南蛮列传下平南僚》中有记载："又有乌武僚，地方瘴毒，中者不能饮药，故自凿齿。"由此可见，早在唐代以前，壮族先民对瘴毒防治已有一定的认识。瘴病重症，可能出现抽搐昏迷、口噤不开等症状，导致药食不能进入。故人们先行凿齿，以便应急时能顺利服药。

四、鼻饮

古代南方壮族人民以及其他一些民族有一种奇特的习俗，即鼻饮。有学者认为鼻饮是模仿大象用鼻饮水的仿生行为。有关鼻饮的记载始于汉代，如《异物志》记载："乌浒，南蛮之别名，巢居鼻饮。"《汉书·贾捐之传》记载："骆越之人，父子同川而浴，相习以鼻饮，与禽兽无异。"到了宋代，周去非的《岭外代答》对鼻饮的方法做了比较详细的描述："邕州溪峒及钦州村落，俗多鼻饮。鼻饮之法，以瓢盛少水，置盐及山姜汁数滴于水中。瓢则有窍，施小管如瓶嘴插，诸鼻中，导水升脑，循脑而下，入喉……饮时必口噍鱼鲊一片，然后水安流入鼻，不与气相激。既饮必噫气，以为凉脑快膈，莫若此也。"由此可以看出，鼻饮流行于壮族聚居地区（邕州溪峒及钦州村落），鼻饮之法，非但饮水，还可饮酒。宋代陆游的《老学庵笔记》记载："辰、沅，靖州蛮有仡伶、有仡僚……邻里共劝，乃受，饮酒以鼻，一饮至数升，名钩藤酒，不知何物。醉则男女聚而踏歌。"这段话描写了当时南方壮族先民以鼻饮酒，不限男女，载歌载舞的热闹场面。清朝陆次云的《峒溪纤志》曰："咂酒一名钓（钩）藤酒，以米、杂草子为之，以火酿成，不刍不酢，以藤吸取。多有以鼻饮者，谓由鼻入喉，更有异趣。"可见，壮族鼻饮之习俗一直延续到清代。

壮族地区夏季炎热多雨，湿热地气和动植物腐臭之气混合而形成瘴毒，素有"瘴乡"之称。从周去非《岭外代答》所记载鼻饮中加入山姜药物来看，鼻饮应是民间壮医所总结的一种针对瘴疾和中暑的防治方法。在壮族地区，至今流传着一种洗鼻及雾化吸入以防病的方法，即煎取某些草药液令患者吸入洗鼻，或蒸煮草药化为气雾，令患者吸入以预防一些时疫疾病。这种方法究其源流，与古代鼻饮不无关系。这种奇特的卫生民俗包含着物理降温和黏膜给药等科学因素，对鼻病、喉病等呼吸系统病证都有一定的疗效。

五、嚼槟榔

槟榔在岭南地区的栽培、嚼食已有很久远的历史。早在东汉时期，杨孚在《异物志》中就有关于岭南越人嚼槟榔的记载。明代王济的《日询手镜》记载："岭南人好食槟榔，横人尤甚。"壮族人过去行聘、结婚，槟榔为必备之物。清代的《白山司志》记载："土人结婚……行聘亦以槟榔为重。富厚家以千计。用苏木染之，每八枚包以箬叶，每二三十叶为一束，缚以红绒。"槟榔作为聘礼，女方只要收下，即表示承认婚约。壮族人民平时待客也以槟榔为先。在广西龙州、防城港、上思、上林和宁明等地的壮族村庄里，盛行着"客至不设茶，唯以槟榔为礼"的习俗。徐松石的《粤江流域人民史》记载："壮人喜食槟榔及蒌叶，现在两粤此风仍盛。"民国的《上林县志》记载："凡交际，亦以槟榔为先。客至，茶话及宴会，俱以槟榔致敬。"从谐音来看，"槟"者，"宾"也；"榔"者，"郎"也。古人称贵客为宾为郎，故以槟榔待客，表示对客人的尊重和敬意。从药用价值来看，槟榔能辟秽除瘴、行气利水、杀虫消积。如唐代刘恂的《岭表录异》记载："槟榔交广生者……自嫩及老，采实啖之。以扶留藤、瓦屋灰同食之，以祛瘴疠。"《平乐县志》说，当地"气多痞瘴，槟榔之嚼，甘如饔飧"。可以说，壮族人民嚼食槟榔的一个重要原因是用槟榔来防治瘴气。

六、居干栏

干栏，是南方少数民族包括壮族的传统民居，由原始人类的巢居逐步演变而成的一种建筑类型，具有鲜明的地方特色和民族风格，在中国古代史书中又有干栏、高栏、阁栏、葛栏和麻栏等名称，应当是由少数民族语言音译而来的。在壮语中，"干栏（gwnzranz）"是对木结构楼居式建筑的称谓，意即"上面的房屋"。"干栏"一词最早见于《魏书》："僚者，盖南蛮之别种……依树积木，以居其上，名曰干栏。"明代邝露在《赤雅》中也说："辑茅索绹，伐木架楹，人栖其上，牛羊犬豕畜其下，谓之麻栏。"明代田汝成在《炎徼纪闻》中指出："壮人……居室茅缉而不涂，衡板为阁，上以栖止，下畜牛羊猪犬，谓之麻栏。"在壮族聚居的广西合浦、平乐、贵港、梧州、钟山、贺州、兴安、桂林、西林、都安等地，发现大量秦汉时期的墓葬，其中出土有陶制干栏建筑模型，说明壮族历史上有"居干栏"的居住习俗。这种干栏建筑一直沿袭到现在。如今壮族一些地区的群众，仍然习惯于使用这种建筑形式。

干栏建筑的主要特征是分上、下两层的楼式建筑，上层住人，下层贮放农具等器物及圈养牛、猪等牲畜，居住面距地面若干米。壮族先民发明干栏建筑，与壮族聚居地——南方的自然环境有关。南方气候温暖潮湿，河流、湖泊众多，森林繁盛，植被覆盖率高，加上森林中湿热蒸郁，使得植物茎、叶腐败，动物尸体腐烂，容易产生致病的毒气——瘴气。另外，森林地区是毒蛇猛兽栖集之地，为了人畜的安全，壮族先民在建筑设计时除考虑避寒暑外，还要考虑能适应这种自然条件。正如《新唐书·南平僚传》说："土气受瘴病，山有毒草及沙虱、蝮蛇，人并楼居，登梯而上，号为干栏。"干栏建筑因地制宜，上层居室住人，通风凉爽，日照充足，适应南方的地理环境和气候变化，既防潮以减少风湿病的发生，又居高能防避瘴气，并且能避猛兽虫蛇之害；下层圈养牲畜，堆放杂物，可以防止牲畜四处乱窜、随地粪便，维护村寨的环境卫生，具有独特的地方民族特色，也充分体现了壮族先民独特的卫生防病智慧。

第四节　壮医药与壮族服饰习俗

服饰，即服装（衣服）和装饰（修饰）。服装包括衣、裤、裙、帽、围巾、手套、腰带、鞋、袜、绑腿等；装饰包括发型、首饰、背包（背袋）等。服装衣着是一个民族最具特色的外在形象，展现了一个民族的精神内涵。

壮族是一个开放包容的民族，在与其他民族的交流过程中，善于汲取汉族等民族的文化，其中壮族服饰也受到较深的汉族时尚元素的影响。如今在一些经济较发达地区，壮族人民衣着已逐渐被汉化，外表上已难以区分出是壮族人还是汉族人，但有些壮族地区的服饰仍保留着自己的民族特色。特别是在桂北、桂西和桂南的偏远山区，由于自然条件的制约，人们与外界交流互通较少，社会生活改变相对缓慢，这些地区的壮族服饰仍然保持着古代沿袭下来的传统特色。勤劳智慧的壮族人民爱生活、爱劳动，也有着爱美的天性，我们可以从壮族传统服饰的材质、式样、颜色等方面感受到壮族人民的审美情趣和生活态度。

一、卉服

壮族服饰材质以麻、棉、竹为主。这种以草木纤维制成的衣服称为"卉服"。壮族人民最早纺织所用的原料为苎麻和葛麻，麻类布是壮族地区使用最久、最广泛的布类，比棉花还要早。据考证，汉代壮族地区即产苎麻布，从宋代开始，苎麻就是广西的传统产品，广西是全国苎麻的重要产区之一。麻布易散热，其所织夏衣，"轻凉离汗"，能适应南方湿热的气候特点。棉织品又叫吉贝布，吉贝（或古贝）即今之棉花。壮族的棉布在唐代就已闻名京师，诗人白居易曾用桂布（即吉贝布、棉布）缝衣，并赞道："桂布白如雪，吴绵软如云。"壮族人民以竹为布，晋代就已出现。到了唐代，贺州等地竹布被列为贡品。宋代的《太平寰宇记》记载："今之僚，布以竹，灰为盐。"这里的"僚"指邕州壮族人民。清代的《嘉庆一统志》记载了平乐、恭城"县妇能以竹作衫"。可见，竹布是壮乡的特产。直到现代，尽管各种合成纤维不断涌现，但麻、棉、竹等仍是壮族服饰的重要原料。这些原料均为可再生的天然产品，由此壮族人民爱护环境、崇尚自然的理念可见一斑。

二、左衽通裙

壮族服饰式样讲究实用与美观。古代壮族地区服饰的特点是男子左衽（衣前襟开向左），女子着通裙。《战国策·赵二策》记载："披发文身，错臂左衽，瓯骆之民也。"《旧唐书》一百八十五卷记载："南平僚，男子左衽，女子横布两幅，穿巾而贯首，名曰通裙。"到了清代，壮族服饰无论男女，头上均挽髻和包头，上身穿短衫，衫长仅及脐，下身穿短裙或百褶长筒裙。近现代壮族服饰式样有以下特征：上衣为右衽无领阑干衣，袖宽，衣长一般仅及腰间，亦有些地方长至膝盖，领口、袖口、襟边以及下摆边缘均镶有各色花边。下身穿长裤、裤脚宽大，在膝盖处绣有一大一小的花边。裤外套短裙，均用五色绒线绣上花纹图案，亦有用蜡染把铜鼓上的花纹图案印在裙上。不穿裙者往往在腰间系上围裙，围裙上用各种颜色的绒线或丝线绣上精美的花纹图案，中年妇女头上均挽髻并有包头的习惯（见石景斌的《壮族服饰介绍》）。壮族服饰的式样特点之一就是衣袖、裤脚宽松，使四肢得到最大限度的舒展，这样更便于在山里行走和田间劳作，讲究实用。另外，服饰上多或绣或染各种花边图案，图案题材主要是花草树木、鸟兽虫鱼、山水流云、日月星辰等自然界当中与人们的生活息息相关的内容，这样的款式既朴素大方，又符合审美的需要，同时也反映了壮族人民热爱大自然，崇尚人和天地万物互相融合的思想。

三、色尚青黑

在壮族传统服饰中，以黑色、蓝色为最具代表性的颜色。黑色是土地的本色，也是壮族服饰的主色调，代表着庄重和严肃。每逢喜庆或祭祀等重大节日，人们都会穿上黑色盛装。至今，这种主色调仍保留在那坡与龙州等地的壮族人民群体中，如百色市那坡县黑衣壮族人民、崇左市龙州县金龙一带自称"布代"的壮族人民。蓝色是最亲近大自然的颜色，在日常生活中，很多壮族人也经常穿着蓝布服装，披戴蓝布头巾，身穿蓝布肚兜或围裙。蓝色素、黑色素是以十字花科植物菘蓝、草大青、豆科植物木蓝、爵床科植物马蓝或蓼科植物蓼蓝等叶子加工提炼而成，俗称"蓝靛"（其主要成分是靛蓝）。用蓝靛浸染出来的布料，具有色调沉着、色彩清新亮丽的特点。《本草拾遗》说，蓝靛"敷热疮，解诸毒"，可见蓝靛具有清热解毒的作用。因此，壮族的蓝黑色服饰具有解毒的作用，可防避蚊虫，适应壮族地区的气候环境特点。

第五节　壮医药与壮族防疫习俗

一、悬艾虎

壮族民间普遍认为，艾可以避邪气，故有悬艾、佩艾禳邪的习俗。对于身体虚弱常患病的小孩，大人常特意缝制内装有艾叶的小香囊佩挂于小孩身上，作用是避邪气以保小孩平安。有些壮族妇女背小孩走远路，也在背带后面插上一根艾枝。凡认为有邪魔入室的人家，也会在大门口外两侧悬挂艾叶。送葬归来时，通常用艾叶就着清水擦手，或用柚子叶煮水洗手以祛邪气。悬艾和饮菖蒲酒是壮族端午节非常重要的一项活动。《靖西县志》记载："五月五日，家家悬艾虎，持蒲剑，饮雄黄酒，以避疠疫。"农历五月初五的清晨，壮族人民在鸡还没有叫之前就要将艾草采摘回来，用艾叶、艾根做成人形或老虎的形状，俗称"艾虎"，悬在门楣的中央；将菖蒲制成宝剑挂在屋檐下。古人认为虎能够吞噬鬼怪，将艾与虎两种避邪物相加，其避邪功能更强。这一天还要用艾叶、菖蒲、大蒜烧水洗澡，并将水洒在房前屋后。其实，这样做是非常符合夏季卫生要求的。端午节后，天气转热，正是各种病菌生长繁殖的时期，此时用中草药煮水喷洒，可有效地消灭、抑制病菌的生长，清洁环境。这与端午节饮菖蒲酒是同一个道理。《常用壮药临床手册》记载，菖蒲"味辛、苦，性微温。调巧坞，祛风毒，调气机，除湿毒，除瘴毒"。可见菖蒲可以化痰、祛湿、润肺、祛风寒，对预防夏季外感病有一定的作用。

二、佩药

佩药习俗起源于远古时代人类以植物（包括一些药物）为衣（即卉服）时，发现某些植物穿挂在身上，有独特的防病治病作用，并作为民族文化传承下来。壮族人素有"卉服"及佩挂绣球、香囊的习俗。宋人周去非在《岭外代答》中记载："上巳日（农历三月初三），男女聚会，各为行列，以五色结为球，歌而抛之，谓之飞驼。男女目成，则女受驼而男婚已定。"这段话大致是说，每逢春节或"三月三"歌节时，壮族青年男女都到野外举行抛绣球活动，以绣球作为青年男女传情达意的信物，不少青年男女以此结为夫妻。最初绣球、香囊的填充物多为木屑、米糠、香草，最早有文献记载的绣球内包有豆粟、棉花籽或谷物等农作物种子。后来人们发现在其中填充某些药物，佩挂以后对预防感冒、强身健体有较好的作用，就逐渐发展成为一种群众喜闻乐见的防病治病习俗。一般来说，佩药部位多为颈项、手腕和胸腹部。如家中有小儿体弱多病，可用苍术、白芷、细辛、藿香、佩兰、甘松、石菖蒲等适量，共研细末，装袋，以丝线佩挂于颈项或戴于手腕，具有强身健体的作用。在疠疫流行期间，取贯众、皂角、薄荷、防风、朱砂、艾叶、石菖蒲各适量，研成极细末，装入小香囊内，挂于颈部前方，能避瘟防病，可作为疠疫流行期的综合预防措施之一。

三、隔离辟秽

古时候，壮族群众家中若有染患疠疫者，都会在居室门前插上红纸标杆，谢绝外人入内，居室内焚烧苍术、白芷、艾叶、柚子皮等以辟秽祛瘴。在传染病流行期间，染病之家常谢绝外人登门，邻村之间暂不来往；若有人从远处归来，常止于村寨之外，甚至数里之遥，待家人提衣更换，并将其换下的衣物或蒸或煮，用意在于隔离邪秽，消除毒邪，防止疫病传染；如有本村人客死外地，尸体不得抬入家门，必须在村口外面搭棚停尸办丧事。这种习俗的形成，是因为古代壮族群众对在外客死者是否由于传染病所致没有办法弄清楚，便统一采用这种拒毒抗病于村外的做法，这对于预防传染病有积极的意义。从隔离辟秽习俗中，我们可以看出，古代壮族人对疠疫等传染病的预防已有一定的认识，并采取了有效措施，从消毒、隔离等方面防止疾病的传染流行。

第六节 壮医药与壮族丧葬习俗

一、壮族的丧葬习俗

壮族的丧葬习俗体现了壮族社会的伦理观念。在壮族人民看来，葬礼是人生中最重要的一个礼仪之一，其形式因地域的不同而有所差异，各有特点，但大体上都包括报丧、装殓、入棺、停柩、出殡、埋葬等，有些地方还请道公做道场念经。壮族人民在死者的葬式上，有岩洞葬、悬棺葬、土葬、屈肢蹲式葬、水葬等。而在壮族民间，普遍采用的葬式还是土葬。

二、捡骨重葬促进壮医对人体骨骼的认识

在壮族的丧葬习俗中，土葬是目前仍然普遍存在的主要葬式之一。土葬分为一次葬（即大葬）与二次葬（即小葬，又叫捡骨重葬）。民国的《上林县志》记载："惟亲者，则为瘗棺于浅土。三年后起土开棺，拾遗骨于瓦坛而寄诸土，谓之小葬。富贵之家，则盛以美材，停诸室外，必择吉地而始葬，谓之大葬。"可见大葬主要是富贵人家葬式，而二次葬（捡骨重葬）是绝大多数百姓的选择。捡骨的日期多在葬后第三年的清明节前后，也有另择吉日的。捡骨时由子女及亲属动手，先由其把颅骨从棺中捧出，他人才能动手。捡骨时先用稻草、碎布、砂纸、刀片等把遗骨擦干刮净，晾在竹筐里。然后依人体自下而上的次序，将遗骨装入"金坛"，颅骨在最上面，盖好后运到家族坟地中，或另择风水宝地下葬，培土堆成圆形坟丘。二次葬体现了壮族人民尊祖和讲究坟山风水的民俗，这一习惯客观上促进了壮医对人体骨骼的认识。

参考文献：

[1] 潘其旭，覃乃昌. 壮族百科辞典 [M]. 南宁：广西人民出版社，1993.

[2] 梁庭望. 壮族风俗志 [M]. 北京：中央民族学院出版社，1987.

[3] 庞宇舟. 壮族医药卫生习俗述略 [J]. 中国民族民间医药，2008（5）：3-5.

[4] 王柏灿. 壮族传统文化与壮族医药 [C]. 全国壮医药学术会议暨全国民族医药经验交流会论文集，2005：17-27.

[5] 石景斌. 壮族服饰介绍 [J]. 中南民族学院学报，1990（1）：26-29.

[6] 巫惠民. 壮族干栏建筑源流谈 [J]. 广西民族研究，1989（1）：89-94.

第六章　壮医药与壮族歌谣文化

第一节　壮族歌谣文化

"歌谣"是民歌、民谣和儿歌、童谣的总称，是伴随着人类语言产生而产生的最早的艺术形式之一，是民间音乐文学的重要体裁之一。在古代，歌和谣既相关又相别，合乐为歌，徒歌为谣，即配合音乐伴奏的谓之"歌"，没有音乐伴奏清唱的谓之"谣"。现代无论合乐与否，统称为"歌谣"。歌谣形式短小，词句简练，讲究押韵，格律上有独特的表现。壮族歌谣是对壮族口头创作有韵作品的称呼，也称山歌，如《中国俗文学辞典》中的表述："山歌主要是我国南方对民间歌谣的总称。"壮族歌谣是一种用有节奏、有韵律的语言来反映思想感情与生产、生活的文学式样，其音调和谐，韵律自然，充满了鲜明的壮族特色，洋溢着浓厚的生活气息；其内容丰富、全面、深刻地反映了壮族的社会历史、时代生活和风土人情等。

壮族聚居的广西被誉为"歌的海洋""民歌的故乡"，被称为铺满琴键的土地。生活在这片土地上的人们以"善唱"闻名于世，人们在歌声中生活，以歌代言，以歌择偶，被誉为具有诗性思维的民族，在漫长的历史发展进程中，在生产、生活实践中，创造出了灿烂的壮族歌谣文化。壮族歌谣文化是壮族文化中历史最悠久的文化之一，是与壮族歌谣相关的一系列文化事象。

一、壮族语言文字

壮族是生活在华南珠江流域的原住民族，聚居范围东起广东省连山壮族瑶族自治县，西至云南省文山壮族苗族自治州，北达贵州省黔东南苗族侗族自治州从江县，南抵广西北部湾，广西是壮族的主要分布区。壮族作为一个民族，其最重要的基本特征就是有本民族的共通语言——壮语。

1. 壮族的语言

壮语是一种有着悠久历史的优美语言，它是壮族人民在共同的生活、生产中创造的。壮语在我国语言分类上属于汉藏语系壮侗语族壮泰语支，以右江—邕江为界，分南部和北部两大方言。南部方言分布在右江、邕江以南地区和云南省文山壮族苗族自治州南部，北部方言分布在右江、邕江以北地区和云南省的邱北、师宗、富宁、广南（北部）以及广东省的连山、怀集等地。每种方言中，又分为若干个土语，北部方言分为七个土语，南部方言分为五个土语。同一方言中的不同土语之间的语音、词汇差别小，可以通话；不同方言的土语差别大，难以通话。

2. 壮族的文字

壮族曾有自己的早期文字符号，由于秦始皇统一岭南后推行"书同文"而未能发展且逐渐萎缩。由于社会交往的需要，在唐代，壮族借用汉字的形、音、义和六书构字法创造了一种与壮语语音一致的"土俗字"，如宋代范成大在《桂海虞衡志》中所言："边远俗陋，牒诉券约专用土俗书，桂林诸邑皆然。今姑记临桂数字，虽甚鄙野，而偏傍亦有依附。"土俗字，汉人称为古壮字，壮族人自称为"sawndip"，就是生字的意思。古壮字由于其构字形式复杂，随意性大，不宜阅读，故没有发展成为统一规范通行的壮族文字，多为壮族巫师、艺人用于书写经书、编山歌、记事、记录壮语地名等。产生于明代、流传于右江河谷的《嘹歌》，就是以土俗字抄本传世的；壮族的创世史诗《布洛陀经书》，也是根据民间不同版本的古壮字手抄本整理出来的。

二、壮族歌谣

1. 壮族歌谣的起源

越人好歌，壮族人民自古就善于用歌来展现自己的生产、生活和抒发自己的情感，其起源最早可以追溯到壮族原始社会劳动时的呐喊，换言之，在原始时代，人类还没有产生语言，就已经知道利用声音的高低、强弱等来表达自己的思绪和情感了。虽然呐喊不能算是歌，但是孕育了壮族歌谣的种子。关于壮族山歌的起源主要有两种观点：一是对偶婚说。对偶婚说认为，壮族山歌文化起源于远古的族外择偶（对偶婚制）活动。二是娱神说。娱神说认为，壮族山歌文化源于古代的民间宗教信仰，古人为了生产和生活的需要，通常祈求神灵保佑，便以歌赞神和乐神。有文字记载的壮族歌谣约产生于汉代，据西汉文学家刘向的《说苑·善说》记载，公元前528 年，在楚国令尹鄂君子皙举行的舟游盛会上，越人歌手对鄂君拥楫而唱了一首《越人歌》。韦庆稳在 1981 年中国社会科学院出版社出版的《民族语文论集》中发表了《〈越人歌〉与壮语的关系试探》一文，指出《越人歌》是借汉字记音的方法记录的，不但语音、语法、词性等与壮语完全一致，而且其格律和押韵方式也与当今流传的壮族歌谣相同，是一首古代壮族民歌。由此可知，悦耳动听的壮族歌谣流传至今已有近 3000 年的历史了。

2. 壮族歌谣的内容与形式

壮族歌谣种类繁多，有诉苦歌（包括长工苦歌、媳妇苦歌、单身苦歌、叹苦歌、怨命歌等）、情歌（包括散歌、套歌、探问歌、赞美歌、讨欢歌、示爱歌、定情歌、交友歌、发誓歌、分别歌等）、风俗歌（包括庆贺歌、祝寿歌、仪式歌、敬酒歌、迎

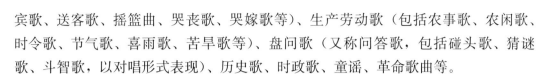

宾歌、送客歌、摇篮曲、哭丧歌、哭嫁歌等）、生产劳动歌（包括农事歌、农闲歌、时令歌、节气歌、喜雨歌、苦旱歌等）、盘问歌（又称问答歌，包括碰头歌、猜谜歌、斗智歌，以对唱形式表现）、历史歌、时政歌、童谣、革命歌曲等。

由于南北壮语方言的差异，壮族歌谣有"欢""西""加""比""论"等不同称呼，形式多样，韵律独特，曲调优美，语言生动形象。"欢"或"比"，多为徵调色彩，常用徵调式和宫调式；"西（诗）""加""论（伦）"多为羽调色彩，常用羽、商调式。

（1）欢

"欢"流行于广西北部红水河两岸及以北区域，其歌词式样繁多，句式和句数多样，讲究腰脚押韵或头脚押韵。其特点是歌词结构简练，重叠复沓，一咏三唱，环环相扣，韵律抑扬顿挫，朗朗上口，便于抒发感情，突出主题，加深印象。无论是吟诵还是歌唱，都富有音乐感，悠扬动听。

（2）西

"西"是流行于广西南部壮族方言区的歌体，从唱词的韵律和结构来看，"西"比"欢"活泼，没有腰脚押韵或头脚押韵的要求，只要求上联（前两句）末字与下联（后两句）末字互相押韵即可。形式结构为两句一联，可长可短，句数不定。其歌词吟唱朗朗上口，韵律铿锵悦耳，多用于对歌。

（3）加

"加"是流行于邕宁、扶绥、大新等汉壮杂居一带地区的歌体，形式短小精悍，旋律强，曲调委婉流利，装饰音较少，多用于表现爱情、生活情感。

（4）比

"比"流行于广西桂北一带的河池、东兰、巴马、融安等地，曲调严格，其歌词多为五字句，讲究腰脚押韵，曲调纤细委婉，装饰音较多。

（5）论

"论"流行于那坡、崇左、大新、宁明、凌云等桂西南的中越边境一带，其音调高亢，旋律跳动大，一曲多变，装饰音较多，曲调委婉多变，富有抒情性，格式多为五言、七言句型，押尾韵，常用于对歌。

（6）多声部山歌

多声部山歌流行于广西6个地区30多个县，唱腔100多种，有二声部和三声部，曲调优雅，织体简单朴素，线条清晰，艺术风格独特，具有高度的思想性，艺术形式比较成熟。

3. 壮族歌圩

歌圩壮语称为"圩欢""圩逢""笼峒""窝坡"等，是在特定的时间、地点举行的群体性的唱歌聚会和社交活动，是群众相互接触、交流思想、传承文化、传播知识及传情达意的场合。据 1934 年编的《广西各县概况》记载，广西有歌圩活动的地方有 26 个县，遍布广西各地。其起源与远古氏族的生产生活方式、节日集会、宗教祭祀、族外婚制等有关。举办歌圩的时间主要在春、秋两季，根据歌圩举办的时间可分为节日性歌圩和临时性歌圩。节日性歌圩在节日期间举行，如"三月三"、蛙婆节、牛魂节、元宵节等，或缘于祈年，或出于某种纪念，基本上是根据当地的岁时农事的时间来开展。这种歌圩规模大，往往有数千人参加，人们歌唱的热情相当高，通常是连唱几天几夜。临时性的歌圩主要有劳动歌会、圩市会唱、婚娶会唱等，与生活联系紧密，其规模较小、人数较少，是人们抒发情感、唱和应答、交流经验、传授知识的场合。临时性歌圩使唱歌不因农忙而消失、停止，也使唱歌不仅仅是人们农闲之时的消遣，而是真正融入人们生活之中，与生活形成了一个密不可分的整体，因而壮族人民的生活总是充满着歌声，人们的精神世界总是徜徉在歌海里。

壮族歌谣尽管缺乏详细的文字记载，但是依靠口头吟诵在民间世代相传，其能够从先秦一直唱到今天，正是借助了遍布壮族各聚居区的歌圩活动。歌圩的存在和发展，对继承和发扬优良的民族传统文化、保证壮族文化的传承起着重要的作用，促进了人们的情感交流和激发人们追求自由和抒发情怀。

第二节　壮医药与壮族歌谣文化的关系

一、壮族歌谣与壮医药的传承

承载文化因素最多的是语言文字，记载壮医药的文字有两种：一种是汉字。公元前 214 年，秦始皇统一岭南，壮族人民结束了其自主发展阶段，纳入中央集权制的统治之下。秦始皇为开发岭南，先后多次向岭南派遣军队、民众，前后共 150 多万人，使得岭南从此为壮汉杂居之地。随着岭南与中原地区广泛的文化交流，壮医药知识传入中原，成为中医药的组成部分，如《素问·异法·方宜论》记载"南方者，天地所长养，阳之所盛处也，故九针者亦从南方来"，这里的"南方"包括了壮族所在地。中医文献与汉文史料有很多有关壮医药内容的记载，如《本草经集注》《肘后救卒方》《岭表录异》《岭外代答》《檐曝杂记》《桂海虞衡志》及广西的地方志、博物志等。另一种是壮族的古壮字。但壮族的古壮字使用范围小，主要用于记录壮族的创世神话、传抄宗教经典、民歌，用来记录、编写民间故事、传说、民谣、谚语和戏剧等，主要使用者是布摩及民间艺人，因此用古壮字记载的壮医药内容是少量的、零散的，至今没有发现专门的古壮字记载的医药书籍。

壮族历史上没有形成本民族规范统一的通行文字，其古壮字使用范围小，而汉字是秦代才传入且不为壮族老百姓所掌握。壮族的历史、风俗、政治、经济、文化、

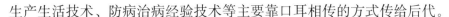

生产生活技术、防病治病经验技术等主要靠口耳相传的方式传给后代。

语言既是文化的组成部分，又是民族文化的活载体。壮族有自己的语言，且早在先秦时代，壮族先民就形成了自成体系的语言文化。壮族人民的语音功能发达，酷爱唱歌，壮族人从咿呀学语就开始用山歌传情达意，高兴时唱，忧愁时唱，人多时唱，独自一人时也唱。人们以生产、生活为背景，因事而发，随编随唱，有感而歌，用歌问路访寨，用歌迎宾接客，用歌寻偶择配……壮家儿女自幼即置身歌海之中，耳濡目染，遂形成幼年学歌、青年唱歌、老年教歌的传统习俗。

壮族歌谣在壮族的发展历史中具有重要的意义，它不仅是人们表达感情、交流思想的工具，而且还肩负着另外一项艰巨的使命——记载历史，如刘锡蕃所言："壮乡无论男女，皆认唱歌为其人生观上之主要问题。人之不能唱歌，在社会上即枯寂寡欢，即缺乏恋爱求偶之可能性，即不能通今博古，而为一蠢然如豕之顽民。"壮族歌谣的题材十分广泛，内容丰富多彩，艺术表现形式多样，生动而深刻地反映了社会生活以及自然界的各个方面。歌曲除抒发感情的"情歌"外，还有讲述历史的"古歌"、传授技术的"劳动生产歌"、自然界的"天文地理歌"、预防疾病的"医药保健歌"、社会的"伦理道德歌"等，充满了壮族人民的知识和智慧。此外，调研中还发现，一些民间壮医把收集来的或自己编撰的壮医歌诀进行分门别类，用来传授给学习者，使之容易记忆。如柳州的老壮医卢金山将自己创编及收集的民间壮医歌谣分成"入门歌诀""药物歌诀""方剂歌诀""肺病方歌""肝胆病秘方山歌"等。

歌谣是诗化了的语言，在壮族医药文化的传承中显得尤为重要。壮族祖辈积累下来的卫生保健知识、疾病诊治方法等能代代延续传播，壮族歌谣这种不受时间地点的限制、通俗易懂易记的诗化语言，起到了十分重要的作用。正如柳州壮医卢金山教授徒弟的歌中所唱："柳州有座鱼峰山，山下有个小龙潭。山脚潭边唱山歌，医药山歌早已传。自从盘古开天地，药王传医又传药。广西歌仙刘三姐，她用山歌唱医药。"

1. 壮族歌谣中的卫生保健知识

衣食住行是健康的重要条件，是卫生保健的重要内容，这些日常生活中的保健内容在壮族歌谣中随处可见，如生产劳动中的"四季农事歌""节气歌""十二月对唱歌""造屋歌"，生活歌中的"十月怀胎歌""十二时辰歌"，情歌中的"赞美歌""离别歌""相思歌"，习俗歌中的"哭嫁歌""盘问歌"，等等。在这些歌谣中讲述了饮食、衣着要随着季节更替而相应变化，房屋的环境、朝向与健康密切相关，妇女怀孕的整个过程的变化及注意事项等有关日常生活方方面面的内容，在歌谣吟唱的过程中，人们可以获得日常卫生保健知识。

（1）述婚姻史，倡对偶婚

壮族的传世史诗《布洛陀经诗》和流传在宜州和金城江一带的《盘同古》揭示

了壮族由杂婚至对偶婚的进步过程。杂婚时代"那时人间还没有伦理，那时家公与儿媳共枕席，那时女婿与岳母共床眠"，同辈兄妹婚时代"只剩下伏羲两兄妹，兄妹两人结夫妻，他俩商量结夫妇，夫妻同居三年整，夫妻同床满四年，妻子怀了孕，怀孕整整九个月，生下儿子像磨刀石，怪儿降生在半夜，伏羲夫妻好奇怪，为何生儿不像人，为何生儿变成磨刀石……"同时《盘同古》指出只有不同族群之间的婚配才利于人类的生存繁衍，告诫人们不可近亲结婚，内容如同现代宣传近亲结婚不利后代繁衍的山歌："非亲婚嫁可以论，真正老表别结婚。科学已经证明过，痴仔大多近亲生。不论家族或亲戚，相互结婚总不宜。如果哪个不相信，苦酒自酿喝一世。有一些人不相信，结婚硬去找表亲。结果生出痴呆仔，既害自己又害人。"

（2）重视孕育，创怀胎歌

生育是关系到种族繁衍的大事，因此在壮族各地区的生活歌中大都有"十月怀胎歌"。十月怀胎歌的唱词概括了胚胎在母体中的生长变化过程，孕妇在胚胎每月生长中的不同变化、反应和生活中的注意事项。这类歌谣对孕妇在怀孕期间及生产胎儿时都有很好的指导作用，如流传在崇左一带的十月怀胎歌："一月怀胎在娘身，一点阴阳造化成；好比草木逢春茂，乾坤造成始由根。二月怀胎在娘身，朦胧血脉裹元精；娘始怀胎吐苦水，方知身上有妊娠。……九月怀胎在娘身，预安产室在房中；走亲访戚娘怕去，担心胎儿半路生。十月怀胎在娘身，娘在房中腹疼频；腹痛阵阵如刀割，头晕眼黑失三魂。……"

（3）房屋建筑，防潮避兽

壮族的传世史诗《布洛陀经诗》中的《造万物》，记载了壮族先民在相当长的时间里是居住在野外的，居住地气候炎热，多雨潮湿，树丛茂密，野兽横行，人们的安全及健康受到严重的威胁。聪明的壮族先民利用高大的树木构木为巢，在树上居住。

歌谣中这么描述"古时还没有造房屋，百姓没有地方睡觉，人们没有房屋居住，夜里走到半路就睡在半路，夜里走到森林就睡在森林里，布洛陀在上面（天上）看见了一切，派下一名巢氏王，让他教人们建住地。那时没有铁和钢，只能在高高的山上砍树，巢氏王把树枝弯下相勾连，用木签来做榫，将茅草盖在屋上面，人在下边居住。造房屋和谷仓，就从那时开始，划分公婆与夫妻。"

巢居这种干栏式的建筑结构，与地面保持一定距离，通风透气、采光良好，具有防潮、防蛇、防兽、防病等作用，是非常适合南方潮湿环境的居住方式。

（4）房屋朝向，依山傍水

壮族人民对与日常生活息息相关的住房十分重视，从建房的选址、落基、材料及房屋的结构、采光等都事先商议计划好，这从流行于右江流域的平果、田东等地的壮族民歌《嘹歌》中可以得到佐证。《嘹歌》中有专门的《房歌》，这是一首从开始商议建房到房子建成的全过程的长歌，包括商议、伐木、开凿、买牛、踩泥、打瓦、烧砖、安磉、合架、围墙、赞房、保宅等十二个部分，是男歌手或女歌手应邀到女方或男方村子做客时对唱的。对房子的建设、作用等各方面进行歌咏的歌谣在壮族各地都有："蛇居有深洞，蛟龙居深潭，为什么起房，为遮雨挡风；狗在窝过夜，猫睡在火旁，为什么起房，为让人安居。"

随着生产力的发展，人们发现房屋所处的环境、方位及建房的时辰等对身体健康都有影响，因此在建房时会慎重考虑上述因素。如"树高鸟就爱，海阔龙就恋，在此建新房，华堂更生辉；树高鸟就爱，海阔龙就住，在此建新房，风来福气到；爹建房坐北，面朝向阳山，爹屯里建房，总不会生病；爹建房坐北，面朝向阳山，爹屯里建房，牛知去知回；爹建房坐北，面向广阔地，爹平地建房，朝向向太阳"，"房屋大门向东方，建房主要靠采光，白天门窗打开了，阴天同样亮堂堂"，"建房靠山靠得稳，才有缘分进屋来"，"建房坐北面南方，六畜兴旺人安宁。建房选得好方向，财丁两旺人欢畅"。

（5）关注气候，防病保健

"立春节气最头先，春寒为过还冷天；惊蛰突然变冷天，老牛最怕这一变；体弱多病放寒冷，体壮也要多保健……白露秋风渐渐起，雨量渐少天气变；立冬过后雨量少，冷风吹拂人身寒……"，"春分有雨病人少，初一翻风又落雨，沿村病疫定然凶；立夏东风吹发发，沿村没有病人魔；季秋初一莫逢霜，人民疾病少提防；重阳无雨三冬旱，月中亢旱病人忙。凑巧遇逢壬子日，灾伤疾病损人民。初一西风盗贼多，更兼大雪有灾病"，"二三月里换节气，鸟换绒毛人换衣，脱掉棉衣穿单件，潇潇洒洒赶歌圩；二三月闷热，穿土布嫌痒，穿洋布嫌粗，穿绸衣凉爽……七月逢立秋，日行渐南斜，夜长日渐短，找长袖来穿；十月北风寒，靠干柴取暖，十月劲风吹，用竹篙拍棉，穿棉衣过年，盖棉被过冬"。这些民歌讲述了气候变化与人们的穿着、疾病的关系，教导人们在气候变化时要注意防病，这与壮医的基础理论"阴阳为本，天、地、人三气同步"的天人自然观是一致的。

2. 壮族歌谣中的壮医基础理论

壮族歌谣中的壮医基础理论零星分散，有的体现在日常的歌圩中，如问："阿哥样样认得清，妹今来问哥分明，开天辟地是哪个，阴阳日夜谁人分？"答："盘古开天又辟地，那时阴阳两边分，白天有了太阳照，夜里又有月亮明。"或日常韵词对答"一天公一地母，公不离母，秤不离砣"，这些虽然还不是壮医的阴阳为本的理论，但是却潜移默化地指导着壮医的临床实践。

另外，有的歌谣是民间壮医在医疗实践中的经验总结，大都掌握在个别壮医的手中，这部分的内容独具特色，指导着壮医的诊断治疗，如"寒手热背肿在梅，痿肌痛沿麻络央，唯有痒疾抓长子，各疾施治不离乡"是壮医药线点灸疗法取穴规律的总结，指出治疗疾病要根据病情，循龙路、火路取穴，发冷、发热、肿块、肌肉萎缩、皮肤病的治疗取穴不一样。百色陈林摘录了其岳父潘振香老壮医一首关于《孩儿发畜病辨证法》的歌诀给笔者："抽兰密肚啼，睡红牙气畜；孩儿察色形，白头沙锁病。"在这首五言四句的歌诀中，体现了潘振香老壮医对婴儿多发疾病的高度概括。他认为婴儿多发畜病（当地壮医将婴儿发病称发畜）及白头、沙锁病，辨证主要观察婴儿的形体及肤色，歌诀后附有所述疾病的表现及辨证和治疗方法。这些歌诀是师傅用以传授徒弟的，其内容有时需要经验总结和歌诀编唱者解释才能让人明白。

3. 壮族歌谣中的药物方剂

稻作民族注重气候等因素对农作物收成的影响，壮医秉承了壮族的实用观念，他们看重疾病的治疗效果，因此非常重视药物功效和方剂疗效，在几千年漫长的医疗实践中积累和总结了壮族地区常见药物的功效并形成独具特色的组方原则。用歌谣记载的有关壮医方剂疗效和药物功效的内容特别丰富，如东兰县的韦炳智医生就将自己收集的部分壮药资料加以整理编辑，书名为《民间医药秘诀》，由广西民族出版社于 1989 年出版，全书共收载 220 味药，按功效分为 17 类，全书以歌诀的形式呈现，如"痧证常用南蛇簕，医治跌打和骨折，含咽根本除骨鲠，瘰病功效也不劣""伤寒可用野芋头，感冒结核疗效优，误服过量易中毒，速饮酸醋能解救"。

歌谣中对药物功效记载的内容大致可分为两种：一种是概括药物功效的共性，如"天上飞禽，补阳益气，水里游物，大补血阴，诸兽胎盘，总是大补，乳汁补津，以骨补骨，肝补肝脏，腰子补肾，血补血液，筋补强筋，以脑补脑，鞭睾茎睾，对应用药，走医绝招""叶茂有毛能止血，草木通心善祛风。叶枝有刺皆消肿，叶里藏浆拔毒功。圆梗白花寒性药，热药根方花色红。根黄清热退黄用，节大跌打驳骨雄。形态识别可辨认，药中五味各分清。辛散气浓解表药，辛香止痛治蛇虫。苦凉解毒兼清热，咸寒降下把坚攻。淡味多为利水药，甘温健脾补中宫"。另一种是阐述单味药物的功效，如"味甘性平土人参，润肺止咳又调经，少乳遗尿痈疖症，病后滋补功效深""患了疟疾不用愁，请君服用一箭球，跌打外敷也有效，身患菌痢把它求""辛酸性平狗仔花，清热消肿顶呱呱，能治疟疾荨麻疹，木薯中毒快用它""狗肝菜长园边地，清热利尿甚急需，小儿痢疾可对症，目赤疮疡效不低"。

二、壮族歌谣对情志的影响

壮族地区生活环境恶劣，有"瘴乡"之称，纵观整个壮族发展的历史，自秦始皇公元前 214 年统一岭南，广大的壮族先民就受到中央政权及本族统治者的双重统治及压迫，生活苦不堪言。他们不断为争取自己的权利而进行抗争，宋代有侬智高起兵反抗，清代有洪秀全领导的金田起义。生活之地的荒凉，山间劳作的艰辛，中央王朝和地方豪权双重统治的压迫，生活在壮乡的人们虽然生活艰辛困苦，但是却充满欢歌笑语，这与他们喜好唱歌有密切的关系。

1. 唱山歌是良好的社交活动

壮族是稻作民族，多居住于河谷盆地或丘陵地带，在相对封闭的地理环境里劳作，难得相互交往。壮族先民长期在岭南的"溪峒"间从事农耕活动，劳动任务繁重，山野空漠，歌声可以帮助人们驱走疲乏，鼓舞劳动士气，提高劳动效率。而生活在群体的社会里，人们需要向外界反映自己的身体和精神，并使自己适应所生存的现实世界。听歌、唱歌活动就是人们实现这种情感交往的桥梁，人们利用农作的间隙、传统的节日、喜庆聚会等时机用歌声来交流，表达、宣泄内心情感，在情感交流中互相同情、理解和支持，促进心理健康。

壮族是一个在歌海中生活的民族，唱山歌是壮族人民交际和表情达意的方式，是他们日常生活的一部分。众多汉文史料对此都有记载，《岭外代答》记载："广西诸郡，人多能合乐。城郭村落祭祀、婚嫁、丧葬，无一不用乐，虽耕田，亦必口乐相之。"在壮乡，人们逢事必唱歌，习惯以歌代言，用山歌来表达他们的喜怒哀乐和对生活的要求、愿望，用山歌来结朋交友、寻找意中人、记录历史文化等，形成了以歌会友、以歌传情、以歌择偶的风俗。

唱山歌为人们搭建了良好的社交平台，在壮乡各地都有规模宏大的定期歌圩。到了歌圩日，人们穿着节日盛装从四面八方赶来听歌、唱歌，用山歌来表达思想、交流感情，歌颂大自然和生活中的美好事物，鞭笞生活中的丑恶现象。壮族人民在歌圩的阵阵欢歌笑语中获得彼此的敬意与友情，获得自我实现的成就感，增强了自信心。

社会的认同和自我肯定是良性刺激，可以使人产生正面的情感或情绪，可以促进身体的气血流通，有利于身心健康。现在很多医院和机构运用歌唱疗法来治疗抑郁症。

2. 歌谣是壮族祛烦怡情的方式

《岭表纪蛮》云："蛮人生活痛苦，居地荒凉，工作繁多，若不以唱歌宣其湮郁，则绝无祛烦怡情之余地。"平时，壮族人民多居住于河谷盆地或丘陵地带，在相对封闭的岭南"溪峒"间从事农耕活动，"处穷独而不闷者，莫过于音声也"。他们在劳动中或独自轻吟或合唱："不得唱歌人会老，唱起山歌转后生；好比后园种韭菜，割它一头又转青。地要翻犁土才松，花要日晒花才红；禾要加肥苗才壮，人要唱歌才威风。姐心就像红薯藤，刘头掐尾种还生；不唱山歌脸苦苦，听到歌声又开心。""炒菜无油菜不软，煮茶无糖茶不甜。做活唱歌驱疲倦，欢欢乐乐过一天。"伴随着歌声，繁重的劳动变得轻松起来，空漠的山野有了生机，歌声帮助人们驱走了劳动带来的疲乏，鼓舞了劳动干劲，提高了劳动效率。

古代壮族居住之地有"瘴乡"之称,自然灾害时有发生。壮族人以山歌来笑对种种艰辛和苦难,化解烦恼,"出门用歌来走路,睡觉用歌当床铺。结亲用歌当彩礼,过年用歌当食物","山歌不唱心不开,大路不走起青苔;路起青苔人跌倒,山歌不唱沤心怀","唱歌好,好比热茶暖透心;唱歌好比抖大气,几多忧愁一扫清","柴火不晒最难烧,人不唱歌容易老,酸甜苦辣任君唱,万般忧愁随风飘","人穷不会穷一世,天冷只会冷一时;寒冬腊月下花种,春来就会开满枝","唱首山歌解心忧,喝口凉水解心头,凉水解得心头火,唱歌解得万般愁"。

"饭养身,歌养心""只有家中断茶饭,哪有人间断歌声"……壮族人民把唱歌看得与吃饭同等甚至更重要,人们将在生产、生活中看到的、听到的、感悟到的情景,随编随唱出来,常常你一问、我一答地进行对唱,如《岭外代答》云:"迭相歌和,含情凄婉……皆临机自撰,不肯蹈袭,其间乃有绝佳者。"歌谣中生动的譬喻和描写,常常给予唱者和听者极大的感动,使貌似单调的生活和劳动充满着浓厚的生活情趣,散发出乐观向上的气息。

3. 山歌吟唱的形式利于调畅气机,宣泄不良情绪

情志病的发病机制为内脏气血,尤其是五脏气机失调。《素问·举痛论》指出:"百病生于气也,怒则气上,喜则气缓,悲则气消,恐则气下,惊则气乱,思则气结。"忧伤、思虑、惊恐等不良情绪憋在心里会导致人体气机升降失调,进而引起脏腑气血失衡,伤及内脏,导致疾病发生。山歌吟唱的形式具有通达血脉、畅通人体气机、振奋精神、疏通不良情绪、防治身心疾病的作用,如《乐书·第二》所言:"音乐者,动荡血脉,流通精气,而正如和心也。"

壮族山歌内容丰富多彩,不仅有情歌、叙事歌、农事歌、生活歌、风俗歌等,还有悲歌和挽歌。悲歌是由于人们感情被压抑、生命安全受威胁、身体被摧残、理想遭破灭与渴望自由生活、生命安全之间的倒错,叩击着灵魂之门,从而抒发出来的一曲曲深沉悲愤与激昂的生命之歌。挽歌也叫哭丧歌,是壮族人民用歌声表达痛失亲人后内心的悲戚,在丧事上唱的歌。

当人们在生活中遭受挫折和不幸,受到打击时,最容易产生悲伤、凄婉、怨怼、哀痛、愤怒等不良情绪,壮族的悲歌就是创作者根据亲身经历,把自己内心世界的感情体验与音乐融为一体,创编成歌曲,以歌为媒介将内心难以用语言表达的情感真切地倾诉出来。有学者认为壮族悲歌的创作和传唱,有益于歌唱者心灵苦闷的发泄,是创作者和传唱者求得心灵解脱和安慰的一种尝试,当歌者完全沉浸在其中演唱时,其内心的苦痛郁闷得到了宣泄,情绪随之发泄,恰如清代吴尚先所言:"七情之病,看花解闷,听曲消愁,有胜于服药者矣。"

唱歌不仅可以消愁解闷,而且还能陶冶性情,如孔子言:"安上治民,莫善于礼,移风易俗,莫善于乐。"音乐是情感的语言,它可以抵达人的心灵、拨动人的神

经，减轻心灵负担，促使人们在优美的旋律中向平和的态度转化。当今社会因生活节奏快、竞争激烈等致情志疾病高发，世界各地如芬兰、德国等组织了"发牢骚合唱团"，合唱团的宗旨是"把烦恼写出来，将牢骚唱出来"，牢骚歌唱完后，情绪得到了释放，人们就会感觉心情愉悦，海阔天空，性情平和。

情志致病是中医病因学说的重要组成部分，是指因喜、怒、忧、思、悲、恐、惊七情变化而导致的疾病。壮医的病因学说是"毒虚论"，认为"毒"邪是发病的重要条件，体"虚"是疾病发生的内在因素，两者相因而为病，是导致人体生病的必要因素。壮医病因学说对情志致病不是很重视，与壮族酷爱唱山歌很少罹患七情所致的病证有关。

参考文献：

[1] 陆斐，王敦. 壮族歌咏文化的诗性思维与民族心理 [J]. 百色学院学报，2010，23 (1)：31－35.

[2] 莫清莲，黄萍，黄海波. 略论壮族民歌在壮医传承中的作用 [J]. 中国民族民间医药，2009 (21)：25－27.

[3] 莫清莲，戴铭，农敏坚. 壮族民歌中的保健医事记载 [J]. 中国民族民间医药，2009 (23)：5－6.

[4] 张声震. 布洛陀经诗译注 [M]. 南宁：广西人民出版社，1991.

[5] 萧凤培. 广西民间文学作品精选：融安县卷 [M]. 南宁：广西民族出版社，1992.

[6] 雷庆多. 广西民间文学作品精选：崇左县卷 [M]. 南宁：广西民族出版社，1998.

[7] 农敏坚，谭志表. 平果嘹歌·长歌集·三月歌 [M]. 南宁：广西民族出版社，2004.

[8] 韦炳智. 民间医药秘诀 [M]. 南宁：广西民族出版社，1989.

[9] 莫清莲，林怡，戴铭. 壮医病因学初探 [J]. 中国中医基础医学杂志，2014，20 (3)：293－295.

[10] 中国歌谣集成广西卷编辑委员会. 中国歌谣集成：广西卷 [M]. 北京：中国社会科学出版社，1992.

[11] 韦苏文. 壮族悲歌论 [J]. 民族艺术，1992 (2)：114－124.

第七章　壮医药与壮族节庆文化

第一节　壮族节庆文化

　　节庆，即节日、庆祝日。节日是相对于常日而言，它是古人通过对天候、气候、物候的周期性转换之观察与把握而逐渐约定俗成的。节庆民俗则是与农业文明发生、发展同步萌芽出现的，最终形成了一系列适应自然环境、调节人际关系、传承文化理念的禁忌、占候、祭祀、庆祝、娱乐等活动项目。不同的时节，有不同的节庆民俗活动，且以年度为周期，循环往复，周而复始。一个民族的节庆文化与该民族所处的自然环境、生产和生活方式、原始信仰有着密切关系，与其所具有的文化与社会功能密切相关。壮族的节日莫不如此，在内容和形式上体现了浓厚的壮族特色。壮族的节日已成为壮族文化的重要特征与标志，凝聚着壮族人民的创造精神与深厚情结，承载着壮族人民对人寿年丰、平安富足生活的不懈追求与期待。

一、壮族节庆分类

　　壮族传统节日大致可分为农耕季节性节日、宗教性节日、纪念性节日三大类。无论是何种类型的节日，其核心都是为了祈祷生产丰收、生活富足、人丁繁衍、家业兴旺、平安幸福。

　　1. 农耕季节性节日

　　壮族是稻作民族，其节庆日自然而然与稻作农业生产活动有着密切关系。这一类节日包括农历一月的蚂蚂节、二月的祭社节、三月的开耕节、四月的牛魂节和拜秧节、五月的农具节、七月的尝新节、八月的跳岭头节、十月的庆丰节等，主要是围绕农事季节来进行的。

　　2. 宗教性节日

　　主要是祭祖性的活动，包括农历三月的扫墓节、布洛陀诞辰节，六月的莫一大王节，七月的迎祖送祖节，等等，每一个节日都要在村寨祠堂或自家厅堂祭祀祖先，反映了壮族的祖先崇拜观念与习俗。

　　3. 纪念性节日

　　主要是纪念先辈和其他历史人物、事件。如"三月三"歌圩节是为纪念壮族歌仙刘三姐，故又称歌仙节；娅拜节是为了纪念宋代一位壮族女英雄娅拜；六郎节是

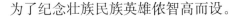

为了纪念壮族民族英雄侬智高而设。

二、壮族节庆文化的特点

壮族的节庆文化历史悠久，源远流长，是壮族传统文化的重要组成部分，在其漫长的形成、发展过程中，逐步展现出自己鲜明的特点。

1. 鲜明的稻作农业特色

壮族地区地处亚热带，雨水充足，适宜水稻的生长。壮族是最早发明水稻种植的民族之一，日常生活、生产活动与稻作有着千丝万缕的关系。壮族有很多节庆活动都是围绕着生产季节和农作节奏来开展的，是稻作文化伴生的。如农历三月开耕节是春耕开始的一种仪式，由村寨中有威望的头人在村边一块水田里，先在田边摆上祭品，焚香祭拜天地，然后牵牛持犁在田间来回犁一道，标志当年的春耕正式开始。此后，各家各户方可开耕犁田。农历四月初八牛魂节是人们为表示对牛耕作之劳的感谢和犒劳，专门给牛休息一天，把牛牵到河里清洗，喂以精饲料，同时清扫牛栏。农历七月初七尝新节，此时田间稻谷接近成熟，人们到田间采摘率先成熟的稻穗回家，三穗挂在厅堂中的祖先神台上，其余脱壳与旧米一起煮成饭，先祭祖先诸神，然后全家享用，因为这是一年中最先成熟的稻谷，故称为"尝新"。农历十月庆丰节，此时晚稻已全部收割并晒干，人们举行隆重的庆祝丰收仪式，祭祀酬谢诸神保佑之功，打扁担、跳春堂舞，以示庆祝。

2. 强烈的祭祖情结

壮族人民认为，祖先死后，其灵魂还在阴间活动，会给人世间的子子孙孙福佑，消灾保平安。在过年过节的时候，人们都在中堂供起祖宗，摆供品，燃香火，焚纸钱。清明时节，到先辈墓前祭扫，摆上酒肉、五色糯米饭，表示对祖宗的思念。农历七月十四鬼节（中元节），烧几套纸糊衣裳，为祖宗的魂灵御寒；烧几沓冥币，给祖宗在阴间使用。平时，杀鸡、杀鸭、煮猪肉，也要敬祭一下祖先。因此，虽说壮族人民也有万物有灵的观念，也崇拜"花神""蛙神"，但壮族人民最信奉的还是自己的祖先。

3. 深刻的饮食文化印记

壮族人过节称"哏节"（gwnciet），"哏"（gwn）就是吃的意思。也就是说，壮族过节是以"吃"为核心。过节时，除了必备酒肉以祭祀祖先诸神灵，祈求庇护，同时还会准备丰盛的酒菜犒劳自己，并宴请亲朋好友。壮族以"吃"为核心的节日习俗，究其原因，除有"民以食为天"的本能因素外，还与壮族的稻作农耕生产方式密切相关。稻作农业耕作技术要求高，生产周期长，劳动强度大，从开始的耕田插秧、中间的施肥灌溉，到最后的收割入仓，其间工序可谓繁杂，每一道工序都要付出艰辛的劳动。加上南方气候炎热，人们头顶烈日在水田中劳作，耗费的体力更大。这时，人们就要适度休整，增加营养，改善生活，才能够继续从事繁重的体力劳动。因而自觉地产生了全民性的、约定俗成的身心休息日，以适应人们休整的需要。在节日这一天，各家各户备有美酒和鸡肉、鸭肉、鱼肉等丰盛菜肴，同时用糯米包粽子或蒸糕点糍粑，犒劳自己。于是，节日成为人们放松身心，安心享受美食，享受辛勤劳作成果的快乐日子，也成了人们的一种期待，一种合家团圆、共享美餐、身心放松、幸福快乐的象征。壮族以"吃"为核心的传统节日，正是在人们的这种期待、享受和快乐中传承下来的。

4. 显著的群众性、集体性

千百年来，壮族先民与大自然进行了长期艰苦的斗争，在生产力低下的环境中，为了获取生活资料，为了自身的生存与发展，形成了群体协作、团结互助的优良传统。壮族最重要的生产习俗是"滚揉"（vunzraeuh）、"多揉"（doxraeuh），意为邀约相助，俗称"打背工""赔工"，是氏族社会集体劳动的遗韵。"多揉"范围很广，耕田、种地、收割、建房子、婚嫁、丧葬等，人们都喜欢用这种形式主动相帮。这种集体协作、团结互助的精神，也反映在节日活动中。壮族的多数节日活动都是以村落为单位进行的，如蚂拐节、"三月三"歌圩节、布洛陀诞辰节、药市节、莫一大王节、庆丰节等。在节日活动中，全村男女老少共同参加，相互分工协作，由村中头人负责组织，由麽公或道公（师公）主持祭祀仪式，然后集体聚餐。通过集体性的节日活动，展现了村寨的经济实力、组织能力、人气和声誉，增强了族群内部和族群之间的凝聚力。

三、壮族主要节庆

壮族的传统节日较多，与其他民族的传统节日一样，都有其起源、发展与演变的过程，许多节日往往伴随着一个个美丽的传说故事，令人神往。

1. 春节

春节是壮族的岁首节庆，也是壮族最隆重的节日之一。壮族的春节，一般是从农历正月初一到正月十五，正月十五那天各家吃了专供祖神的"母粽"（特大粽子）后即告散年，意即新年节期聚庆终止。也有部分地区的新年节庆活动延至正月末，故通常又将整个正月作为庆新春节期，称为"过正月""吃正月"，壮语"cieng"（"正月"的简称）意即春节。

大年初一，是壮族一年中最隆重的节日。鸡鸣第一遍时算是新的一天开始，这时就要起床迎新年，穿好新衣、新鞋后，先给祖宗牌位烧香，点蜡烛，摆放贡品，然后燃放鞭炮。放炮后，小孩向长辈"恭喜"，长辈给小孩一些压岁钱和鞭炮。无论男女老少，均盛装打扮，喜气洋洋。新媳妇和姑娘们争相奔向溪河泉边，挑新水，喝"伶俐水"，据说谁先得到新水，谁就会变得聪明伶俐。家族内和邻里间相互串

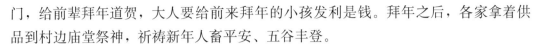

门，给前辈拜年道贺，大人要给前来拜年的小孩发利是钱。拜年之后，各家拿着供品到村边庙堂祭神，祈祷新年人畜平安、五谷丰登。

在大年初一，各地壮族都有许多禁忌。如禁止扫地，认为此日扫垃圾出门，是家财外流的预兆；禁见鲜血，大部分壮族人认为，大年初一见鲜血不吉利，故禁止杀生。因此，除夕时就要把大年初一要吃的鸡肉、鸭肉、鱼肉准备好；禁止借债、催债，一些壮族地区认为，春节期间借债或被人催债，预示当年生产、生意不吉利，如果要借债或催债，需在除夕晚上以前和农历正月十五日以后进行。

春节期间，壮族人民还开展丰富多彩的文化娱乐活动。跳春堂舞（或打春堂），壮语叫"特郎"或"谷郎"（dwklongj），是壮族人民在春节期间用来庆贺新年、预祝丰收的舞蹈，至今仍流行于马山、都安、武鸣、上林、忻城、天等、平果等地。跳春堂舞时，最初是用捣米的木杵与春米木槽互相敲打，名曰"谷郎"（壮语"谷"是"做"之意，"郎"为春米槽）。后来为了方便，用扁担来代替沉重的木杵，用长板凳来代替笨重的木槽，因此有的地方又直呼为"打扁担"或"打虏烈"（"虏烈"即打扁担发出的声音）。舞者男女不限，人数不定，各执扁担，围绕板凳，上下左右，边唱边打，围观者在一旁喝彩助威，气氛非常热烈。其他活动还有舞狮、打铜鼓、武术等。

2. 蚂𧊅节

蚂𧊅（即青蛙）节是东兰、巴马、凤山、天峨、南丹等县壮族地区春节期间的一个习俗节日。壮族传说中掌管风雨的是蚂𧊅女神。每年的大年初一至初二，红水河沿岸壮族村寨通过祭祀她，祈求年年风调雨顺，岁岁五谷丰登，四季人畜兴旺。相传，蚂𧊅女神是雷王的女儿，掌管雨水，使得大地风调雨顺。有一年，壮家有个叫东林的青年，因为丧母而痛苦不堪。他听到屋外蚂𧊅"呱呱呱"地叫个不停，一时烦躁难耐，就用热水把蚂𧊅浇得死的死、伤的伤、逃的逃。从此，蚂𧊅不叫了，天也不下雨了，人间便开始大祸临头。东林吓坏了，去求神祖布洛陀，得到神训应向蚂𧊅女神赔礼道歉。于是，东林赶紧在大年初一敲起铜鼓，请蚂𧊅女神回村过年，并为死去的蚂𧊅送葬。后来，人间又重新得到蚂𧊅女神的保佑，风调雨顺。从此，当地的壮族人民年年要过蚂𧊅节，祭祀蚂𧊅。

蚂𧊅节的活动大致可分为三个阶段。第一阶段为"找蚂𧊅"。每当农历正月初一黎明，人们就敲着铜鼓成群结队去田里找冬眠的蚂𧊅。据说，先找到蚂𧊅的人是幸运的，被誉为雷王的女婿"蚂𧊅郎"，成为该年蚂𧊅的首领。第二阶段为"孝蚂𧊅"和"抬蚂𧊅游村"。人们把这只蚂𧊅接回村，放入由黄金老楠竹精心制作的小棺内，再将小棺放入"花楼"中，指定两名歌手抬着装蚂𧊅的"花楼"，由孩子们簇拥着游行于全村各户，并一路传唱祈求风调雨顺、人寿年丰的"蚂𧊅歌"，然后拿出年糕、粽子、糍粑、米饼、彩蛋、白米饭、钱等让大家分享。从农历正月初一到正月底，白天孩子们抬着蚂蚂游村，到每家每户贺喜；晚上，则抬到蚂蚂亭下，人们跳"蚂蚂舞"和唱"蚂蚂歌"，以示为蚂蚂守灵。第三阶段为"葬蚂蚂"，此为蚂蚂节活动的高潮。正月底这天，人们选择吉时，众人由"蚂蚂郎"带领，抬着蚂蚂"花楼"送到坟地安葬。下葬前，由主祭人挖开前一年的蚂蚂坟，验看当年蚂蚂的遗骨，据其颜色预测当年的年景。如果蚂蚂的骨头呈金黄色，便预示当年是好年景，这时全场欢声雷动，铜鼓齐鸣；如果蚂蚂骨头呈灰色或黑色，便表示当年年景不好，于是人们就烧香祈求消灾降福。接着举行新蚂蚂的下葬仪式。葬礼之后，男女老少一起围着篝火唱歌、跳舞，送蚂蚂的灵魂上天。

3. 花婆节

传说壮族始祖母姆六甲是从花丛里走出来的，她掌管着人类生育繁衍的花园，专门为妇女赐花送子，人们尊之为赐花婆婆，妇女怀孕生育就是花婆婆赐予花朵的结果。后来姆六甲主管赐花送子之事，故其被奉为花婆神。农历二月廿九日（一说为农历二月初二）为花婆神的诞辰日，届时，壮族妇女备办鸡肉、鸭肉、鱼肉和香烛纸钱到花婆庙中举行隆重的祭祀仪式，并举办花婆施粥、放花灯、巡游等民俗活动，然后成群结队到野外采花来戴，祈求生育和保佑小孩健康成长。没有生育的妇女，是日要到野外采花来戴，以求花婆神赐花送子。若日后怀孕，为使小孩出生后有灵魂，需请师公到野外念经求花，还要在路边小沟做架桥仪式，把花从桥上接过来。小孩出生后，要在产妇床旁安上花婆神位，定期祭拜。

4. 清明节

清明节是祭扫祖坟的节日。壮族人民相当重视清明节，该节是继春节、鬼节之后祭祀亲人的隆重节日。壮族人民祭祖先，扫墓必以三牲供祭，大户人家则联宗祭祖，在坟山大摆宴席，凡过路者均被请去宴饮。一般扫墓均在清明节前后15天内进行。清明节期间，五色糯米饭、糍粑或艾叶糍粑是壮族人民必不可少的美食。壮族人通常会制作五色糯米饭，用以祭祖、招待亲友。过去，即便是穷人，没有大鱼大肉，清明上坟祭祖的时候也一定会摆放一碗香甜的五色糯米饭来祭拜逝去的亲人。

5. "三月三"歌圩节

农历三月初三又称"三月三"歌节或"三月三"歌圩，是壮族的传统歌节。歌圩节的来历说法不一。据说，在唐代，壮族出了个能歌善唱的刘三姐，她聪明过人，经常用山歌来歌颂劳动和爱情，揭露财主们的罪行，财主们对她又恨又怕。农历三月初三那天，趁刘三姐到山上砍柴时，财主派人砍断了山藤，导致她坠崖身亡。后人为纪念刘三姐，于农历三月初三、初四、初五连续唱歌三天，形成歌圩。又有一说，在桂中偏北的融水苗族自治县安陲乡樵花岭一带，每年农历三月初三是这里的会期，已有几百年历史。传说刘三姐从三江侗族自治县去柳州市，船经樵花岭，唱了三天三夜的歌。为了纪念她，每年农历三月初三就定为赶歌圩的日子。歌圩节这一天，家家户户做五色糯米饭，染彩色蛋，欢度节日。歌圩节一般持续两三天，地点在离村不远的空地上，村民们用竹子和布匹搭成歌棚，接待外村歌手。对歌者以未婚男女青年为主体，他们以歌传情，以歌为媒，以歌求偶。如果男女双方情投意合，就互赠信物，以示定情。歌圩规模大小不一，小的歌圩有一两千人，大的歌圩可达数万人之多。人们到歌圩场上赛歌、赏歌，人山人海，歌声此起彼伏，热闹非凡。歌圩所唱涉及内容也很广泛，有天文地理、神话传说、岁时农事、社会生活、伦理道德、恋爱婚姻等各个方面，几乎无事不歌。此外，歌圩上往往举行抛绣球、碰彩蛋、抢花炮、板鞋竞技、跳竹竿舞等有趣活动，还有壮戏、师公戏、采茶戏和其他歌舞表演。抛绣球主要是娱乐活动，也做定情信物。当姑娘看中某个小伙子时，就把绣球抛给他。在现代，抛（投）绣球是一种集体性的体育运动。碰彩蛋是互相取乐承欢，亦有定情之意。1985年，广西壮族自治区人民政府将"三月三"定为广西文化艺术节。

6. 牛魂节

壮族人民认为牛并非人间凡品，而是天上的神物。传说牛于农历四月初八诞生于天上，因此这天是牛王的诞辰日。远古时期，陆地上没有草木，岩石裸露，黄土遍地，尘沙弥漫，人类生活受到极大的影响。牛王奉玉帝之命来到人间播种百草。玉帝指示它每三步撒一把草种，可它却一步撒三把草种。由于撒种过多过密，使得满山遍野杂草丛生，连人类耕种的田地也长满了杂草，禾苗受到损害。于是，玉帝便罚它在人间吃草，并替人类出力耙田犁地。这样牛便在人间以草为食，耙田犁地，一年到头辛苦劳作，赢得了人们的尊敬。人们感激它的付出，便在每年农历四月初八牛王诞辰日祭祀牛魂。于是，便有了牛魂节。牛魂节又叫作牛王节、脱轭节。这一天，牛主人给牛休息，各家各户把牛梳洗干净，把牛栏修整一新。寨老们对全寨耕牛评头品足，激励大家爱护耕牛。家家蒸制五色糯米饭，用枇杷叶包糯米饭喂牛。主人在牛栏外安个小矮桌，摆上供品，点香烛，祭祀牛魂。

7. 药王节

农历五月初五为药王节，亦称药师节、药市节和端午节，是壮族的传统节日。传说药王是壮医药神，他发现药草，为人治病，还向众人传授种药、采药、治病的知识。壮族地区较大的村寨都立有药王庙，于每年农历五月初五药王节祭祀药王并进行采药防病活动。如广西隆胜各族自治县一带壮族群众此日上山采回乌桕、田基黄、葫芦茶、元宝草等草药煮水洗澡，据说可使皮肤光洁，不生疥疮。靖西市的壮族地区则在这天开设药市，专卖各种草药。药市这天，交易摊位有2000个左右，赶市者达30000多人次，上市的草药品种多达数百种，主要有黄花倒水莲、虎杖、苏木、骨碎补、十大功劳、大罗伞、小罗伞、金不换、绞股蓝、石菖蒲、大血藤、吹风藤、土甘草、土牛膝、土党参、土当归、救必应、丢了棒、九节茶、金果榄、田

七、岩黄连等壮族道地草药材。壮族民间习俗认为，药王节的草药，根肥叶茂，药力宏大，疗效最好。这一天人们到药市上饱吸百药之气，可以预防疾病。这天，百姓还喜欢到药市上买药、认药，既可防病治病，又可增长知识。此外，药王节这一天各家各户还包"羊角粽"，做艾叶糍粑，在屋里熬醋液，烧柚子皮，在门边插艾草、菖蒲，以驱邪逐疫。

8. 六郎节

六郎节于每年农历六月初六举行，是壮族的传统节日，又叫过小年，亦有的称"六郎节""七郎节"。节日期间，三天不做任何农活（和春节一样），村村寨寨、家家户户宰鸭杀鸡，做五色糯米饭，进行祭祀活动，极为热闹、欢快。相传，壮族英雄侬智高突破敌人重围以后，六月里经过的地方在六月过节，七月里经过的地方在七月过节。宋朝皇帝十分忌恨侬智高，严禁人们纪念他。于是，壮族人民把六月节称为"六郎节"，七月节称为"七郎节"，以此纪念民族英雄侬智高。酒肉饭菜备办就绪之后，祭祀活动开始。先由寨主在村头祭献壮族首领侬智高，尔后各家各户可在门前摆上竹榻祭献、祈祷。这天晚上，还要举行"驱鬼"的活动。活动以村为单位，杀鸡、鸭等和用谷草捆成形形色色的魔鬼，敲锣打鼓，由"仆摩"念咒语进行驱赶。在某些壮族村寨还举行隆重的体育活动，如抢花炮、打篮球、赛马等。这一天，壮族妇女做五色糯米饭，互相比较所染的颜色，看谁的颜色最鲜艳。第二天还要将自己所做的五色糯米饭背回娘家"拜年"。

9. 莫一大王节

莫一大王节是广西柳江、龙江两岸壮族的传统节日，也称五谷庙节，于每年农历六月初二举行。莫一大王是壮族民间师公教神灵系统中一个富有民族特色的土俗神，号曰"通天大圣"。传说农历六月初二为莫一大王诞辰，因其拯救壮族人民有功，且保佑五谷丰收，壮族人民感其恩德，故于村前建庙宇、在家中立神位供奉。每年行小祭，供祭鸡肉、鸭肉、猪肉；隔六年一大祭，大祭必全村寨集资杀猪宰羊。届时每家派一人参加，在莫一大王庙举行盛大的祭祀仪式，由村寨头人主持，请道公诵经祈祷。祭时按一年12个月，分别将猪和羊的肉、肝、肠、骨头等不同部位做成12道菜，逐一摆在供台上。待12道菜供齐，即可焚纸行礼。祭毕，将每道菜平均分给各人品尝。

10. 鬼节

农历七月十四是壮族的祭祀性节日，俗称"鬼节"，又叫"七月半""七月节""中元节"。这是壮族仅次于春节的大节。这个节日的活动内容包括祭祖和祀鬼。相传农历七月十四是壮族始祖布洛陀逝世的日子，故人们世世代代在这一天祭奠始祖。从农历七月十四开始大祭，供桌上摆满猪肉、整只鸡、整只鸭、米粉、发糕、糍粑、糯米饭，一直摆到农历七月十六。每次吃饭之前，得先把供品热一下，只有祭过祖，

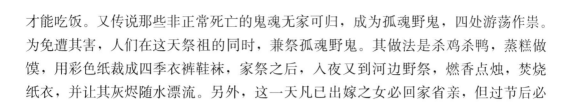

才能吃饭。又传说那些非正常死亡的鬼魂无家可归，成为孤魂野鬼，四处游荡作祟。为免遭其害，人们在这天祭祖的同时，兼祭孤魂野鬼。其做法是杀鸡杀鸭，蒸糕做馍，用彩色纸裁成四季衣裤鞋袜，家祭之后，入夜又到河边野祭，燃香点烛，焚烧纸衣，并让其灰烬随水漂流。另外，这一天凡已出嫁之女必回家省亲，但过节后必须回去，当夜不能在娘家留宿。

11. 擂背节

在桂西一带擂背节又称为"布侬"，是壮族的传统节日。"擂背节"，壮语称为"吟勾到"，"吟"即吃的意思，"勾到"即新谷来到的意思，"吟勾到"即新谷来到了，尝尝新。因为在吃新谷、尝新米的节日晚上，青年男女都要举行擂背活动，所以又称"擂背节"。擂背节在每年农历七月十五举行。家家户户宰鸡杀鸭，做豆腐，蒸新米饭，供祭祖宗，合家欢宴，并用米饭喂狗和猫，以示不忘其守家捕鼠之劳。晚饭后，青年男女打扮一新，相聚在村旁的晒场或草坪上，在月光下或篝火旁举行擂背活动。男女互相挑逗嬉戏，你踩我的脚尖、我碰你的脚跟，进而我擂你的背、你擂我的背。男擂女的背道"吟勾到，扭勒俏"，女擂男的背念"吟勾到，扭勒保"。老人小孩也来围观助兴，满场欢声笑语。按习俗，男先擂女的背，表示男方先看中女方；若女先擂男的背，表示女方爱上了男方；若双双互擂，表示互相爱慕。这时，如果男女双方互有爱慕之情，便会互相追逐跑出场外，到村头寨边对歌、吹木叶，窃窃私语，倾吐情话，互赠情物，播下爱情花种。

12. 中秋节

农历八月十五俗称中秋节、仲秋节、团圆节。壮族有过"八月十五"的习俗。壮族人民认为，每年农历八月十五，月亮是一年中最圆、最亮的一天，是一个很吉利的日子，天上地上，都很安乐祥和。这一天，在外的游子都要赶回家与家人团聚，共享天伦之乐。家家户户吃月饼，蒸粉做糕，杀鸡宰鸭，做丰盛的晚饭，赏月、祭月、拜月，祈求团团圆圆、和和睦睦。各地还有不少的娱乐活动，如广西德保县、靖西市一带，壮族人民这天过"歪囊海"请月娘下凡与民同乐。桂西、桂北的男女青年择地举行歌会，对歌传情，因此很多地方把农历八月十五称为中秋歌节。孩子们则用柚子皮做面具、花灯，打陀螺，踩高跷，扮高公矮婆，尽情玩耍。

13. 祝寿节

壮族有"九九归一，百岁成仙"的说法，农历九月初九这天主要是给老人祝寿，也叫祝寿节，是老人寿辰活动的延续和补充。没有老人的人家也过节，有老人的人家则特别讲究。儿子要给老人剃头、穿新衣服；已出嫁的女儿都要回来，并带一只鸡、几斤米，俗称"补粮"，给老人添粮增寿。席间，子女儿孙先给老人喂饭，然后才进餐，以示孝敬。若老人在这年满60岁，子孙们要杀鸡宰鸭为其祝寿，并给老人添置一个寿米缸，以后每年农历九月初九都要向米缸内添米，直至装满为止，谓之寿米。此缸米只有老人生病时才煮来吃，但不能吃完。

14. 庆丰节

农历十月间，晚稻谷全部收割完并晒干，人们举行隆重的庆祝丰收仪式，祭祀酬谢诸神保佑之功，打扁担、跳春堂舞，以示庆祝。是日，各家各户准备丰盛菜肴，宴请亲朋好友，谁家客人来得越多，宴席就越热闹，这家主人就越高兴，这预示着来年收成更好。

15. 年晚

大年三十又称年晚，即腊月三十，这是壮族人民一年当中最繁忙而又最热闹的节日。这天，男女老少全家欢聚一堂，煮出初一那天吃的米饭，叫"压年饭"，这是预祝来年五谷丰登的意思。晚上，各家各户杀猪宰鸡，包粽子，做年糕，做米花糖，煎馍，缝制新衣，张贴春联，等等。入夜，以猪头、阉鸡、果品隆重祭祖，全家人一起吃年夜饭。然后大人围在火边，除夕守岁；小孩尽兴游戏，通宵不眠。各户在门前悬挂鞭炮，待鸡鸣时燃放，以鸡啼第一声时最先点响爆竹者为最吉祥，俗称"压鸡嘴炮"，并在火灶边摆放供品迎接灶王爷归来。之后，每鸡啼一遍，就燃放一阵爆竹，直至天明。

第二节　壮医药与壮族节庆文化的关系

一、壮医阴阳学说与中元节的渊源

农历七月十四是壮族的祭祀性节日，俗称"鬼节"，又叫"七月半""七月节""中元节"，是壮族仅次于春节的大节。这个节日的活动包括祭祖和祀鬼。顾名思义，"鬼节"因节日活动内容与"鬼"有关而得名。相传农历七月十四是壮族始祖布洛陀逝世的日子。壮族民间还有传说，说人死后变成鬼，都要到阴间去，只有到农历七月初七至十五才能"放假"回到人间探望亲人，故人们世世代代在这一天祭奠远祖。又传说那些非正常死亡的人的鬼魂无家可归，成为孤魂野鬼，四处游荡作祟，常抓人做替身。为免遭其害，人们在这天祭祖的同时，兼祭孤魂野鬼。因南方有水的地方居多，据说，江河是贯穿阳间和阴间的地方，祭拜祖宗时，所用的纸钱、衣物是要靠鸭子驮过奈何桥的，因此在"鬼节"一定要吃鸭子。久而久之，吃鸭子就成了过"鬼节"不可缺少的一项内容。其实，壮族地区地处亚热带，每年农历七月正是雨季，常常继发山洪，因而经常有人跌落山崖、溺水而亡。"野鬼"之说，是老一辈为了告诫人们（特别是莽撞的青少年）不要到山溪、河流附近去玩耍，免得发生意外，惹祸上身。

"中元"源于道家的"三元"之说。道教经典称农历正月十五为上元，农历七月十五为中元，农历十月十五为下元。按阴阳之说，月朔（初一）与月望（十五）是阴阳交感的日子。月朔之日，阳气、阳神、天神、生命之神居于主宰地位；月望之日则阴气、阴神、地祇刑杀之神统驭一切。依此推理，祭祀女神、月神、刑杀之神及祖先亡魂的日子便安排在月望。

壮族聚居和分布地区处于亚热带，虽然年平均气温较高，但是四季仍较分明。日月穿梭，昼夜更替，寒暑消长，冬去春来，使壮族先民很早就产生了阴阳的概念。加上与中原汉族文化的交流及受其影响，阴阳概念在生产、生活中的应用就更为广泛，自然也被壮医作为解释大自然和人体生理病理之间种种复杂关系的说理工具。明代的《广西通志》卷十六记载，壮族民间"笃信阴阳"。著名壮医罗家安在其所著的《痧证针方图解》一书中，就明确以阴盛阳衰、阳盛阴衰、阴盛阳盛对各种痧证进行分类，作为辨证的总纲。从壮族重视农历七月十四"鬼节"来看，壮医阴阳学说的渊源与壮族人民日常生活当中的节庆习俗不无关系。如生者与逝者，所处的境界即分为阳间与阴间，所谓"阴阳相隔，人鬼殊途"；祭祀祖先的日子也选在阴气、阴神主事的月望之日即中元节；就连过中元节所吃的鸭子，也有着其独特功能——沟通阴阳两界的使者。可见壮医阴阳理论并非凭空而来，它来源于壮族人民对自然界的认识，来源于壮族人民的生产生活、思想理念，有着深刻的壮族文化基础。

二、壮医三气同步理论与农耕性节日

壮族是典型的稻作民族，日常的生活、生产活动在很大程度上离不开稻作这个主题。壮族的农耕季节性节日大多顺应自然界的变化，围绕着生产季节和农作节奏而巧妙安排。如农历一月过完年节（春节），休整完毕，农历二月即进入春耕时节。春耕结束后，农历三月即是歌圩节的欢娱时刻了，这时候人们载歌载舞，愉快享受农闲。春耕过后，人们感激牛在春耕中的辛勤劳作，便在牛王诞辰日农历四月初八这天祭祀牛魂，给牛休息。于是，农历四月便有了牛魂节。农历十月，晚稻谷已全部收割完并晒干，人们举行隆重的庆祝丰收仪式，祭祀酬谢诸神保佑之功。于是便有了农历十月的庆丰节。

壮族人民早就认识到，人是自然界的一员，必须与大自然和谐相处；但人是万物之灵，人只要善于认识、掌握、利用自然规律，就能解决与自然界的矛盾。于是自然界有四季更迭，寒来暑往，便有了农作活动的春耕夏种、秋收冬藏。从壮族农耕性节日的安排可见，壮族人民不仅认识并掌握了自然界的运动规律，而且也顺应着自然界的运动规律安排作息，反映了壮族人民那种张弛有度、应时而作的自然生活规律。这是壮族人民"人与大自然和谐相处"思想的体现。

我们从壮族人民这种在生产生活上"崇尚自然，顺应自然"的理念，可以看到壮医"人不得逆天地""人必须顺天地"的三气同步的端倪。天、地、人三气同步，是根据壮语"人不得逆天地"或"人必须顺天地"意译过来的。壮医认为，人与天地须同步运行，人不得逆悖天与地，此即三气同步。就人体内部而言，其上、中、下三部分，亦即天、人、地三部分，需保持协调平衡，身体才能健康无病，亦即三气同步。壮医关于三气同步的概念，最先是由广西名老壮医覃保霖先生在《壮医学术体系综论》一文中首次提出。接着，著名壮医专家黄汉儒教授对三气同步的理论进行了系统地阐述，主要用于说明人与天地之间的相互关系及人体内部之间的相互关系。

壮医三气同步的理论源于壮医对天地的认识，与壮族先民对天地起源的看法及当时壮族先民朴素的宇宙观有关。天地二界必须保持同步平衡，才不会有自然灾害；再联系到人界，则人、天、地三者之间，需保持同步平衡，人才不会生病。其实壮族先民早就自觉或不自觉地遵循这个规律，并且应用于农耕活动的安排当中，正如壮族《传扬歌》中所唱，"正月到二月，耕田抢下种""春风二三月，耕耘正当时，早种苗禾壮，晚种收枯枝"。人们既要顺应农事活动的自然规律，又要发挥主观能动性，改造自然，安排好生产，才能获得丰收。只有真正做到"物我合一"，粮食才会增产丰收，人民才会健康平安。

三、壮医药的应用与药王节

壮族人民很早就有同疾病及一切危害健康的事物做斗争的历史。在壮族众多的节庆活动中，我们也可以找到防病祛邪的内容。

药王节是壮族众多节日中壮医药内涵最丰富的节日，它包含了壮族群众对疾病防治的认识，对药物的栽培和采摘，对药物的功能、用法的认识等内容。在药王节活动中，以靖西端午药市历史最为悠久，影响最大。据考证，靖西端午药市始于宋朝，盛于明清。清代的《归顺直隶州志》记载："五月五日，家家悬艾虎，持蒲剑，饮雄黄酒，以避疠疫。"当地壮族群众认识到，农历五月初五正值仲夏，气候炎热而湿气重，这种气候条件有利于毒虫滋生，易于引发疠疫流行。这个季节也是一些植物根茎成熟的时候，是采药的好时节，药物能发挥其最佳效果。农历五月初五，家家户户将艾草采摘回来，用艾叶、艾根做成人形或老虎的形状，俗称"艾虎"，悬在门楣的中央；将菖蒲制成宝剑挂在屋檐下，还要用艾叶、菖蒲、大蒜烧水洗澡，并将水洒在房前屋后。壮族的这一节日习俗，是有一定科学道理的。艾，《中国壮药学》载其能逐寒湿，理气血，止痛止血，并富含挥发油，可产生奇异的芳香，有驱蚊蝇、虫蚁的作用。《常用壮药临床手册》载，菖蒲有调巧坞、祛风毒、调气机、除湿毒、除瘴毒等功用。大蒜也有解毒杀虫的作用。因此，用艾叶、菖蒲、大蒜烧水洗澡，并将水洒在房前屋后，对居住环境有消毒杀虫的作用，可切断疾病的传染源，是符合夏季防病治病的卫生要求的。药市这天，交易摊位达 2000 个左右，赶药市者达 3 万多人次，上市的药材品种多达数百种，主要有黄花倒水莲、田七等道地壮药，对壮族地区道地壮药的开发利用有促进作用。

四、壮医养生保健与节庆活动

1. 饮食保健，防病治病

壮族的节庆文化与饮食文化是紧密结合的。节日期间，"吃"是核心内容，可以说壮族的节日，是"舌尖上的节日"。这既突出了"民以食为天"这个永恒的主题，又反映了壮族节庆文化的一个显著特点。壮族节日饮食文化丰富多彩，其中还包含一定的食疗保健内容。如春节期间家家户户必备的粽子，以传统的板栗猪肉粽最具代表性。包粽子用的粽叶——柊叶具有清热利尿，治音哑、喉痛、口腔溃疡以及解酒毒等功效。经过大半天的熬煮，粽叶中的药用成分已充分融入糯米当中。栗子性温味甘，有养胃健脾、补肾壮腰、强筋活血、止血消肿等功效。因此，节日期间吃粽子，除了可以享受美味，补充丰富的营养，还具有粽叶、板栗等药食两用食材相应的保健功效。五色糯米饭是壮族人民在节日招待客人的传统美食，特别是在农历三月初三几乎是家家户户必备。五色糯米饭因糯米饭呈黑、红、黄、紫、白 5 种颜色而得名，壮族人把它看作是吉祥如意、五谷丰登的象征。五种颜色所用的染料均是天然植物染料，如黄色染料用山栀子或姜黄，黑色染料用枫叶，红色染料、紫色染料是用同一品种而叶状不同的红蓝草（壮语叫"gogyaemq"）经水煮而成。《中国壮药学》记载，山栀子"苦寒，清热解毒，泻火，凉血止血，利尿"，姜黄"苦辛温，破血行气，通经止痛"。《常用壮药临床手册》记载，红蓝草"味苦、辛，性寒，调龙路，清热毒，祛风毒"。此外，红蓝草还有生血作用，清代《侣山堂类辩》曰"红花色赤多汁，生血行血之品"，《本草纲目》里说枫叶"止泄益睡，强筋益气力，久服轻身长年"。因此，经常食用五色糯米饭，可清热解毒、补血强筋骨、延年益寿。由此，壮族人民独特的养生保健智慧可见一斑。

2. 心理健康，精神安慰

壮族节庆活动中的一个重要内容就是祭祖拜神。壮族人民认为祖先的灵魂会影响到子孙后代，并且相信去世的祖先会继续保佑自己的后代，因此有了对自己祖先、对壮族始祖布洛陀的崇拜。在科学技术极其落后的先古时期，壮族先民认为青蛙是一种能呼风唤雨的神灵物；同时，每年春天，青蛙开始叫的时候，人们就知道播种插秧的季节到来了。由于青蛙有这种"能力"，于是它就成了壮族先民的崇拜对象。人们对青蛙图腾的崇拜是祈求风调雨顺，获得丰收；拜花婆神是为了求子；对祖先的崇拜是表达亲情和怀念，希望庇佑子孙后代……这些祭祀活动，使人们得到心理上的安慰、精神上的净化，使人们对未来充满希望，对生活持乐观态度，有利于健康生活。

3. 休闲休整，恢复体力

不懂得休息，就不懂得工作，现代人更是强调劳逸结合。而勤劳智慧的壮族先民，很早就自觉地在繁重的稻作生产之余，借庆祝节日之际，品美食，访亲友，叙亲情，使身心得到休整，使体力得到恢复，为下一阶段的劳作而准备。年轻人在过节之时，也通过对歌、擂背、抛绣球等文体活动，找到自己心仪的伴侣，使得青年男女精神愉悦、阴阳协调、心理健康、家庭幸福。在这些节日活动中，自始至终，无论男女老少，到处都是欢声笑语。在笑声中，在欢呼雀跃中，人们情绪得到宣泄，心情无比愉悦，忘却了忧愁和烦恼，有助于人的健康长寿。

4. 强身健体，益智怡情

壮族的节日往往伴随着丰富多彩的体育活动。传统的体育节目如大年初一舞狮、"三月三"歌节抛绣球、抢花炮、跳竹竿舞、板鞋比赛等。如今，壮族各村寨大都建有篮球场，节日期间经常举行篮球比赛。这些活动容易开展，器械简单而富有趣味性，易于普及，故受到广大壮族人民的欢迎。具有民族特色的体育活动，既能强身健体，又能益智怡情，体现了壮族人民对运动养生的重视，也体现了壮族人民热爱生活、乐观向上、团结奋进的精神。

参考文献：

[1] 覃彩銮. 壮族节日文化的重构与创新 [J]. 广西民族研究，2012 (4)：66 - 72.

[2] 潘其旭，覃乃昌. 壮族百科辞典 [M]. 南宁：广西人民出版社，1993.

第八章　壮医药与壮族饮食文化

壮族是我国人口最多的少数民族，壮族的饮食文化受地理环境、气候条件、风俗习惯以及所在的社会环境等因素的影响。壮族地区食材广泛，壮族人民喜食土生土长的绿色食品，创造出了丰富多彩的饮食文化。这些食品不仅用于充饥和维系生命，而且还具有满足味觉、强壮身体、防治疾病的作用。在长期的历史发展过程中，壮族的饮食文化和壮医药紧紧联系在一起，相互融合、相互影响、相互促进。

第一节　壮族饮食文化的特点

壮族是一个典型的稻作民族，其作物栽培非常丰富，同时壮族居住地处亚热带地区，终年湿润多雨，百谷皆宜，粮食品种多种多样，一年四季瓜果飘香。由于得天独厚的自然环境及壮族人民的勤劳智慧，使壮族人的食物十分丰富，并逐步形成悠久的壮族饮食文化。壮族的主食有稻米、玉米、芋头、红薯、木薯、荞麦、黑饭豆、白饭豆和绿豆等。玉米品种齐全，其中糯玉米是壮族培育的优良品种之一，可以用来做粽子和糍粑，和糯米一样可口。壮族的传统肉食有猪肉、鸡肉、鸭肉、鱼肉、鹅肉、羊肉、牛肉、马肉以及山禽野兽等。壮乡的蔬菜种类繁多，有萝卜、豆、瓜、竹笋、蘑菇、木耳、白菜、芥菜、包菜、蕹菜、头菜、芥蓝菜等。壮族人对山货的食用有特别的爱好，以竹笋、银耳、木耳、菌类最为名贵。壮族地区素有"水果之乡"的美名，水果种类繁多，宋代《桂海虞衡志》就记有120多种。壮族人爱吃的水果有甘蔗、金橘、柚子、碟子柑、扁桃、菠萝、波罗蜜、香蕉、荔枝、龙眼、黄皮、橄榄和芒果等。壮族人过去的酒水主要是自家熬酿的米酒、白薯酒和木薯酒，酒精度数都不高，其中米酒是过节及待客的主要酒水。

壮族地区动植物资源十分丰富。在古代，壮族先民就把天上飞的、地上跑的、水中游的、地里长的各种可食动植物做成各类食品。在漫长的历史发展过程中，壮族的饮食习惯形成了自身的显著特点。

一、喜食糯食

壮族是以大米为主食的民族，广西地区是野生稻的故乡，壮族先民是最早栽培水稻的民族之一。最迟在汉代，壮族先民就确立了水稻的主粮地位。稻谷按米质可分为籼稻、粳稻、糯稻三大类。其中，籼稻米和粳稻煮熟后不黏，而糯稻米煮熟后较黏。与大多数以大米为主食的民族相比较，壮族喜欢食用糯米制成的食品，在壮族的主食结构中糯米所占的比例也是比较大的。壮族主要用糯米制作节日食品，如粽子、糍粑、米糕、五色糯米饭、汤圆、油团等。其中，最具壮族民族特色的当属粽子和五色糯米饭了。

壮族称粽子为"粽粑"，所制的粽粑花样繁多。在广西宁明县，春节时壮族群众往往制作一种大得惊人的粽粑，这种粽粑用芭蕉叶子包成，内放一条剔去骨头的腌猪腿，足有八仙桌那么大。这么大的粽粑是用于除夕祭祖的。祭祖完毕，同族人共同分食这只大粽粑，以示大家同心同德，和睦美满。在云南省文山壮族苗族自治州，壮族群众喜欢在节日制作"马脚杆粽"。这种粽子是用长 30 厘米、宽 10～15 厘米的大粽叶包成，其形状一头粗大，另一头细长，很像一只带蹄的马脚，所以人们称之为"马脚杆粽"。制作马脚杆粽时，要先将糯米淘洗后浸泡半个小时以上，把头年的干粽叶烧成草灰，与滤干的糯米均匀混合，再拌以火腿丝、枣子、猪肉、盐（或糖）等，最后包上粽叶，入锅水煮而成。这种马脚杆粽色泽灰黄，口感滑腻，味道鲜香，既可热食，又可冷食，保质期较长，不仅是当地壮族群众节日的必备之品，也是青年男女赶集、赶歌圩、赶花街互相赠送的常备礼品。

五色糯米饭，又称花色饭、花糯米饭、五彩糯米饭、五色饭等，是壮族"三月三"节庆必备食品。农历三月初三，家家户户做五色糯米饭，以纪念歌仙刘三姐。五色糯米饭是用红蓝草、黄花、枫叶、紫番藤的根茎或花叶捣烂，取汁分别浸泡于糯米中（留一份米未泡色），然后蒸熟而成，其颜色分别呈红、黄、黑、紫、白五色。人们常将五色糯米饭捏成饭团，不同颜色的饭团陈列在一起，鲜艳夺目。彩色糯米饭的色彩原料不仅起着色的作用，而且也起到调味的作用，不同的彩色糯米饭有不同的香味。糯米饭经着色处理后，不易馊，不易坏，起到了防腐、保鲜的作用。彩色糯米饭除普通食用外，不同颜色的糯米饭还具有不同的作用，如黄色的糯米饭是壮族群众在上坟、接鬼和送鬼时使用的。

除制作节日食品外，人们还用糯米做一些特殊风味的主食，如南瓜饭等。南瓜饭是将一个老南瓜切开顶部作盖，挖掉中间的瓜瓤，将泡洗好的糯米、腊肉等放入瓜中，加适量水拌均匀，盖上瓜盖。将南瓜放于灶上，用文火将瓜皮烧到焦黄，再用炭烬火灰围住南瓜四周，使之熟透，然后将瓜剖开而食，风味独特。

同其他民族一样，壮族人民还用糯米酿酒。刘恂的《岭表录异》记载了唐代时壮族先民酿酒的方法："别淘漉粳米，晒干，旋入药，和米捣熟，即绿粉矣。热水溲而团之，形如餢飳。以指中心，刺作一窍，布放簟席上，以枸杞叶攒罨之。其体候好弱，一如造曲法。既而以藤篾贯之，悬于烟火上。每酝一年用几个饼子，固有恒准矣。南中地暖，春冬七日熟，秋夏五日熟。既熟，贮以瓦瓮，用粪扫火烧之。"明清以来，酿酒在壮族地区十分流行，稍富之家，几乎户户酿酒。除纯度较高的酒外，

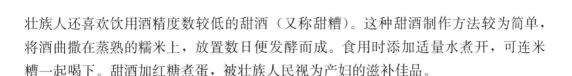

壮族人还喜欢饮用酒精度数较低的甜酒（又称甜糟）。这种甜酒制作方法较为简单，将酒曲撒在蒸熟的糯米上，放置数日便发酵而成。食用时添加适量水煮开，可连米糟一起喝下。甜酒加红糖煮蛋，被壮族人民视为产妇的滋补佳品。

二、喜食生食

壮族喜食生食的传统十分悠久。生食品既有植物，也有动物，甚至是活的动物。唐代时，壮族先民即生食用蜜饲养的活小老鼠，唐代的《朝野佥载》卷二载："岭南獠民好为蜜唧，即鼠胎未瞬，通身赤蠕者，饲之以蜜，钉之筵上，嗫嗫而行，以箸挟取啖之，唧唧作声，故曰蜜唧。"到了近代，壮族生食、半生食的传统得到了继承。民国时期徐松石在《粤江流域人民史》中谈到壮族的饮食时，称壮族"喜欢半生半熟。樊绰《蛮书》说夷人食物有猪羊猫犬驴骡豹兔鹅鸭等，但食法与中土略异，因为他们不待烹熟，皆半生而食。此种风俗也与今日两粤的人士相类……鱼生和生菜的生食已不待论，就是一般蔬菜和鸡肉、鸭肉、牛肉等，烹者亦以略生为主"。在壮族的生食品种中，最有名气的当属生血和生鱼片。

壮族人民常吃的生血有猪、羊、鸡、鸭等动物的血，认为常吃生血能增血补气。有学者认为，此习俗来源于早期人类对血液的神秘观念，是待客的礼俗之一。在生血中，壮族人民以生羊血为贵，认为它最滋补。清代陆祚蕃在《粤西偶记》中说左江的山羊"生得剖者，心血为上，余血亦佳"。壮族人民食生血的方法：将尚带热气的生猪血、生羊血、生鸡血、生鸭血倒入干净的盘中，不停地搅动，不让其凝结，把用各种佐料炒熟的肉和下水趁热倒下去，拌匀使血凝结，即可食用。

生鱼片又叫"鱼生"，是壮族节日待客的佳肴。清光绪的《横州志》记载当时人们制作、食用生鱼片的方法：剖活鱼细切，备辛香、蔬、醋，下箸拌食。现在壮族人食用生鱼片时，一般是将鲜嫩肥美的鲤鱼去鳞、刺，洗净后切成小薄片，拌入芝麻油、食盐、味精、葱、蒜、姜等，另备醋、黄皮酱、酱油等，食用时可根据个人口味，夹生鱼片蘸醋、黄皮酱或酱油吃，鲜嫩可口。会吃的人还加花生、芝麻及芫荽、椿芽一起吃，生脆鲜嫩，凉润爽口。

三、喜食腌食

壮族人民非常喜欢食用各种腌制食品。民国时期刘锡蕃在《岭表纪蛮》第四章记载："腌菜一物，为各种蛮族最普通之食品。所腌兼有园菜及野菜两种，阴历五六七月间，蛮人外出耕作，三餐所食，惟有此品，故除炊饭外，几无举火者。"壮族常用作腌菜的蔬菜有白菜、芥菜、萝卜、豇豆、刀豆、番木瓜、辣椒、姜、笋、薤等。其中，腌笋尤其出名，清代《白山司志》卷九记载："四五月采苦笋，去壳置瓦坛中，以清水浸之，久之味变酸，其气臭甚，过者掩鼻，土人以为香。以小鱼煮之，为食中美品。其笋浸之数年者，治热病如神，土人尤为珍惜。"

壮族不仅腌制各种园生、野生蔬菜，而且也腌制肉类鱼虾。民国时期的《同正县志》记载："西部山麓诸村远隔市廛，每合数村共同宰一猪，将分得肉和糯米粉生贮坛中，阅十余日可食，不须火化，经久更佳，名曰'酸肉'。"民国时期的刘锡蕃在《岭表纪蛮》第四章亦记载："若屠牛豕，即以其骨合菜并腌，俟其腐烂，然后取食。"用鱼腌制的鲊是壮族腌菜的典型代表，壮族制鲊的历史非常悠久，宋代周去非《岭外代答》卷六记载："南人以鱼为鲊，有十年不坏者。其法以及盐面杂渍，盛以之瓮，瓮口周为水池，覆之以碗，封之以水。水耗则续，如是故不透风。鲊数年生白花，似损坏者。凡亲属赠遗，悉用酒、鲊，唯以老鲊为至爱。"

四、喜食酸辣食

生活于我国西南地区大山里的少数民族普遍嗜好酸辣食品，在民间往往有"三天不吃酸，走路打孬蹿""食不离酸""不辣不成菜""没有辣椒待不了客"之类的民谚。

壮族和西南地区的其他少数民族一样，也非常喜食酸辣之物。如云南省文山壮族苗族自治州的壮族人民特别喜欢喝酸酸的老扒汤。老扒汤的做法：将煮饭的米汤冷却，入缸，把洗净的青菜、白菜、甘蓝或其他菜叶切成小块，拌盐，放入坛内冷水汤中，封缸贮存一两日后，缸内的米汤和菜叶经发酵变酸，成为酸汤和酸菜；用酸汤和酸菜加肥厚的火熏腊肉块或油炸腊肉块煮汤，就成了老扒汤。也可根据各人喜好和具体备料情况，加豆腐和其他配料做成各种菜汤，作佐餐菜肴。老扒汤鲜酸爽口，可解暑。在插秧时节到农历八月这段天气较热的时间里，老扒汤是壮族人餐桌上经常出现的当家菜。腌制酸菜的酸汤煮沸后冷却，还可作为解暑饮料，清爽提神。

壮族人民喜食酸辣之物，是与他们的生活环境和物产有关的。壮族人民多生活于潮湿多山的地区，多吃酸辣，可以驱寒散湿；同时，壮族人民食用糯米较多，而糯米性黏不易消化，故也需要多食酸辣刺激胃肠，促进消化吸收。

第二节　壮族饮食礼俗

饮食礼俗是人们在饮食生活中所形成的各种礼节，是礼最外在的表现形式和严格规范下所支配的活动之一。汉代经学大师董仲舒的《春秋繁露·天道施》言："好色而无礼则流，饮食而无礼则争，流争则乱。"同其他民族一样，壮族在长期的饮食生活中也形成了一套丰富多彩的饮食礼俗。

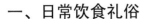

一、日常饮食礼俗

同其他少数民族相比较，壮族受汉族传统文化的影响是比较大的，因此敬老爱幼、上下有序、男尊女卑等传统观念在壮族的日常饮食礼俗中有所反映。如进餐时，老人往往受到特别的尊重，给老人盛饭时，要用双手从老人侧背把碗递上；饭后，要给老人递上茶水或清水漱口。壮族认为鸡鸭的心、肝营养丰富，胸、尾肥嫩，因此人们食用鸡、鸭时，要把心、肝、胸、尾留给老人食用。又如壮族进餐时往往采取男女分桌而食，以免违犯"男女授受不亲"的古训。餐桌席位也有比较严格的规定，家长夫妇坐正位，子女坐旁位，媳妇坐下位。

二、待客饮食礼俗

壮族是一个好客的民族，这在古代文献中多有反映，如明代邝露《赤雅》上卷记载："人至其家，不问识否，辄具牲醴，饮啖，久敬不衰。"清代闵叙《粤述》记载："（客）至，则鸡黍礼待甚殷。"民国的《上林县志》记载："亲友偶乐临存，虽处境不宽，亦须杯酒联欢，以尽主人之谊；倘远客到来，则款洽更为殷挚。"龙州一带的壮族有"空桌留客"的风俗，即家有来客，主人便张罗酒菜，并在厅堂摆好饭桌餐具，表示已约客人吃饭，客人不能拒绝，若客人执意要走，便会扫主人面子。

在许多地方，壮族村寨任何一家来了客人均被视为全寨的客人，往往几家轮流请吃饭，客人要轮流吃一遍，不吃者为失礼。只有各家都尝一点，才算领了情、尽了礼。壮族宴客时，要让年老的客人、贵客与主人一起坐正位。招待客人的餐桌上必须备酒，方显得隆重。酒宴上，人们有喝"交杯酒"的习俗。壮族喝"交杯酒"，其实并不用杯，而用白瓷汤匙，两人从酒碗中各舀一匙，相互交饮，眼睛真诚地望着对方。为了表示对客人的尊敬，每上一道菜，主人都要先给客人夹一筷菜后，其他的人才能下筷。宴席上，壮族人是不会让客人的碗见底的，客人碗里往往被好客的主人夹满了菜，堆得很高。在壮族主人眼里，菜堆得越高表示越尊敬。有的壮乡，甚至用一根筷子穿起几块肉，往客人嘴里塞，名曰"灌肉"。有的初到壮乡的客人，怕吃不完剩下难为情，尽量把碗中的菜吃光，结果越吃主人就越往碗里夹菜，主人见客人吃不完才高兴，觉得尽到了礼；如果客人碗里的饭菜吃光了，便觉得食物不够丰盛，招待不周。

三、人生礼仪食俗

在婚嫁、丧吊、寿诞等人生礼仪活动中，饮食活动往往具有不可替代的重要作用和含义，因此人们格外重视这些人生礼仪活动中的食俗。在各种人生礼仪活动中，婚嫁活动最为隆重，其饮食习俗也始终贯穿于从恋爱定亲到拜堂成亲整个婚嫁过程。

在广西靖西、德保、那坡、大新等地，男女恋爱一段时间后，到翌年正月初，女方家庭要办一桌丰盛的筵席款待新上门的女婿，当地称为"考婿宴"。在考婿宴上，女方家长特邀本村一位德高望重、见多识广的前辈考问女婿各方面的知识，有农业方面的，有日常生活方面的，也有宗教历史方面的，等等。这种考问的方式一般是在自然、融洽的进餐过程中进行的。考婿宴上准女婿的表现将直接影响到男女双方是否订婚。

在壮族的订婚礼仪中，有以槟榔做聘礼的风俗，清代《白山司志》记载："婚姻不用庚贴，但槟榔一盒、戒指一对送，谓之吃。"槟榔果呈长椭圆形，橙红色，壮族平时有食槟榔以助消化的习俗。宋代罗大经的《鹤林玉露》和清代的《白山司志》中均记载壮族人民喜食槟榔的原因是为了御瘴。壮族人民以槟榔做订婚聘礼，除因槟榔好吃之外，还因为它与"宾郎"谐音，古人称贵客为"宾"、为"郎"，以槟榔做聘礼，有尊敬女方的意思。

在红水河和柳江沿岸的一些地方，新娘上轿前要坐在堂屋中间，背朝香火，由一个父母、儿女双全的人把夫家送来的一碗饭端在手上，司仪高颂："一碗米饭白莲莲，糖在上面肉在间。女家吃了男家饭，代代儿孙中状元。"周围的人答："好的！有的！"端碗的人轻轻地把碗里的一根葱、一只鸡腿、一块红糖拨过一边，给新娘扒三口饭，她吃三口吐三口（弟妹用裙子接住），接着又把一把筷子递给她，她从自己肩上递给后面的小辈，自己却不得朝后看，表示永不后顾。

在婚嫁宴席上，壮族实行男女分席，但宴席一般不排座次，人们可以不论辈分大小坐在同一桌上就餐。壮族婚宴还有入席即算一座的礼俗，即不论年龄大小，哪怕是妇女怀中尚在吃奶的婴儿，也可得到一份菜肴，由家长代为收存，用干净的阔叶片包好带回家。这些礼俗体现了壮族平等相待的观念。但在有些壮乡，婚宴时男宾坐高席，女宾坐竹簟，反映了当时壮族社会对妇女有一定的歧视，如今这种现象已经很少见了。

除婚嫁饮食礼俗外，壮族的其他人生礼仪食俗也很丰富。如广西大新县安平一带的生子"三朝礼"颇为独特，届时外婆家要送1担糯米和20个鸭蛋。婿家请全寨小孩来绕着房子喊："俏（指婴儿）来啊，耕田去啊，种地去啊！……"喊完后，每个小孩可得到一团糯米饭和一个鸭蛋。在桂西一些地方，60岁以上的老人做寿酒时，其长子"须行反哺之礼，以饭菜喂之"。

四、节日饮食礼俗

壮族的节日饮食礼俗也有一些独特的内容，如春节时人们要吃粽粑，一般不吃青菜，认为春节吃青菜来年田里就会长草，影响庄稼收成。"三月三"是壮族的重要节日，除吃五色糯米饭外，壮族还有吃五色蛋的习俗。五色蛋是把鸡蛋（或鸭蛋、鹅蛋）分别染成五种颜色，每人吃一个有色蛋，小孩每人还要在胸前挂一串五色蛋，作为碰蛋游戏之用。中秋节时，壮族人家也有赏月、吃月饼的习俗。孩子们在这天

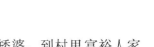

往往用柚子皮自制成各种奇形怪状的鬼脑壳，化装成高公、矮婆，到村里富裕人家桌上取食月饼。青年男女则结伴到田地里象征性地偷回一些瓜果蔬菜，俗称"偷青"，认为吃了这些偷来的瓜果蔬菜可以明目。

第三节　壮医药与壮族饮食文化的关系

一、壮医三道论与壮族饮食文化

壮医认为，人体内的谷道、水道和气道及其相关的枢纽脏腑均为人体生命活动营养物质化生、贮藏、输布、运行的场所，它们之间分工合作，互相配合，各司其职，滋养全身，从而实现了天、地、人三气同步，保证了各种生理活动的正常运行。谷道是食物消化吸收及精微输布的通道，气道是人体一身之气化生、输布、贮藏的处所，水道则是人体水液化生、贮藏、输布、运行的场所。壮族地区清新的空气、优质的水源及天然的绿色食品，对谷道、气道和水道功能的正常运行发挥了重要作用，从而提高了人体对疾病的抵抗能力，使人体维持健康的常度。壮医认为，五脏聚集精华，滋荣体质；六腑敷布水谷精微，扬清舍浊。五脏六腑的功能主要依靠"三道"来调养，而在壮族民间，尤其重视对谷道的调理。

壮族民间长寿老人众多，这与他们饮食合理有节是密不可分的。壮医非常重视对谷道的调理，与中医学的"脾胃为后天之本"不谋而合。壮族地区饮食有"五低"（低脂肪、低动物蛋白、低盐、低糖、低热量）和"二高"（高维生素、高纤维素）的特点，人们多以粗粮素食为主，长期食用土生土长的绿色食品。如巴马的黄珍珠玉米就具有营养丰富，脂肪、蛋白质含量比较高等特点；烹饪菜肴所用的火麻仁油是目前世界上唯一能溶于水的植物油。此外，他们还有饮食清淡、不挑食、不偏食等良好习惯，食物摄入的热量也比较低。他们合理的饮食搭配和良好的生活习惯对保证谷道的通畅和功能的正常发挥有着重要作用。人们也常以谷道功能是否正常来衡量人体的健康状况。

二、壮医药膳与壮族饮食文化

壮医药膳是在壮医药理论的指导下，由药物、食物和调料三者精制而成，用以防病治病、强身益寿的美味食品，具有浓郁的地方特色和民族特色。

壮医在全面分析患者的症状、病因、体质的基础上，结合环境、季节合理运用药膳进行食疗。食补的原则为春升、夏清淡、秋平、冬滋阴。壮医药膳的烹调特别讲究保持食物和药材的原汁原味，使食物与药材的性味紧密结合，更好地发挥治疗、保健作用。烹调方法有蒸、煮、炖、炒、煲汤等，制作药膳时，还加入一定的调料，增加药膳的色、香、味，增强食欲。

瓜果是常用的原料，用于制作各种民族特色的瓜果药膳，如山楂糕、菠萝盅、石榴汁。此外，壮族人民对米饭的做法也多种多样，竹筒饭、生菜包饭、五色糯米饭享誉海内外。

如今，壮族人民在传统药膳的基础上，又推出了具有民族特色的现代药膳，品种不断增加，如药膳罐头、保健饮料、药膳糖果、药膳点心、药酒等，受到越来越多的海内外来客的欢迎。壮医药膳将为人们的防病治病、延年益寿做出更大的贡献。

三、壮医养生与壮族饮食文化

壮医养生是在壮医理论的指导下，壮族人民在长期医疗活动中形成的独特养生经验总结。药补不如食补，壮医养生尤为重视饮食在强身健体、预防疾病、增进健康、延缓衰老方面的作用。

壮医擅用血肉之品补体虚。虚是指由于先天不足或后天失调，或疾病耗损引起人体正气不足，致脏腑功能衰退而出现的各种临床表现。壮医的虚证主要包括老年病、慢性病和急性病邪毒祛除之后的恢复期症状等。壮族认为人为万物之灵，动物药为血肉有情之物，同气相求，故用来补虚最为有效。古往今来，壮族就深谙此道，喜欢用肉食和动物血来强壮和进补身体。壮族的传统肉食有猪肉、鸡肉、鸭肉、鹅肉、羊肉、牛肉、马肉、鱼肉等。羊肉，《中药大辞典》中记载其可以"益气补虚，温中暖下。治虚劳羸瘦，腰膝酸软，产后虚冷，腹疼，寒疝，中虚反胃"。鱼生营养丰富，味鲜香甜可口，壮族民间在每年中秋节，家家户户都做鱼生吃。动物血如猪血、牛血、鸭血、鸡血、羊血、鹅血等，本身就有补养气血的作用。羊血，味甘、苦，性凉，具有解毒、凉血止血、活血化瘀的作用，可治野葛等植物药中毒、肠风下血、吐血、血崩、胞衣不下、跌打损伤等；壮民杀猪时用猪血及碎肉拌上优质糯米，佐以葱、蒜，灌入洗净的猪肠中，用细线扎成一节节，入锅煮熟即成。这种用猪血制成的"龙棒"，又称为"血糯肠"，可做主食，补虚效果不错。又如广西名菜"三七鸡"，经常进食可起到治疗营养不良性贫血，预防瘀阻性痛经的作用。除此之外，还有一些动物有补虚的功效，如乌骨鸡、麻雀、老鼠、蛇等。乌骨鸡味甘、性平，能补益肝肾、补血养阴、退虚热，故可治疗肝肾不足、虚劳、阴血不足诸证，以及阴虚内热、糖尿病、妇女崩中带下虚损诸证；用麻雀配合羊肉做食疗药膳，可以治疗因胞宫寒冷而引起的不孕症；如子宫虚冷无子者，可用山羊肉、麻雀肉、鲜益母草、黑豆，互相配合做饮食治疗；对颈肢节胀痛，历年不愈，每遇气候变化而加剧者，壮医主张多吃各种蛇肉汤；对于肺阴耗伤而干咳者，喜用猪肉或老母鸭、鹧鸪肉煲莲藕吃。壮医不仅对虚证如此，而且对挟瘀之证，有时亦配血肉之品，除用扶正祛瘀之品外，常与山药牛肉粥同服，以增强扶正之功效。

　　壮医擅用各种药酒防病强身。壮族世代居住五岭之南，山岚瘴气盘郁结聚，不易疏泄，阳盛阴凝，蕴湿化热，挟痧带瘴，常易猝发。气候炎热，阴湿多雨，故很多疾病皆与湿邪有关。《本草拾遗》中记载，白酒"通血脉，厚肠胃，润皮肤，散湿气"。壮族人民的祖先精通酿酒之道，自家酿制米酒、糯米甜酒、红薯酒、白薯酒和木薯酒，酒精度数都不太高，适当饮用，均有祛湿除瘴、温通经脉、消除疲劳的效果。其中，米酒是逢年过节接待客人的必备之品，在米酒中配以鸡胆称为"鸡胆酒"，配以鸡杂称为"鸡杂酒"，配以猪肝称为"猪肝酒"。饮鸡杂酒和猪肝酒时要一饮而尽，留在嘴里的鸡杂、猪肝则慢慢咀嚼，既可解酒，又可当菜。红薯酒可以起到预防高脂血、高胆固醇的作用。糯米甜酒可以起到补气养血的作用。在壮族地区若有客人到，习惯先敬糯米甜酒，以示欢迎。还有以广西特产水果龙眼为原材料制成的龙眼酒，能起到补血益智、养心安神的作用。用余甘果来酿酒，对防治高血压、高脂血症有一定的效果。蛤蚧酒最能体现壮族特色，蛤蚧味咸、性平，有补肺肾、定喘咳、助肾阳、益精血、下淋漓、通水道的功用。取蛤蚧成品与白酒共同密封泡制，经过加工后做成蛤蚧酒，可以起到补肺定喘、温肾壮阳的作用，对治疗肺肾阳虚之喘咳、慢性支气管炎等有很好的疗效。壮族人民还把蛤蚧酒作为保健治疗并举的药酒来经常饮用。此外，三蛇酒也属于药酒。三蛇酒是用特殊处理的过山龙、扁头风、金环蛇或银环蛇加入一些草药浸泡好酒而成，是一种名贵的药酒。用眼镜蛇的蛇胆兑白酒，可以起到很好的祛风湿、除湿毒的作用。

　　壮医擅用各种饮品解毒防病。壮医毒虚致病理论是壮医学独具特色的病因病机学说，壮医认为毒是引发疾病的主因。由于壮族地区特殊的气候和地理环境，毒不仅指一些有形的毒物（如蛇毒、虫毒、毒草、毒树等），而且也指无形之毒（如热毒、火毒、风毒、湿毒等），还泛指一切致病因素的总称。壮族地区气候炎热，烟瘴易发，在此生活的人们往往有极易上火、易阳胜动火、易感湿热等体质，故能清热消暑、除瘴祛湿的饮品才是壮族地区的特色饮料。壮族人民喜欢用槟榔、山楂叶、米酸水制成饮料。春夏之际，疾病流行，壮族家中往往备有槟榔，用来煮水饮用，可以消除瘴气。壮族民间还常用晒干的山楂叶浸泡于开水中，待冷却后饮用，是止渴解暑的常用饮料。在壮族农村，家家自制米酸水，用来浸泡辣椒、豆角、嫩笋、蒜头等。炎暑时节，饮用些米酸水，不仅可止渴解暑，而且还可防治肠胃疾病；菜肴中加入些米酸水，可使人增加食欲。用余甘果果肉晒干制茶即余甘果茶，除对防治高血压、高脂血症有一定的效果外，还可防治支气管炎、咽喉炎等。壮族传统的夏天清凉饮料是凉粉果汁，这些饮料清凉甜爽，饮用后口渴马上缓解。接骨茶、桂皮茶、甘蔗水等用药简便、精专，可以起到很好的清热祛火的作用。由于壮族地区湿热交蒸，壮族人民易染湿气，有祛湿热作用的木瓜汤、木瓜盅等亦是深受壮乡人民喜欢的祛湿凉茶。鸡骨草、狗肝菜直接用水煮煎服，能起到解热毒、除湿毒、退黄的作用。玉米含谷胱甘肽，有抗癌的作用。广西巴马长寿之乡的壮族人民除把玉米作为主食外，还经常用玉米煮汤代茶饮。

参考文献：

[1] 冯秋瑜. 壮族饮食文化特点 [J]. 中国民族医药杂志，2009 (11)：77-79.

[2] 刘朴兵. 壮族饮食文化习俗初探 [J]. 南宁职业技术学院学报，2007 (12)：1-4.

[3] 唐振宇，庞宇舟，蓝丽霞，等. 壮医养生法则初探 [J]. 中国中医基础医学杂志，2015 (1)：21-22.

[4] 朱华. 中国壮药志 [M]. 南宁：广西民族出版社，2003.

[5] 叶庆莲. 壮医基础理论 [M]. 南宁：广西民族出版社，2006.

[6] 蓝毓营. 壮医毒虚致病学说初探 [J]. 中华中医药杂志，2010，25 (12)：2147.

第九章　壮医药与壮族人居文化

第一节　壮族人居文化的演变

壮族及其先民的居住条件与特有的自然环境及生产力水平有着密切的关系。壮族居住房舍就地取材，早期因势而居，从岩居穴处，巢居树宿，发展成为干栏建筑。

一、岩居穴处

岩居穴处是早期人类最先开拓的居住形式。岭南山多，洞穴也多，故使岩居穴处有了更多的自然环境条件。《隋书·南蛮传》记载："南蛮，类与华人错居，曰蜒、曰獽、曰俚、曰僚，俱无君长，随山洞而居，古先所谓百越是也。"宋代《太平寰宇记》记载，宜州"山川险峻，人民犷戾……礼仪俗殊，以岩穴居止"。岩居穴处以蔽风雨，是人类最简便的居住形式。

二、巢居树宿

在原始社会时期，壮族先民主要靠采摘果实、狩猎来维持生活。"僚依山林而居，无酋长版籍，蛮之荒无常者也，以射生食物为活，虫豸能蠕动者皆取食"，由于岭南地区潮湿多雨，地势不平，毒蛇猛兽以及其他自然灾害经常威胁人们的生命安全。为了生存，壮族先民在同自然界做斗争的过程中，不断寻求最佳的居住环境。为了避免毒蛇猛兽的袭扰，逐渐形成了择高而居的方式。《韩非子·五蠹》有云："上古之世，人民少而禽兽众，人民不胜禽兽虫蛇，有圣人作，构木为巢，以避群害，而民悦之使天下，号曰'有巢氏'。"晋人张华在《博物志》中明言："南越巢居，北溯穴居，避寒暑也。"《水经·温水注》记载："秦余徙民，染同夷化，日南旧风，变易俱尽。巢居树宿，负郭积山，榛棘蒲薄，腾林拂云。"《林邑记》记载："……朱吾县浦，今之封界。朱吾以南有文俍人，野居无室宅，依树止宿，鱼食生肉，采香为业，与人交市，若上皇之民矣。"《天下郡国利病书》记载，蜀中"今山谷中有俍，但乡俗构屋高树，谓之阁阑"。《隋书·地理志》（下）记载，俚人"巢居岩处，尽力农事"。《宋史·良吏》记载："又俚民皆巢居鸟语。"文俍人即俍人、俍人、俚人均是壮族先民的一种别称，有树宿的习俗。

91

三、干栏建筑

随着生产力水平的提高，壮族先民从树宿逐渐演变成择高而居的形式，发展为居干栏建筑。干栏建筑是壮族地区现存的形态较为原始古朴的一种民居建筑形式。这类建筑主要分布在远离城镇、交通不便的山区村寨中。《旧唐书·西南蛮传·平南僚》记载："人并楼居，登梯而上，号为干栏。"《新唐书·南蛮传·平南僚》记载："山有毒草、沙虱、蝮蛇，人楼居，梯而上，名为干栏。"随着人们开始饲养牲畜，干栏上层住人，下层圈牲畜。宋代范成大在《桂海虞衡志》记载："居民苦茅，为两重棚，谓之麻栏，上以自处，下蓄牛豕。"早期的干栏建筑以竹木为架，上覆茅草或竹。随着社会的进步、经济的发展，干栏建筑的材料从竹木向土瓦、砖石转变。

干栏建筑从其结构来看，又可分为全楼居高脚干栏、半楼居干栏、低脚干栏、地居式干栏、横列式干栏等5种类型。从使用的建筑材料来看，又有全木结构、木竹结构、石木或砖或夯土混合结构、砖石或夯土结构等4类。

1. 全楼居高脚干栏

这类干栏民居是壮族地区现存的最原始古朴的一种建筑形式，主要分布于广西北部的龙胜各族自治县、三江侗族自治县、融水苗族自治县，中部的忻城县和西部的靖西市、西林县以及东部的贺州市等壮族聚居的山区村寨，其中以龙胜各族自治县的龙脊十三寨最为普遍，保留得最为完整、典型。其房屋多建在山岭的陡坡上，并依次辟坡而建，多为独家而立，或两家连为一体，鳞次栉比，檐柱相对，但整个村寨无一定布局和界定，每一村寨由20~50座房屋组成。其建筑的特点是全木结构和高脚楼居，即在高坡上开辟的房基上立木为柱，穿斗架梁，设檩铺椽，合板为墙，屋顶盖小青瓦（也有的用杉树皮或茅草覆盖），呈悬山式或半歇山式。内部辅板为楼，第一层架空，形成高脚木楼，围栏圈养猪牛和堆放杂物；第二层为人居，内以木板分隔成间，设木梯而上；第三层通常为半阁楼式，铺以木板，用以置放粮食和杂物，每层高2.0~2.4米。

2. 半楼居干栏

这类干栏建筑通常与全楼居木结构高脚干栏建筑同处在一个村寨里，而且梁架结构亦与前者基本相同，不同的是，此类干栏房屋依陡坡辟地而建，前三进间底部立柱架空，形成高脚干栏楼房，人居住在以铺板为面的第二层楼上，而后两柱则立于突兀而起与第二层楼板面齐平的台面上，与木楼下的地面高差约2米，使居室面形成四分之三为楼板、四分之一为地面的格局，故名"半楼居干栏"。此外，有些地方的半楼居干栏的后部以石块或泥砖为培，形成木石或砖混合结构。

3. 低脚干栏

低脚干栏指干栏的架空底层降低至1米左右。这类干栏建筑主要分布于广西西

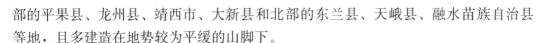

部的平果县、龙州县、靖西市、大新县和北部的东兰县、天峨县、融水苗族自治县等地，且多建造在地势较为平缓的山脚下。

4. 地居式干栏

这类干栏建筑以融水苗族自治县的壮族村寨较为常见。其特点是在开辟平整的地面上立柱穿斗架梁，搁檩辅椽盖瓦，以四面拼板为墙，也有的砌土砖为墙，悬山顶，一般三开间、二进间，内部沿立柱用木板相隔成间；一般分上、下两层，下层即地面为居住面，上层为木板楼，用以放置粮食杂物。因地形所限，人们常在屋前的高台下立以木柱，用以支撑外伸的檐檩和屋檐，并且在柱之间连枋设栅，构成走廊；或沿门前地面辅板设栅，构成望楼或走廊。其廊下架空仍保留着传统的干栏建筑的一些遗迹。

四、地居式建筑

地居式建筑又称硬山搁檩，广泛分布于交通方便、与汉族杂居的城镇及其附近的广大农村。其形式和结构多样，且因地区不同而有所差异，但是其基本结构仍是大同小异，均为土墙（或石或砖）木檩小青瓦，悬山顶，并流行三开间主房的院落式，分上、下两层，人居下层（即地面居），上层为半楼或满楼，中间厅堂为明间。有些地方的地居式房屋局部还保留穿斗木构架的遗迹。如忻城县宁江一带的壮族居民，其厢房的隔墙筑至山尖处，近前檐墙部分留空，上方以穿斗木构架支托斜梁，其斜梁延至前檐，檐外以挑托檩，这是将传统的干栏式迴廊内缩的结果。

第二节 壮族住宅的特点

一、壮族住宅布局

壮族住宅的内部布局都严格遵循一个规矩，即以神龛为中心，火塘辅之。神龛在家中是至高无上的，它居于整个房子的中轴线上，显示出祖先崇拜的庄严、家族传统的威力，求得祖宗的灵光普照全屋。在神龛下面设一张八仙桌，桌上设置香案，以供香火。生人不许乱动香案，惹是生非，亵渎祖宗，否则将受斥责或引起主人的不快。八仙桌两侧设两个座位，左侧供一家之主专坐，其他人不许越位，冒犯家长尊严，右侧则是客坐。另一个重要部分——火塘，可置于厅堂的一侧或后部，位置仅次于神龛，因为这里是人们饮食的地方。壮族人民一般都在火塘、灶头附近设置祭坛祭祀灶王爷，以求得福光不熄，五谷丰登。住宅后半部为生活区，约占少半。前半部为举行庆典和社交活动的厅堂，两边是厢房，与厅堂相通的厢房是客房。主人卧室在后半部及与厅堂隔开的厢房。其中，神龛后面一般不让人住，要住也只能是一家之主。壮族住宅布局示意图见图 9-1。

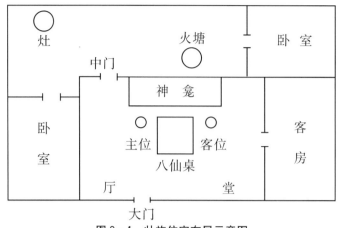

图 9-1 壮族住宅布局示意图

干栏房屋的平面布局,特别是全楼居干栏和半楼居干栏的面积较宽大,一般多为六逢五往,一侧有披厦,面阔 20 米左右,进深 10 米左右,入口处设在房屋底层一侧,而后沿木梯登上第二层,大门口建有一长约 7 米、宽约 2.5 米的望楼,旁侧置放有木凳,可供人们外出进屋前挂放雨具和小工具,或稍作休息用。屋内厅堂与大门相对,并向两侧扩展相通,间无隔板,长约 18 米,宽约 8 米,两侧各设有一火塘,其家人通常在右侧火塘炊煮,左侧火塘一般在婚丧和其他喜庆之日宴请宾客时才使用。如此宽敞的厅堂,便于人们举行集会、设宴和其他集体活动,而无须到户外(户外也极少有宽敞的平地)。常用的火塘一侧的壁面上都修设有壁龛,可放置炊器和饮食器具。后侧和左侧均以木板分隔成间,用作卧室或储藏室。其平面布置颇为考究,区域布局亦较严格。

如龙胜一带壮族的住宅从前厅进入堂屋,面对祖宗神位,神位的背面安排卧室。正中卧室住父辈(家公),左边房住母辈(家婆),怕妇女"亵渎"祖宗。如若正中卧室及左边房住的是家公、家婆,则家婆房有小门与家公卧室相连。右边房住儿媳。厅左、右两侧的房间为子女居住,儿子居右侧房间,女儿居左侧房间(以后结婚在外,回家时仍住此间)。这个布局有个明显的特点,就是夫妇异室。龙脊十三寨的房子布局,在右角的梯子旁边有女孩房,突出于卧室前面,这有利于她们和小伙子交往。龙胜一带壮族的住宅示意图见图 9-2。百色一带的干栏式住宅中间为厅,厅的后半部做厨房,左厢房、右厢房做卧室。左厢房前半部分为父辈居住,左厢房、右厢房的后半部分为儿孙住。如果分家,长子住原屋,表示继位,其他兄弟择地另建。

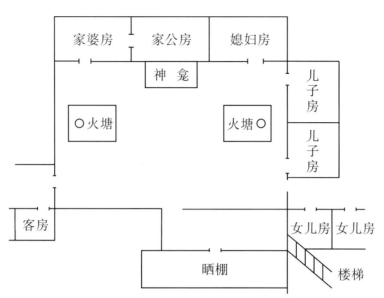

图 9‑2　龙胜一带壮族的住宅示意图

天峨县白定乡壮族住宅厅堂的神台和两个火塘也是"品"字形分布，但卧房分布与龙脊的不同，家长房不在神台后面，而是在左后角。神台后面为普通房，儿媳或女孩都可以住，说明桂西边远山区受男尊女卑的影响是比较小的。

此外，旁侧增建的披厦亦设有望楼和迴廊，可供乘凉用。在一侧的前面还设有以木竹建成的晒台，凡收成的谷物均可放在晒台上晒干，无须在外寻地晾晒。在房屋四周的板墙上，有序地开设窗口，既便于房间通风，又利于采光，保持室内空气通畅，光线明亮。厅堂和火塘处皆为明间，另一侧没有阁楼，并以木板分隔成间，多用作储藏室，也有作为卧室，以备客人多时使用。因此，住宅在生活起居方面可以自给自足，一家人的日常生活，包括晒谷、春米、饮水、炊煮、饮食、宴客、集会等活动，均可在家中进行。

低脚干栏和地居式干栏房屋的面积就相对窄小，也较低矮，远不及全楼居高脚干栏和半楼居高脚干栏那样高、宽敞和实用，一般为三开间，面阔 13 米左右，进深约 10 米，结构较简单，建筑造价也较低，出入也比较方便，可基本满足一家人的生活需要。

壮族人民认为，大门是招财进宝之门户，是拒鬼魅于门外的关口，因此大门一般都开在正中央，与祖宗的神龛相对，有借祖宗的神灵护佑大门带来福气之意。但各地的风俗又各有不同，有些地方则认为"开门见山，祖宗不安，人丁不旺"，大门不开在中间，而开在靠左一侧；有些地方则不开后门，意为财不外流，倘若要开后门，也不能和前门同在一条直线上，以免财从前门进，后门出。从如此繁多的习俗可以看出，大门关系一家人的祸福，因此壮族人民在门框上贴上镇邪之符，或悬挂八卦镜、镜子及剪刀之类辟邪之品，拒鬼怪于门外，求得一家的平安。

随着人们生活水平的提高，壮、汉民族的交融，现在很多壮族人都住进现代化的楼房中，干栏建筑也随着时代的变迁而慢慢减少，但是住宅布局等依旧保存着壮族人民一些特有的习俗。

二、壮族土司官署、祠堂

壮族地区的土司制度，等级森严。土司对壮族人民建造住房有各种限制，不准其造高质量的住宅，以显示土司贵族与平民在住房上的等级差别。清代，上映、向都等地的土司规定平民不能用雕龙画凤来做装饰，台阶不能高过土司的房屋。因此，土司的屋宅无论是从规模布置，还是从质量装修来说，远非平民房可比。

明清的土官土司参考了汉族官宦人家的生活方式，构建了具有民族特点的土司衙门建筑群，至今保存较完好的有道光年间修建的忻城土司衙门和乾隆年间修筑的土司祠，它们的特点是在壮民族传统文化的基础上，接受了中原文化的影响，建筑布局模仿汉营造制式按一定的轴向展开，官舍并用，前衙后府；砖木结构，雕梁画栋，油漆彩画，显示了壮、汉两族建筑技术的融合。

忻城土司衙门是我国乃至亚洲现存规模最大、保存最完整的土司建筑之一，被誉为"壮乡故宫"。土司衙门建筑群占地40000多平方米，由衙门、宅第、官塘花厅、寺庙、祠堂、陵园等组成。土司衙门始建于明万历十年（1582年），全部为砖木结构。木构件均采用珍贵木材制作，天面飞檐翘脊，落地门式屏风，彩绘浮雕、镂空花窗、朱漆梁柱、气势轩昂，吸取了明代先进的建筑营造艺术与结构的优点。土司衙门由照壁、前门、头堂、长廊、二堂、三堂、后院组成，在其左右还分布有东辕门与西辕门、东花厅与西花厅、东厢房与西厢房、兵舍、监狱等，祠堂则由照壁、大门、祭堂和后堂组成。整个布局以土司衙门为核心，前门临街，门前为宽廊，廊柱有清代同治年间广西著名书法家郑小谷撰写的阴文楹联："守斯土，莅斯民，十六堡群黎谁非赤子；辟其疆，利其赋，三百里区域尽隶王封。"大门两侧是八字跨街牌坊，称东辕门、西辕门，门楣上横额分别浮雕"庆南要地""粤西边隅"8个字。衙门东面20米是莫氏祭祀祖宗的祠堂，占地1470平方米，始建于清乾隆十八年（1753年），因毁于兵燹，于道光二十七年（1847年）重建。分前、中、后三进：前进是正门；中进为正厅，两侧分别设有客房，前后镂刻贴金花窗，工艺精巧，装饰豪华；后进安放莫氏历代宗亲牌位。祠堂东侧有风格独特的三清观，西侧为鳞次栉比的官族府第，住着和土司最亲近的弟妹及叔侄等家庭成员。其间配置有士兵练武场和诊疗室等伺服系统。官府西侧建有关帝庙。由于严格的等级制度，两庙附近安排了土司的韦、刘、杨三姓亲戚居住，再往外才是民众的住宅和城墙。土司衙门南边有造型别致的"半月亭"和专供土司修身养性的"龙隐洞"，北有亭榭、石桥和环布奇花异木的土司官塘，西北安置有肃穆的土司家族陵园。所有建筑的整体造型都与土司衙门建筑风格协调和谐。

第三节 壮族房屋的建造与壮族村落

一、壮族房屋的建造

壮族房屋的建造一般包括选址、择吉、建造、落成庆典等过程。按照壮族习俗，上述每个环节都有相应的祭典活动，以求吉利。房址以宽敞、向阳并有所依托的地方为好。河谷平原的则要避开低洼地带，选择较为隆起的地方，因为南方易涝，地势高则免于水患。尽可能靠近河流、沟渠或水塘，以便于汲水和洗涤。房屋方向一般是坐北朝南或是坐西朝东，这并不十分讲究。

择吉方面，壮族建造新房，一般都避开农忙季节，以便邻里乡亲都可以前来帮忙；同时也避开雨季，这样便于施工，房基坚实，有质量保证，建起的房子牢固。择吉还包括开工动土要选择人和、财和、丁旺三吉利的日子。一般备好材料，选好时辰后，即可开工。

壮族工匠制造屋架不放大样，全凭师傅传授的经验，有严格的规格和尺寸比例。大型的干栏一般宽 16 尺（约 5.33 米）、长 32 尺（约 10.7 米）、高 24 尺（约 8 米），小型的干栏长、宽、高分别为 24 尺（约 8 米）、12 尺（约 4 米）、16 尺（约 5.33 米）。一般都是三进到五进。木匠根据木材的长短粗细，计划好高度和进深，就可以断木截枝，凿眼削榫。干栏的外山墙为四柱一梁，内山墙为三长柱一短柱一梁，短柱立于横梁之上，顶端驾着脊檩。椽子用一排雕成立鱼形或花瓶形的短柱支撑。每个斜面立短柱 5～7 根，从下往上排列，呈山形，用小横梁与中柱相连。这四柱一梁和若干小短柱用榫连接在一起，就构成了一面完整的山墙。若干山墙（至少是两面外山墙，一面内山墙）立在预先制好的柱基上，用榫连在一起，就成了一座干栏的骨架。榫和眼要求角度不差，大小合适，不用一颗铁钉，可以随时拆开，运到新地址重新立起后，完好如初，有很高的工艺水平。若是穷家，用大毛竹做梁柱，无法做榫，只好用藤条或竹篾捆绑连接，柱子须埋入地下。房顶一般盖苦茅或鱼鳞瓦。墙面一般以竹皮编织而成，家境好一些的用木板，大户人家则用红砖砌墙。

在制作房架的同时，石匠要做房基。干栏房基比较讲究，前半部为干栏下层，一般高 2.5～3.0 米；后半部垒成台基，夯上土，是烧火做饭的生活区。柱础用青石刻成，带花纹。富裕之家还要用很多长条石，垒成十多级的台阶，而穷家就只能准备木梯子。

房基准备好了，还要择吉日，才能立柱、安梁、架椽檩。在壮族人的观念里，立柱、安梁、接檩被认为是十分庄重的事情，不得冒犯任何鬼神，尽管它们无影无踪。不仅要请道公卜吉日、择良辰，而且还要供祭、念经、祷告。此外，还有很多禁忌，如上梁时辰不能逢午，据说逢午意味忤逆，将来子孙不孝；也不能鸡斗狗咬，鸡不能上梁，因为这意味着鸡飞狗跳，全家不宁。这一天，全村喜气洋洋，像过年过节一般，各家的劳动力都主动到场相助，抬梁扶柱，递檩架椽。后生爬到架上，用木槌把榫打入榫眼。欢笑声、木槌声、吆喝声交织在一起，在山谷中回响，十分热闹。如果主家手头拮据，同寨各家及亲友还要送些米和肉，热情相助。立好骨架后，单等上梁时辰，时辰一到，大梁披红挂绿，在鞭炮声中徐徐上升，对榫，敲打入榫眼，然后主客同入宴席，举杯相敬。人们散去之后，主家自己再选"北风杀"日之外的日子盖瓦，编竹墙，修整内部，这得需要几个月到半年左右的时间。

干栏房屋建成，被认为是大吉大利的喜事。乔迁之日，亲友云集，主家要大加庆贺一番。此时的头件大事，是庄重地把神龛、牌位、香炉迁到新居，杀猪宰鸡祭祖，并请师公喃摩（诵经念咒）。法事庄重而热烈，充满了对未来的憧憬和期待。之后，亲友和主人喝交杯酒，祝贺主人人丁安泰、六畜兴旺、百事顺利。

最后，是新房落成后的绿化工作。搬进新居后，通常要种植竹木果树于干栏四周，既美化环境，又增加收入。独家独院者，还种植带刺的箣竹，围成防盗篱笆，以保证居家安全。

二、壮族村落

壮族是个稻作农业的民族，村落的形成与农业生产和发展有关。壮族定居点一般都选在河流大转弯或大河与小河交汇处，河面宽阔，水流缓慢，背山靠水。水生生物丰富，利于捕捞，生活有保障；一旦山洪暴涨，退可上山，以保安全。附近要有较开阔的平地，有田可耕，涝不淹，旱能引水灌溉，适宜稻谷生长，能确保过上"饭稻羹鱼"的生活。

壮乡多崇山峻岭，丘陵绵延，河网众多，大小谷地和平峒分布于山岭河谷之间，可供开垦。土地、水源、气候的有利条件利于稻作农耕，壮族的村落就坐落在这些谷地或平峒里。壮族"无河不住，无田不居"和依山傍水择居而住。从秦始皇打开岭南通道以后，中原人士为避战乱迁来岭南，形成壮、汉杂居的格局。汉族一般都相对集中在交通便利的城镇附近，与壮族根据农耕需要在谷口和河溪上游建村落形成鲜明的对比，故有"汉人住街头，壮人住水头"之说。

壮族村落靠山近水，背北向阳，村前面有开阔的农耕用地，后面有挡住北风的高山。这种村落选址、朝向、定位选择逐渐模式化，世代传承，建成了壮乡星罗棋布的村落，有其科学道理。

壮族村落的大小，视附近的可耕作农田面积而定。高山地区山多地少，村落的规模小，分布稀疏；在丘陵和平峒则规模较大，分布也密集。村落的房子由干栏组成，从山脚依缓坡一幢一幢地往上建，直达山腰。干栏方向一般是坐北朝南或者坐西朝东，这并不十分讲究，而是讲究根据山弄峒场的形状，选择一处视野开阔、清流环绕的地方建造。道路依房屋排列自然形成。

壮族很重视村落内的植树造林美化工作。村落四周围有竹林,壮族人喜欢在自己干栏的四周,用荆棘编成篱笆围上一圈,篱笆和干栏之间的环形空地是院子,可以为菜圃和果园,种上青菜、木瓜、木棉、柚子、柑橘、黄皮、龙眼、芭蕉、桃、李,使干栏周围绿地如茵,果木遮天,竹丛掩映,别有一番情趣。

第四节　壮族人居文化与壮医药的关系

壮族先民根据壮族地区的地理环境及气候条件,形成了具有本民族特点的人居文化,特别是为了预防疾病、避免虫兽伤害、利于卫生和保健,发明了干栏建筑。

干栏建筑是壮族人民为了适应南方地区炎热多雨、地面潮湿、瘴气弥漫和毒虫猛兽横行的自然环境而发明建造的一种居住形式,满足了人们的生理和心理需要。干栏建筑有以下特点:一是防避瘴气。壮乡被称为"瘴乡",诸多史书、地方志都对壮族地区的瘴气论述颇多,瘴气和瘴区成为死亡毒气、死亡之乡的代名词。据说古代凡有被贬官吏、文人、军士都视"瘴乡"为畏途,十去九不归。壮族先民十分注重未病先防,并在长期的生活和实践中总结出一些颇具特色的预防瘴气的方法,干栏建筑就是为预防瘴气而建造的。二是避免潮湿。壮族居住地地处亚热带,气候炎热、潮湿、多雨。《素问·异法方宜论》记载:"南方者,天地所长养,阳之所盛处也,其地下,水土弱,雾露之所聚也,其民嗜酸而食附。故其民皆致理而赤色,其病挛痹……"由于气候潮湿多雨,易犯"挛痹"之疾,干栏楼居建筑背坡而筑,人居高层,干燥通风,可以减少风湿病的发生。三是防范虫兽袭击。干栏建筑底层架空,离开地面,可以防范毒蛇猛兽的袭击,减少虫兽引起的伤害。四是卫生保健。干栏建筑"人居其上,牛犬豕居其下",既可人、畜分离,又使得通风、采光良好,冬暖夏凉,居住起来很舒适。这些特点使其成为经济适用的民居建筑形式,体现了壮族同胞顺应自然、师法自然,与自然环境和谐共存的生态审美观。

参考文献:

[1] 覃彩銮. 壮族传统民居建筑论述 [J]. 广西民族研究, 1993 (3): 112-118.

[2] 陈丽琴. 那坡壮族干栏建筑的生态研究 [C]. 玉溪: 中国艺术人类学论坛暨国际学术会议——艺术活态传承与文化共享论文集, 2011.

[3] 梁庭望. 壮族风俗志 [M]. 北京: 中央民族学院出版社, 1987.

[4] 袁少芬. 当代壮族探微 [M]. 南宁: 广西人民出版社, 1989.

[5] 范阳, 丘振声. 壮族古俗初探 [M]. 南宁: 广西人民出版社, 1994.

[6] 覃尚文, 陈国清. 壮族科学技术史 [M]. 南宁: 广西科学技术出版社, 2003.

第十章　壮医药与壮族舞蹈、体育文化

　　壮医药是壮族人民在历史上创造和沿用的传统医药，具有明显的民族性、传统性和区域性，其形成和发展与壮族舞蹈、体育有着密切的关系。壮族舞蹈、体育文化是壮医药文化的重要组成部分。壮族人民在长期的生产生活实践中形成了丰富多彩、独具特色的传统舞蹈和体育形式。这些在传统民俗活动中呈现出来的舞蹈和体育形式对促进人类的健康有着十分重要的作用，具有畅通气血、宣泄导滞、疏利关节、增强体质、防病保健、延年益寿等作用，成为壮族传统的养生保健方法。

第一节　壮医药与壮族舞蹈文化

一、壮族舞蹈文化

1. 壮族舞蹈文化源流

　　壮族人民喜好舞蹈，能歌能舞，创造了形式多样的舞蹈艺术，且历史悠久。早在先秦时期，古骆越人就创造了精彩纷呈和别具地方民族风格的舞蹈，这在广西左江崖壁画以及铜鼓上就可窥其一斑而知全貌，代表着壮族舞蹈的灿烂历史。在规模宏大、气势雄伟的左江崖壁画上，人物图像众多，而且一律做双手肘上举、双脚叉开，为半蹲姿势，排列整齐，队形多变，有呈横排、纵排的，也有众多的人物围成圆圈，其动作整齐划一。这样的队形分组排列，而每一组画面都有一个形体高大、身佩刀剑、头戴羽毛或高髻的正身人像，其身旁或前面画有一面内带芒星的铜鼓或羊角钮钟图像，这是典型的集体祭祀舞蹈场面的形象反映，是舞蹈过程中对其代表性舞姿的定格式写照。据研究，位于画面中心形体高大、装饰与众不同的正身人物，既是氏族部落的首领和主持祭典的巫师，同时也是集体舞蹈的领舞者，其旁侧的铜鼓或铜钟，是形成节律和伴奏舞蹈的乐器。整个画面展现的是众人在巫师的带领下，随着激昂洪亮的鼓乐节奏狂欢起舞。

　　壮族原始的舞蹈多为模拟动物形态而创作。据民族学家考究，拟蛙舞是左江崖壁画所展示的舞蹈的主旋律。其舞蹈主要是通过双手的曲肘上举和两脚的叉开弓步，上下对称，构成蛙跃姿势。这种拟蛙舞蹈，隐含着古骆越人对蛙神的崇拜，以祈求功利。

　　拟鹭舞是壮族古代另一种极富地方特色的舞蹈。在广西贵港市出土的铜鼓身上就饰有拟鹭舞。舞者的装束精致独特，头戴插有鸟羽的华冠，身穿以羽毛为饰的长裙，裙前同幅略过膝，后幅则拖曳于地。舞时身体重心稍偏后，上体微微昂起，双手向左右或前后轻盈摆动，双腿叉开，似做行步状，而头、胸、身保持相应的协调姿势，似鹭鸟之形，是舞蹈过程中一种典型的舞姿瞬间定格式造型的形象写照。表演者以2～3人为一个小组，共有8个小组。这些相对独立的舞蹈小组同时翩翩起舞，步伐轻盈婉转，动态一致，无疑就是一种多姿多态的大型集体舞蹈。这种拟鹭舞体现了壮族先民对鹭鸟的崇拜，希望能获得鹭鸟的灵性，以弥补自身能力的不足。可见，原始的壮族舞蹈是作为构成人类活动、构成社会生活的必要媒介而存在的，与现代舞蹈更多的是表演性和娱乐性的不同。

壮族是我国最早种植水稻的民族之一，壮族地区早期农业的特点是以稻作为本。壮族所居的岭南地区，气候温暖，雨量丰沛，河流密布，水源充足，土地肥沃，非常适宜稻谷的生长。壮族人民对舞蹈艺术有着深厚的感情和深切的感受，他们在长期的生产生活实践中，通过深入地观察和提炼，创作了多种反映生产劳作的舞蹈。如壮族著名的扁担舞、铜鼓舞、春堂舞、绣球舞、捞虾舞、采茶舞、竹竿舞等，大多模仿劳动动作，主题鲜明，舞步雄捷，诙谐活泼，感情逼真，反映了壮族人民的农耕劳作过程，充分体现了壮族劳动人民勤劳的特性以及倔强和爱憎分明的性格。这些舞蹈大部分经久不衰，至今仍很流行。

2. 常见壮族舞蹈及其分类

壮族自古精通歌舞，壮乡处处皆歌海，"刘三姐"享誉海内外。壮族对舞蹈也有深刻和独到的研究，壮族民间的舞蹈有300多种，形式多样，内容丰富，涉及宗教祭典、祈神求福、驱鬼攘灾、劳动生产、歌抒社交、生育婚丧、节日娱乐等社会生活的各个方面。按其性质划分，壮族传统舞蹈大致可分为宗教性舞蹈和娱乐性舞蹈两大类。宗教性舞蹈具有浓厚的宗教气氛和明显的宗教目的，其内容多与祈神驱鬼、攘灾求安有关，娱神性较强，在壮族传统舞蹈中一直占据主导地位，对人们的社会生活及思想观念产生深刻的影响，如道公舞、铜鼓舞等。娱乐性舞蹈包括自娱性舞蹈、表演性舞蹈及壮戏舞蹈，多在节日或喜庆活动期间举行。舞蹈的形式和主题主要有模拟生产劳动舞和拟兽舞两类。如壮族各地流行的捞虾舞、捕鱼舞、撒秧舞、插田舞、收割舞、舂米舞等，属于模拟生产劳动舞；舞狮、舞龙、舞春牛、彩蝶舞、金鸡舞、蚂蚜舞、斑鸠舞等，属于拟兽舞。

（1）春堂舞

春堂舞源自壮族的舂米劳动，以舂米为主题，以敲击声伴舞，节拍鲜明，于春节期间举行表演，庆祝新年的到来，预祝来年粮食丰收。刘恂的《岭表录异》记载："广南有春堂，以浑木刳为槽，一槽两边约十杵，男女间立，以春稻粮，敲磕槽弦，皆有偏拍。槽声若鼓，闻于数里，虽思妇之巧弄秋砧，不能比其浏亮也。"春堂又称

"谷榔"，表演者以妇女居多，常多人持木杵闱聚于盛有稻谷的大木臼边，以优美的动作挥动木杵撞击木臼，声如木鱼，运杵成音，轮番把稻谷舂成米。

（2）扁担舞

扁担舞又称打扁担，流行于广西马山、都安、东兰、邕宁、南丹等地，每年农历正月初一至元宵节期间表演。表演者以妇女为主，人数不定，但均为偶数，有四人、六人、八人、十人、二十人不等。

扁担舞是从舂堂舞发展而来，源于壮族舂米的劳动生活。扁担舞最初是用一块木板，盖在舂米槽上并用扁担敲打。因此，打扁担在壮语中又叫"谷榔"。因石槽太重，不易搬动，于是慢慢改为用长条凳。现代扁担舞多用板凳、扁担或竹竿为道具，板凳为木制，扁担和竹竿为竹制，表演形式多样，或分立于长凳的两边敲打凳子，或互击扁担。表演者随着扁担敲击板凳和扁担互击发出的音响节奏而舞，边打边唱边舞，时而双人对打，时而四人交叉对打，时而多人连打；有站打、蹲打、弓步打、转身打等，轻重、强弱、快慢错落有致，模拟农事活动中的赶牛下地、耙田、插秧、收割、打谷、舂米、纳布等动作过程。扁担舞不但能增强体质，而且运动步调一致，动作优美，行走灵活，协调自然，节奏强烈，声响清脆，深受壮族人民的喜爱。

（3）铜鼓舞

铜鼓舞是壮族古老的舞蹈形式之一，历史悠久，源于古代民间的祭祀活动，早在壮族地区的左江崖壁画上就有以铜鼓作乐的形象，后用于娱乐和礼仪活动。

铜鼓舞以壮族闻名的民间乐器铜鼓为道具，击鼓伴舞，自娱自乐，流传于广西东兰、都安、马山等地，大都在春节和庆丰收时表演。《唐书·南蛮列传》记载："击铜鼓，吹大角，歌舞以为乐。"明代汪广洋的《岭南杂咏》有"村团社日喜晴和，铜鼓齐敲唱海歌"的记载。

铜鼓舞表演时，一般由7人以上组成舞队，其中4人敲铜鼓，1人打皮鼓，1人舞竹筛或雨帽，1人舞竹筒。铜鼓两面或四面成套，两面铜鼓的各由2人共敲一鼓，称一公一母；四面铜鼓一组的，4人每人各敲一鼓，称二公二母。

舞蹈的内容多为农业生产活动过程的再现，如开场、春耕、夏种、秋收、冬藏、迎春等部分，用舞蹈形式表现出来，给人以鼓舞、向往，充满生机。

（4）绣球舞

绣球舞是壮族民间舞蹈，早在宋代就已盛行于壮族民间，主要流行于广西德保、靖西、田东、田阳、龙州、天等、大新、都安、马山等地。

绣球是广西壮族青年男女的爱情信物，每逢春节或"三月三"歌圩，壮族青年男女便会齐聚对唱山歌表达爱情。如果壮族少女钟情于某个男青年，便会将布鞋、毛巾等礼品系在自己亲手精心绣制的绣球上，载歌载舞，将绣球抛向意中人。男青年得球后，亦载歌载舞，将礼品回敬女方。绣球舞即源于此，多在歌圩中进行。绣球舞集舞蹈和体育娱乐于一体。抛绣球时，有转球、摇球、抛球、接球 4 个舞蹈动作。

（5）采茶舞

采茶舞主要流行于广西玉林等地，是民间自娱性舞蹈，于春节期间表演。通常由一男二女表演，歌舞结合，男的称茶公，女的称茶娘，道具分别有钱尺、彩扇、手帕、彩带等。主题主要是表现人们的生产劳动过程，有时插入反映青年男女爱情的故事情节。其动作朴实大方，富有幽默感。茶公常用颤腿、屈膝做矮桩动作，舞步轻快潇洒。手中的钱尺在表演"开荒舞"时可当作锄头，表演炒茶时可做拉风箱状，动作诙谐，富有情趣。茶娘多表现羞涩含蓄、细碎轻盈的舞步，多用"十字步""踏步转"，手中彩扇轻挥疾拢，犹如云朵飘舞、柳絮轻扬，舞姿婀娜，仪态万千，充分表现出少女的天真烂漫、活泼可爱。舞时载歌，或配以鼓乐，场面气氛热烈，具有较强的娱乐性。

3. 壮族舞蹈文化的特点

舞蹈艺术是伴随着人类社会生产和生活同步产生的，同样壮族舞蹈也是在壮民族心理素质和文化内涵的基础上，伴随着壮民族的形成发展而成为人们日常生活中不可缺少的文化意识形态。因此，壮族舞蹈风格植根于壮族社会的政治文化、宗教文化和生存环境。

（1）崇拜图腾

壮族舞蹈具有浓烈的原始气息，展现出较为突出的原始风貌。追根溯源，壮族舞蹈是在原始巫术与自然崇拜的氛围中产生和成长的。壮族自古重巫，素以信鬼好巫而著称于世。《九歌》《楚语》等古籍中对壮族先民信奉多神教、崇尚巫术宗教的风俗均有记载。壮族舞蹈与巫师祭祀酬神活动密切相关。远古时候，壮族先民的生产力水平十分低下，对自然界的各种现象，诸如地震、洪水暴发、火山爆发等，甚至日常生活中的日出、日落、刮风、下雨、雷鸣、闪电等无穷变化的大自然奥秘无法解释，特别是对人在夜间做梦和生老病死更是感到神秘莫测。因此，他们便开始无边无际的幻想，笃信万物有灵、灵魂不灭和信奉多神。壮族民间崇拜的神灵多而杂，有自然神、社会神、守护神等，崇拜仪式也随诸神的功能不同而不同。巫师祭祀敬神时总是边跳边唱，乐神消灾祈福。

壮族的很多舞蹈均与壮族的图腾崇拜密切相关。如壮族地区左江崖壁画上描绘的拟蛙舞就是古骆越人对崇拜物蛙神的亲近和娱乐，以祈求功利。而汉代铜鼓上记载的拟鹭舞则体现了壮族先民对候鸟鹭鸟的崇拜，希望能获得鹭鸟的灵性，达到预知气候变化、飞越高山、遨游长空和避凶趋吉的目的。流传于壮族民间的铜鼓舞和蚂蚜舞的起源与壮族崇拜蚂蚜、模仿蚂蚜形态有关，而且铜鼓舞与蚂蚜舞大多与蚂蚜歌节祭祀蚂蚜同时举行。

（2）反映劳作

壮族人民热爱劳作，并把生产生活动作舞蹈化。扁担舞、舂堂舞、捞虾舞、采茶舞等，大多模仿劳动耕作中所使用的工具及动作，伴随着鼓乐欢快的节奏，模拟劳动过程中典型的象征性动作，表达欢度佳节、庆祝丰收和向往幸福生活的心境。扁担舞模仿用扁担在舂米槽上敲打；舂堂舞则以木杵撞击木臼，模拟把稻谷舂成米的劳作过程；采茶舞则以茶山、茶篮等为道具，反映茶乡壮族姑娘双手采茶、拣茶和在茶叶丰收归途中追扑蝴蝶的形象。再如壮族的手巾舞，是以手巾为道具，手巾在壮族生产生活中常用来揩汗、裹头、包东西等，表现了壮族人民丰富的劳作生活。

（3）传情达意

壮族青年在劳作之余，常以歌舞表达自己的情感，其中以绣球舞最为常见。绣球舞以爱情信物绣球为道具，在对唱山歌中找到意中人后，青年男女便将绣球互抛给意中人。绣球舞的原意是在歌圩上男女双方互送礼物，把这些礼物和石块包起来，甩的时候才不容易偏离方向，因而古代壮族称之为"抛帕"，后来则改用爱情信物绣球。竹竿舞也是壮族青年男女在节日里常跳的舞蹈，这种舞蹈须多人配合方能完成，跳舞者的双腿轻巧地在竹竿间穿梭，善于跳竹竿舞的小伙子往往因为机灵敏捷、应变自如而博得姑娘们的青睐。竹竿舞配以音乐伴奏，能促进人们对音乐节奏的理解，协调运动，增强韵律感，成为人们交流思想、抒发情感的有效方式。

舞蹈文化以肢体作为符号，与特定的民族的生产方式和生活方式相适应。纵观壮族舞蹈，无一不深深地蕴含着壮民族的历史生态烙印。随着壮族社会经济水平的提高及政治、文化的进步，人们的神权观开始异化，壮族舞蹈逐步向世俗化、生活化发展。如今，舞蹈大多选择在一定的节日场合进行，多以增进友谊，交流生产生活经验、交流感情为目的，这些民族舞蹈的自娱社交活动，大大地丰富了壮乡文化生活。

二、壮族舞蹈文化对壮医药的影响

舞蹈是文化的基本形态之一。壮族人民能歌善舞，创造了丰富多彩的民间舞蹈，可以说，这些舞蹈对壮族的医疗保健和运动医学的发展做出了重大贡献。

1. 壮族舞蹈促进了壮医药的萌芽和发展

在原始时代，壮族地区社会生产力极其低下，巫风盛行，人们信仰鬼神，哪怕是患了疾病，治疗也是以巫术的形式进行。当时，举凡狩猎、祭祀、祈祷、医疗等活动大都是通过舞蹈来进行的，古代壮族的拟蛙舞、拟鹭舞、铜鼓舞等无不留下巫师祭祀的印记。医巫同源、医巫并存的壮族地区的文化发展特点，对壮医产生了重大的影响。但由于年代久远，且缺乏文字记载及实物见证，只能根据民俗民风窥其大略。古时壮巫分巫婆和魔公，主家有病痛或灾难，请巫婆和神对话，问明病灾的缘由，再择吉日请魔公行法事，杀畜禽敬祭，劝离仙，禳解厄难，舞刀剑，烧油锅，镇妖赶鬼，这就是巫医活动。壮族民间传说三界公能驱邪除魔，保境安民，奉为医神，而立庙定期祭祀。在旧社会，壮医对某些疾病确有较好的疗效，但往往以巫医的形式出现，如刘锡蕃的《岭表纪蛮·杂述》记载，"蛮人以草药医治跌打损伤及痈疮毒外科一切杂疾，每有奇效，然亦以迷信出之""予尝见一患痈者，延僮老治疾，其人至，病家以雄鸡、毫银、水、米、诸事陈于堂。术者先取银纳袋中，脱草履于地，取水念咒，喷患处，操刀割之，脓血迸流，而病者毫无痛苦。脓尽，敷以药即愈"。可见，这些巫医往往懂得一医一药，在其施以巫术的同时多兼以药物治疗，而巫医治病均通过巫术以舞蹈的形式进行。这在新中国成立前，特别是在边远山区的壮族民间更是如此。巫术充满了迷信色彩，虽然有碍于医学的发展，但是在医巫同源、医巫并存的古代壮族地区，巫术对于壮医药的萌芽和发展具有积极的作用。

2. 壮族舞蹈促进了壮医医疗保健意识的形成

舞蹈通过肢体动作表达思想情感，增强体质，促进壮族人民的医疗保健和防病意识的形成。壮族先民自远古以来就生息在岭南地区，该地区气候炎热、山多林密、交通不便，生存条件非常恶劣，出于生存的本能，他们不断地寻求有利于自身健康的生存方法。在长期的实践中，他们逐渐体会到舞蹈是一种有益身心健康的活动，能增强体质，使性格变得开朗，身体变得柔软，让体质得到改善。因此，在劳作之余，空闲时间，或节日里，人们便会唱歌跳舞，或模仿狩猎，或模仿劳作，或模仿动物，以交流感情，放松情绪，因而对壮族地区的疾病谱有着重要的影响。壮族人较少患内伤杂病，尤其是情志方面的病更少，这与他们喜好歌舞有密切的关系。

3. 壮族舞蹈促进了壮医治则的形成

壮医对气有深刻的认识，对气极为重视，认为气是构成人体本原的原始物质，人体是由气构成的。气又以动为顺，以畅为治，认为人体内天、地、人三部之气必须保持动态的协调平衡（即稳态）才能达到健康状态。壮族舞蹈均有一定的动作套路，它的动作兼顾到手、头、颈、胸、髋、腿等部位，对舒畅心情、畅通气血很有帮助，因而能起到很好的调气作用。故舞蹈自古就受到壮族人民的青睐，壮乡处处皆歌舞，通过唱歌跳舞调节、激发和通畅人体之气，使之正常运行，与天、地之气保持同步，从而保持身体健康，逐渐形成调气治疗原则。如今，调气原则成了壮医防治疾病的重要原则，为壮族地区人民群众的健康做出了重要的贡献。

第二节　壮医药与壮族体育文化

一、壮族体育文化

1. 壮族体育文化源流

壮族体育与壮族民俗有着十分密切的关系，其深深植根于壮族文化及生活习俗之中，有的体育活动是以民俗的形式进行和发展的，有的体育活动则是依附民俗来开展，成为壮族传统民俗的重要组成部分。民俗体育运动在壮族人民的生活中很早就已经出现，反映了壮族人民的生产实践、社会生活、种族繁衍以及宗教信仰，如斗牛就是一项颇具壮族特色的民俗体育运动，反映了壮族人民的农耕生产方式。壮族是一个典型的稻作农耕民族，早在新石器时代，红水河上游流域就出现了稻作农业。壮族自古生活在岭南地区，该地区山地较多，广西俗语道："高山瑶，半山苗，汉人住在平地，壮侗住在山槽。"耕田种地是壮民族的生存之道，人们至今一直保持着以稻作为主的农业生产方式，形成了一个质态相同、内涵丰富的稻作文化（即"那文化圈"），牛便是壮族主要的农业生产工具，因此与牛相关的体育运动项目随之诞生。据《布洛陀经诗》记载，布洛陀造牛后，便教壮族先民用牛耕田、耙地代替人耕，牛耕田、耙地需要力气，为了知道哪一头牛力气大又灵活，布洛陀就教人们用斗牛来评定。《布洛陀经诗》是一部中国少数民族古籍，成书于明代，经诗中的布洛陀被壮族奉为创世神、始祖神和宗教神，是布洛陀创造了天地万物。经考证认为，广西敢壮山是布洛陀文化遗址和壮族始祖及珠江流域原住民族的人文始祖布洛陀的故乡。可见，壮乡斗牛体育活动很早就已产生，并一直沿袭至今。每到农闲时节，在广阔的山坡、田野随处可见斗牛比赛。

壮族人民在长期的生产生活中，造就了勇于探索和热爱劳动的实践精神。壮族人民勤快爱劳动，逢年过节或有喜庆活动，都要开展抛绣球、赛龙舟、拾天灯、打壮拳等传统健身体育活动，通过体育锻炼增强体质，磨砺意志，预防疾病，这些体育活动自然就成了壮族人民的传统养生保健方法。

2. 常见的壮族民俗体育活动

壮族人民在长期的生产生活中，逐渐形成了自己独特的传统体育活动。这些活动丰富多彩，既是劳动之余的文娱活动，也是壮族人民养生保健、增强体质的手段。常见的壮族民俗体育活动有抛绣球、赛龙舟、拾天灯、打壮拳、抢花炮、对唱山歌、舞狮以及板鞋竞技等，下面介绍一下抛绣球、赛龙舟、拾天灯、打壮拳。

（1）抛绣球

抛绣球是壮族人民喜闻乐见的传统民俗体育项目，在壮族地区广为流行。抛绣

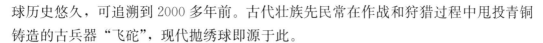

球历史悠久，可追溯到 2000 多年前。古代壮族先民常在作战和狩猎过程中甩投青铜铸造的古兵器"飞砣"，现代抛绣球即源于此。

抛绣球如今用来传情达意、娱乐身心、竞技强身。道具绣球多是用手工做成的彩球，以圆形最为常见，也有椭圆形、方形、菱形等。绣球大如拳头，内装棉花籽、谷粟、谷壳等，上、下两端分别系有彩带和红坠。壮族人民在茶余饭后互相抛接以娱乐身心，起到沟通感情的作用。而在每年春节、"三月三"、中秋节等传统佳节，壮族人民都要成群结队举行歌圩，在引吭高歌之中，青年男女互抛绣球，表达情意。

由于颇具民族性、趣味性和简易性，经改编后，抛绣球已成为广西少数民族传统体育运动会的竞赛项目，同时也是全国少数民族传统体育运动会的表演项目。

（2）赛龙舟

赛龙舟是壮族传统民俗体育项目，主要在壮族地区的梧州、南宁等地流行。赛龙舟也是壮族端午节举行的传统习俗活动。关于其起源，有多种说法，可追溯至原始社会末期，有祭曹娥、祭屈原、祭水神或龙神等祭祀活动。赛龙舟先后传入日本、越南、英国等，是 2010 年广州亚运会正式比赛项目。目前，赛龙舟已被列入国家级非物质文化遗产名录。

赛龙舟于每年的端午节举行。龙舟大小不一，一般是狭长、细窄，船头饰龙头，船尾饰龙尾。桡手人数不一，每船数十人不等。比赛规则是在规定距离内同时起航，以到达终点先后决定名次。

（3）抢天灯

抢天灯是壮族独特的传统体育活动，在壮乡广为流传，一般在喜庆节日和丰收时节举行。抢天灯的道具是天灯，壮族习俗认为天灯象征吉祥和长寿。天灯古而有之，古代用天灯告知村民土匪的行踪，后来就逐渐演变成了追抢天灯的民俗娱乐活动。

抢天灯比赛时，常以村寨为单位组队参赛，选手数十人不等，多是各村寨中身强体壮者。道具天灯的制作简单，以竹子为架，外糊一层纸，底部放上小油灯，形如水桶。天灯做好后，将天灯内油灯点燃，随着灯内温度升高，天灯便会升空飘荡，此时各参赛队选手奋力紧追，甚至跋山涉水，直待油灯熄灭天灯下降落地即可抢取，以首先拿到天灯者为胜。

（4）打壮拳

打壮拳是壮族传统体育活动，也是独特的拳种，历史源远流长，可追溯到 2000 年前绘制的广西壮乡的左江崖壁画。据《宁明州志》记载："花山距城五十里，江上峭壁画有赤色人形，皆裸体，或大或小、或持干戈、或骑马。而且沿江两岸崖壁上如此类者多有。"在左江崖壁画典型画面中，人物形象身高体壮，正面形似站桩姿态，双膝微弯成平马步，双肘微屈上举呈莲花掌，是人体站得最稳的功式，重心自然凝聚于气海丹田，是一种典型的功夫动作形象图。壁画中还展现有环首刀、剑、长枪、手镖、山弩以及竹箭等器械。聪明的壮族先民以壁画描述为主题，开发出一套健身活动——打壮拳，刀、剑等则成了打壮拳惯用的武术器械。壮拳的拳术套路有数十种，其动作彪悍，形象朴实，功架清晰，沉实稳健，拳刚、势烈、多短打、擅标掌、少跳跃，打拳时结合使用壮语发音，借声气摧力。现代壮拳又演变出各种不同的流派，使众多群众受益。

3. 壮族民俗体育的特点

壮族民俗体育活动具有丰富的文化内涵，表现出民族性、传统性、地域性、娱乐性、多样性等特点。随着社会的发展与历史的变迁，一些传统体育活动逐渐失去了原来的娱乐实用的目的，演变为表演性和竞技性都很强的体育运动。如抛绣球最先是寓意壮族两性交往文化，象征幸福的爱情生活；如今的抛绣球，则更多的用于表演和娱乐。又如赛龙舟，原本是端午节祭曹娥、祭屈原、祭水神或龙神等祭祀活动；如今的端午赛龙舟体育活动，则众舟搏击江面，江岸人山人海，锣鼓呐喊不绝于耳，具有显著的体育竞技性。

二、壮族体育文化对壮医药的影响

体育，壮语叫"哑咛"，即经常活动的意思。壮族人民勤快爱劳动，男女老少都喜爱体育。逢年过节或有喜庆的活动，壮族人民都要开展抛绣球、赛龙舟、拾天灯等传统健身活动。壮族体育文化对壮医药的影响是多方面的。

1. 壮族体育促进了壮医理论的形成

壮族体育文化蕴含着丰富的壮医学思想，并促进了壮医理论的形成。早在先秦时期，壮族聚居地广西崇左一带的左江崖壁画，就有典型的功夫动作形象图，著名壮医专家覃保霖认为，左江流域在一个回归年中，由芒种经夏至回到小暑前后，都有特定时刻，太阳正临当地子午线天顶，使天、地、人同在一宏观引线上，此时练功符合天体力学的宏观理论，练功效果最佳。覃氏将其命名为"壮医乾坤掌子午功"，深受后人的追捧。广西著名的体育项目打壮拳即源于此。

壮医乾坤掌子午功强调自然界天、地、人三同步，促进了壮医的人与自然界天地的"三气同步"学术理论。壮医三气同步理论是壮医的核心理论，是壮医独特的天人自然观，源于壮族先民对天地起源及宇宙的朴素认识，用以阐释自然界天、地、人三部之气与人体内天、地、人三部之气的内涵、相互关系及其运动变化规律，是壮医用以解释人体生理病理现象以及指导防治疾病的一种说理工具。"三气同步"理论认为，自然界的天、地、人三气是同步运行的，而人体又分为上部天、下部地和中部人，三部之气也是同步运行的。在生理上，只有人体的天、地、人三部与自然界（天、地）同步运行，制约化生，生生不息，人体才能达到健康境界，否则，百病丛生。

2. 体育活动丰富了壮医药养生保健的内涵

壮医药在预防疾病方面，积累了丰富的经验和知识。体育活动一直是壮医重要的养生保健方法，壮族先民喜好传统体育项目，很早就意识到通过体育锻炼既能疏通道路、调和气血、平衡阴阳、调心安神，还能增强体质，预防疾病。板鞋竞技、抛绣球、赛龙舟、拾天灯等传统健身活动都是壮乡人民喜闻乐见的体育项目，"体育强身"一直是壮医预防疾病的有力武器。通过体育锻炼，人体的肌肉筋骨得到了锻炼，可以宣泄导滞、疏利关节、磨砺意志，有效促进新陈代谢，促进气血流畅，增强体质，使身体不易受致病因素的侵害和干扰，使人与自然环境、社会环境和谐一体，从而达到强身健体、防病治病、益寿延年的目的。因而体育锻炼成为壮医防治疾病的有效方法，大大丰富了壮医药养生保健的内涵。

参考文献：

[1] 张声震. 壮族通史 [M]. 北京：民族出版社，1997.

[2] 黄汉儒，黄冬玲. 发掘整理中的壮医 [M]. 南宁：广西民族出版社，1994.

[3] 李坤荣. 壮族铜鼓舞起源 [J]. 民族艺术，1988 (1)：194 - 199.

[4] 覃彩銮. 壮族舞蹈文化研究 [J]. 民族艺术，1997 (3)：123 - 136.

[5] 宋宁. 壮医三气同步自然观的内涵及其应用 [J]. 中医杂志，2013，54 (14)：1183 - 1185.

[6] 庞宇舟，宋宁. 壮医"治未病"初探 [J]. 中国民族医药杂志，2008，14 (7)：5 - 6.

[7] 李美康，宋宁. 壮医治未病思想探析 [J]. 中国中医基础医学杂志，2014，20 (8)：1034 - 1035.

[8] 覃乃昌，郑超雄，覃德清，等. 红水河文化考察与研究 [J]. 广西民族研究，2000 (2)：77 - 79.

[9] 宋宁. 从花山壁画看壮医治未病医学思想 [J]. 辽宁中医药大学学报，2008，10 (10)：49 - 51.

第十一章 其他医药文化对壮医药的影响及反思

第一节 其他医药文化对壮医药形成和发展的影响

壮医药 2000 多年的发展历史是一个不断总结本民族自身防病治病经验，同时不断吸收其他外来民族的医药文化，从而不断发展和完善的过程。

一、中医药对壮医药的影响

对壮医药形成和发展影响最大的莫过于中医药，一方面因为迁入广西的汉族人口最多，另一方面是中医药理论形成的年代较早，相对于壮医药而言，中医药具有先进性，而壮族对于先进文化的吸收和趋同也符合社会发展规律。中医药对壮医药的影响主要有以下三个方面。

1. 阴阳调和说

阴阳调和是中医的核心理论之一，包含了阴阳一体、阴阳对立、阴阳互根、阴阳消长和阴阳转化五个方面。中医认为，世间万物相生相克，人体只有阴阳平衡，方能保持健康。壮医援入了阴阳说，却没有像中医那样高度概括并运用于整个基础理论和诊疗体系，而是简单理解为生病过程中阴盛阳衰和阳盛阴衰两种转化情况，没有与五行相生相克联系在一起。一般来说，正盛毒重者或疾病的初期，多表现为阳证；正虚毒轻者或疾病的后期，多表现为阴证。

2. 君臣佐使说

中药方中各味药君臣佐使，各司其职，这是以成员在社会秩序中的地位高低、职责来对应药物的主次和作用的。壮医药方类似于中药方的君臣佐使说不同的是，"君臣佐使"关系变成了"波乜"关系。由于壮族地区自古远离中原行政中心，社会秩序较简单，社会结构以各"都老"下的家庭为主，"都老"对各家各户无行政权力，只是以个人威信和凝聚力来感召村民，因此家庭结构在壮族地区中占非常重要的地位，而家庭主要成员的关系"波乜"也相应地被引入了壮医药的组方关系。

3. 经络腧穴说

中医认为人体存在着十二经脉和奇经八脉，这些经络具有沟通上下表里、联系脏腑器官与通行气血的功能，腧穴是人体脏腑经络之气血输注、会聚于体表的部位。

当身体发生病变时，可以在经脉循行部位上取穴，通过针灸推拿等方法，刺激穴位，调整经络气血运行，从而使身体恢复正常。与此相应的是，壮医认为人体内存在着"龙路"（即血液运输系统）、"火路"（即神经系统）两条封闭道路，这两条道路在人体体表网结，而结点即穴位。壮医通过外治法刺激穴位，可以使两路去除瘀滞，运行顺畅，从而达到防病治病的作用。与中医经络相比，壮医的两路更能体现壮族人民朴素直观的思维方式。壮医的外治法吸收了中医的取穴经验，把一些中医的穴位纳入了取穴范围。如壮医在用药线点灸法治疗泄泻症时，一般取壮医特有的脐周穴，但是如果对伴有胸闷呕吐者，则加灸中医特有的内关穴或足三里穴。

二、道教医学对壮医药的影响

道教是中国土生土长的宗教，历代道家们对修道成仙与延年益寿的执着探索，使得道教在医学领域取得了许多成就，对中国传统医学产生了深远的影响。道教对壮族文化的影响远非佛教和其他宗教对壮族文化的影响所能及的。道教医学对壮医药的影响主要有两个方面。

1. "天人合一"思想

"人法地，地法天，天法道，道法自然"是道家的核心理论，道教医学认为人是一个小乾坤，是天地自然的一部分，人应顺应天地自然的关系和规律，使之达到天人合一的境界才能延年祛病。与此相应的是，壮医认为人禀天地之气而生，人体也是个小天地，其生老病死受天地之气涵养和制约，如人体之气能与天地之气同步，则可以保持健康状态，反之则发生疾病。由此可见，壮医病因病机理论的精神实质在于尊重自然、适应自然和把握自然，与道家医学的哲学思想是一脉相承的，是道家道法自然在医学领域的具体应用和发挥。

2. 信仰治疗

传统医学往往蕴含着强烈的哲学和宗教色彩，疾病的信仰治疗，可以理解为利用患者的宗教信仰来治疗生理或心理疾病。道教笃信神仙，相信通过符咒、祈禳能够为人除病去灾。道教符咒、祈禳在壮族地区的盛行有极为深厚的文化背景。壮族先民的信仰以万物有灵和多神崇拜为基础，相信无论是自然灾害还是人的病痛都与灵魂有关，因此巫医并行、神药两解在相当长的一段历史时期内成为壮族人民的主要治疗方式。进入宋代以后，面对巫医的极端盛行，宋王朝实行了倡医禁巫的政策，多次颁布了禁巫的法令，为医学的发展扫除了障碍。壮医学也在这一时期逐渐从巫医中独立出来，走上了理性发展的道路。宋太平兴国初年，范旻知邕州兼水陆转运使，一方面下令禁巫，另一方面拿出自己的薪俸买药给患者治病，愈者千计。他还把验方刻石置于厅壁，使当地人认识到医药的重要性并逐渐信医信药。在宋王朝的极力推行下，受汉文化影响较大的广西北部、东部地区病不求医，但祀鬼神的风气逐渐得到革除，而广西的西部地区到新中国成立前巫医一直占有重要地位。

三、佛教医学对壮医药的影响

佛教医学是以古印度有关疾病、医疗、药方之学为基础，以佛教理论为指导的医药学体系。古代壮族人民通过海上丝绸之路广泛地与海外国家进行交流。据考证，广西的佛教是在汉代末年经由海上传入合浦，再由合浦沿交广通道在广西内地传播的。佛教传入广西后，在壮族原始宗教的影响下迅速世俗化、实用化。据《广西通志·宗教志》统计，唐代时期广西共建有佛教寺院45座，宋代时期广西共建有佛教寺院131座。伴随着佛教文化在广西的传播，佛教医学也渗透到壮医药体系中。壮医对佛教医学的吸收是有限的，佛教医学对壮医的影响仅限于诊疗手段，而非核心理论，这一点与道教医学不同。佛教医学对壮医药的影响主要有两个方面。

1. 瘀滞致病说与外治疗法

佛教医学通过饮食、练习、草药、按摩和冥想等来保持三大生命能量的平衡，从而保持人体健康状态。推拿按摩在佛教医学里占有非常重要的地位，它认为人体经络中流动的能量如果出现堵塞和障碍，就会出现健康问题，指压按摩相应部位可以帮助调整经络中的能量，使其正常地流动，并清除流动渠道的瘀滞，起到治病保健的双重作用。壮医认为，当人体龙路、火路出现瘀滞筋结时，气血运行受阻，导致身体对应部位出现病证。壮医经筋医术就是通过手指触摸，查找导致两路运行受阻的筋结病灶，然后通过按摩、针刺、火罐等消除筋结病灶，达到通痹、理筋整复、祛病止痛的效果。

2. 芳香驱邪说与香药治疗法

佛教医学非常重视香药的治疗作用，认为"香"是弟子与佛陀之间的媒介。焚香熏嗅，以香药涂抹、洗浴，以香料入药，均具有消灾祛病之功效。秦汉时期，海外的奇香异药经海上丝绸之路源源不断传入中国。五代时期李珣根据自己的亲历亲见著有《海药本草》一书，该书收录了很多来自东南亚、西亚的香药，如丁香、乳香、茅香、迷迭香、降真香、甘松香、安息香、蜜香等。海外香药的大量输入，丰富了中医药宝库。北宋的《太平惠民和剂局方》载有医方788个，其中卷一《治诸风》载医方89个，海外香药占20%。壮族地区盛产各种芳香植物药，民间认为香药可驱邪避秽，广泛采摘用于防病保健，具有大众化和非专业化的特点。壮族香药外用时，主要用于佩挂和熏洗。香药佩挂是针对不同的病证在身上佩戴不同的香药。壮族一些地区直至20世纪70年代初期，香药佩挂仍是人们防病保健的重要手段，特别是年幼体弱者更为常见，所用香药均为本土野生采摘。香药熏洗广泛用于各种皮肤不适，特别是在每年春夏之交瘴气盛行的时节，家家户户采艾叶、柚子叶、侧兰、石菖蒲等芳香开窍、化湿行气之物置于房门屋檐下，并用之煎水洗浴。壮族地区一般外出遇有污秽或认为不吉之事，也要用柚子叶等芳香之物煎水洗浴或洗手以辟秽。除香药佩挂和香药熏洗外，壮族在日常饮食中广泛使用各种芳香植物如八角茴香、肉桂、芫荽、辣蓼、蒌蒌、紫苏、小茴香、薄荷、香茅等以行气健脾，去腥气。壮家人喜爱的鱼生宴必配新鲜芳香植物，光是各种芳香配料就有七八种。壮族还喜用各种姜，如山姜、蓝姜、黄姜、砂姜（山柰）等。

第二节　其他医药对壮医药影响的客观条件

壮医药 2000 多年的发展是一个变迁的过程，内部变迁是由于壮族地区经济社会发展和人们对自然界、人体自身认识的提高，从而促进了壮医药的发展；外部引发的变迁是由于外来文化的吸收和融合，改变了壮医药的发展轨迹。由于缺乏文字记载，今天我们从错综复杂，你中有我，我中有你的各传统医药体系中很难准确判断当年它们相互影响的具体年代、内容和形式，但是可以肯定，壮族地区便捷的交通条件、大规模的人口迁徙和文化往来对壮族文化发展形态的影响是巨大的，而文化形态的改变，势必会引起卫生习俗、诊疗方法和手段的改变。

一、便利的交通

古代陆地交通由于山川阻碍，河流成为连接东西南北的交通要道。壮族地区水路纵横交错，四通八达，自古以来就是南北民族迁徙和货物来往的主要通道。公元前 214 年，为了解决出征岭南的补给问题，秦始皇派人开凿灵渠。灵渠的建成是广西历史发展的一个里程碑，对壮族地区的经济社会发展产生了深远的影响。灵渠通航后，中原船只经湘江、灵渠，进入红水河、南盘江、柳江、南流江、西江等，西抵云贵高原，南下北部湾出海口，东达广州，成为中原地区和西南地区出海的重要通道。汉代时期，广西的合浦、贵港、梧州已发展成为重要的商业贸易港口城市，尤其是合浦成为海上丝绸之路的起点站。从合浦发船，可自南海沿北部湾西行，经印度东岸到达斯里兰卡，形成一条穿过马六甲海峡而贯通两大洋的航线。唐宋时期，连接宜州、田东、南宁、钦州几个地方，经钦州出海的水路成为我国与海外其他国家往来的便利通道，钦州因此成为国内外商贸的重要港口。《岭外代答》记载："凡交趾生生之具，悉仰于钦，舟楫往来不绝。"便捷的交通，为壮族地区经济发展、文化繁荣提供了良好的条件。

二、民族的迁徙和交流

从距今 50000 年的旧石器时代起，壮族祖先就生活在祖国南疆。1965 年，桂林市甑皮岩发现 18 具人类骨骼化石，在 14 个人头骨中，有 6 个在顶骨处有人工凿穿的孔。这种现象与山东大汶口文化遗址出土的 5000 年前穿孔人头骨相似，与古代西方医学的开颅术是否有关联？是不是由于史前人类迁徙和交流产生的行为？这些问题由于缺乏资料，难以考证，但是从《尚书》《诗经》《逸周书》《墨子》等史籍考查，都有岭南或广西与内地交往的记载。从秦汉时期起，中原地区因戍兵、躲避战乱以及经济重心的南移，迁入广西的人持续不断。《史记》记载，公元前 214 年，秦始皇置桂林郡、南海郡、象郡，"以谪徙民五十万人戍五岭，与越杂处"，为了使士兵们安心驻守，又"使人上书，求女无夫家者三万人，以为士卒衣补。秦皇帝可其万五千人"。1273 年，蒙古南侵，当地居民为躲避战乱大举南迁入广东、广西、福建等地。除此之外，朝廷命官、贬官、商人以及流放到广西的有罪之人增多，据《汉书》《资治通鉴》等记载，从西汉阳朔元年（公元前 24 年）至新莽（公元 23 年）几十年间，因罪迁徙到合浦郡的达 11 人之多。除中原人民的南迁外，壮族、侗族、苗族、瑶族、傣族、仫佬族等民族之间不断迁徙分合，形成了各民族交错聚居的状态。

大量的人员迁徙和交流，带来了文化上的交融碰撞。中原文化以其先进性和较强的渗透性，很快就被壮族人民接受和吸收。根据壮族地区考古发现，广西在秦汉时期出土的文物中，有许多与中原文化共同的特征，如凤是楚文化中最常见、最具特色的装饰形象，合浦望牛岭西汉墓出土的 1 对铜凤灯，是汉文化渗透到广西的实物证据。改土归流后，许多流官在壮族地区建校办学，吸收壮族子弟学习儒家文化、四书五经，使儒家忠、信、仁、义、礼、智等行为规范在壮乡渐成风气，涌现了一批具有较高文化修养的学者，如明代进士韦昭、韦广、张煊、李文凤等均为宜山（今宜州）人。然而，中原文化在广西地区的发展是不平衡的，主要集中在广西的东北部、中部、东南部，而西部受中原文化影响不大。

除了中原文化，佛教文化也对壮族文化产生了一定的影响。考古发现，广西合浦、贺州、贵港、梧州、桂林、昭平等地的西汉墓出土了较多的琉璃、玛瑙、琥珀、水晶等物，尤以广西环北部湾沿岸的合浦汉墓发现最多，这些物品也是佛经上记载的佛教"七宝"，推测来自印度及其周边地区。因此，可以推测西汉时期佛教已经从海路传入了广西地区，在唐代达到了兴盛，此后缓慢发展。佛教的传入，对壮族先民的宗教信仰产生了一定的影响，如相信万物有灵、为死者超度等。然而，佛教对壮族文化的影响是有一定限度的，壮族只是从实用的角度对佛教文化进行了选择性的吸收和改造。

第三节　其他医药文化对壮医药影响的反思

一、其他医药文化对壮医药的负面影响

文化的形成本身就是一个不断吸收、改造、融合外来文化的过程，壮医药在发

展中大量吸收、改造、融合了其他民族医药的成果。诚然，受生产力水平和认识水平的影响，历史上有一些错误、唯心的观点对壮医药的发展造成了负面的影响，如道教医学的符咒、祈禳与壮族的原始宗教结合后产生了广泛的影响力，在很长一段历史内阻碍了壮医药前行的脚步。但是从壮医药的整个发展轨迹来看，外来医学文化与壮医药文化的结合，还是极大地丰富和发展了壮医药本身。

二、其他医药文化对壮医药的冲击

壮医药文化在发展的过程中由于文化的不自信，容易在吸收外来文化过程中迷失自我，从而逐渐湮没自身的优势和特色。在大量中原汉人南迁后，壮族的一部分人接触了先进的中原文化，深感敬仰，一方面积极学习传播中原文化，另一方面受中原汉文化中心论的影响，对自身民族文化习俗嗤之以鼻。在壮族聚居的广西南部地区上思、宁明、扶绥一带，20世纪50～60年代还有许多群众会用针挑、针刺、捏痧等方法治疗一些常见病，但是在先进的西医面前自惭形秽，认为自己的行为是迷信的、不科学的，不再积极为群众治病。壮族历史上缺乏统一的文字，各地语言差异很大，医药的传播和发展存在很大的困难，因此民间的一些医方医术在其他医药文化的强势渗入下逐渐失传，许多医方医术除零星记载于其他民族的记载之外，已无从考查。当然有一些治疗方法和手段不能适应社会的发展，已不能为群众服务的例外，如古代壮医用陶针和箭猪毛作为针刺用具，现在已被先进的器具所代替；壮医喜用野生血肉之品如山瑞、蛇、穿山甲等入药，现在已不符合国家保护野生动物的政策要求。因此，正确认识壮医药的发展历史以及在整个医学体系中的地位，辩证地看待壮医药与其他民族医药文化的关系，应该是每一位壮医药人应有的思想认识。

参考文献：

[1] 廖国一. 佛教在广西的发展及其与少数民族文化的关系 [J]. 佛学研究，2002 (1)：228－239.

[2] 范宏贵，顾有识. 壮族历史与文化 [M]. 南宁：广西民族出版社，1997.

[3] 朱名遂，谢春明. 广西通志·宗教志 [M]. 南宁：广西人民出版社，1995.

[4] 冯立军. 古代中国与东南亚中医药交流 [J]. 南洋问题研究，2002 (3)：8－19.

第十二章　壮医药文化的传承和发展

壮医药是壮族人民在漫长的生产生活实践中形成和发展起来的独特民族医药，是我国传统医药的重要组成部分。当前，传统医药文化在经济全球化的浪潮下面临着前所未有的挑战，西方医学凭借着科技上的优势，近百年来在全世界范围内迅速应用，有2000多年沉淀的壮医药在这场文化洗礼中如何把握机遇和挑战，争取得到更大的发展，为人类的健康做出自己的贡献，是必须认真思考的问题。

第一节　壮医药文化传承和发展面临的主要问题

新中国成立后特别是改革开放以来，在党和国家的关怀下，壮医药有了长足的发展，建立了自己专门的科学研究、临床、教学机构，壮医药已成为广西医疗卫生体系的重要组成部分，壮医药服务的可及性得到提高。壮医药文化在民间也得到了进一步的宣传和推广，如"三月三"歌圩节、农历五月初五靖西端午药市等。但是，壮医药在传承和发展中也面临着一些亟待解决的问题。

一、不能正确认识壮医药文化在历史发展中的地位

壮医药发展在历史上曾达到较高水平，并对中医药的发展产生过一定的影响和促进作用。如《黄帝内经·素问·异法方宜论》记载有"故九针者，亦从南方来"，广西武鸣马头乡出土的2枚西周时期的青铜针灸针也印证了这个历史记载。壮族先民在治疗暑热、各种痧瘴毒病等方面积累了较丰富的经验，形成了一整套疗效显著、地方特色浓厚的诊疗方法。如在汉代，壮族先民就知道吃薏苡仁、嚼槟榔可防治痧瘴。从晋代起就出现了岭南俚人使用毒药和解毒药的文献记载，中原地区对壮族的解毒药尤为推崇，史上记载的如陈家白药、玳瑁血、曼陀罗花等。在壮族地区的医疗实践入载汉史典籍的同时，壮族地区的药材也源源不断地输送到中原地区，如田七、肉桂、罗汉果、蛤蚧、莪术、广豆根、八角茴香、龙眼肉等在中医药中占有非常重要的地位。一方面，壮族地区的医疗实践丰富了中原地区的医药文化；另一方面，传入壮族地区的中医药与壮医药文化相融合，逐渐形成了独树一帜的"八桂中医学术流派"，丰富和发展了中医药文化。壮族地区植被丰富，四季花开不败，国医大师班秀文善用花类如素馨花、凌霄花、玫瑰花、佛手花等治疗疾病，疗效显著；广西针灸流派受壮医针刺的影响，在取穴、进针、留针等方面颇具特色；广西韦氏

中医骨伤整脊流派，融入了民间壮医治疗骨折筋伤的经验和手法，在脊柱损伤退行性疾病方面具有较大的学术影响力。然而，遗憾的是，壮医药文化的璀璨光芒曾一度湮没在历史的尘埃中。从秦始皇统一岭南起，壮族地区就纳入了祖国统一发展的格局，由于经济文化发展滞后，加之语言文字障碍，许多汉族官员对壮族地区的医疗行为和生活习俗难以理解，往往视之为"蛮夷"并加以否定。一些历史记载为了迎合人们的猎奇心理，对壮族地区的人情风俗进行了夸张、带有偏见的描述。封建社会历代统治者对壮族人民的文化和教育实行压制和禁锢，赵翼《檐曝杂记》记载："土民虽读书，不准应试。恐其出土而脱籍也。"1932 年，桂系军阀在三江设立"改良风俗委员会"，规定当地族人一律改穿汉服，不得相约唱山歌及约期坐夜等。受此影响，壮族地区文化教育落后，壮族人很少了解本民族的历史文化，历史虚无主义思想严重，一些医疗卫生习俗往往与愚昧、落后等联系在一起，壮医药文化只能在民间曲折艰难地发展。诚然，在壮医药文化发展过程中，受到生产力水平和认知水平的局限，曾不可避免地带有民间宗教信仰和唯心主义的色彩，"巫医并行，神药两解"在较长一段时期内盛行，但是我们要看到其中精神和信仰治疗的积极效果，同时认识到巫医并行是人类社会发展到一定阶段的产物，是人类对自然界认识不足、敬畏自然的共同心理历程。

新中国成立后，党和国家为少数民族传统文化的发展扫清了障碍，壮医药也得到了一个广阔的发展平台。我们应该全面系统地认识和了解壮医药，辩证地看待壮医药发展中的问题，既要看到它积极和成就的一面，也要看到它消极和局限性的一面，大胆实践，去伪存真，扬优弃劣，使壮医药文化更适应社会的发展和满足人民的需要。

二、民间积累的大量宝贵壮医药经验面临失传

壮族人口众多，分布地域广泛，历史上延续了 1000 多年的"分而治之"土司制度，使壮族地区分割成一块块或大或小的土司领地，壮族各部落形成了各自为政、互不影响的文化生长格局。壮族地区地形地貌复杂，医疗卫生习俗也各有不同，如桂西北地区山高林密，四季分明，在驱寒祛湿方面积累了以各种药酒和油茶为代表的养生文化；桂东南地区炎热多湿，在降火祛湿方面积累了以凉茶、煲汤和刮痧为代表的养生文化。可以说，壮族民间蕴藏着十分丰富的医药文化宝藏，这些宝藏是壮族人民几千年临床实践经验的积累，由于 20 世纪 90 年代以前没有形成系统的理论，未被典籍所录载，目前挖掘整理这些医药宝藏面临着一些不容忽视的问题。首先是语言障碍，"百越"的族源加上 1000 多年的土司制度使广西成为中国方言种类较多的省区，同为壮族，不同县、乡之间语言无法交流沟通的情况屡见不鲜。许多民间医师只能用方言说出药名或病名，没有相同语言背景的研究人员很难准确地翻

译。其次是由于壮族民间医师用的多是家传方子，不愿公开示人，而当前大量年轻人离开乡土，远离了自己的民族文化。随着民间医师这个群体的年岁渐老，大量流传在民间的没有进入医药典籍的孤方、验方、奇方将有可能永远消失，这将是一个历史的遗憾。

三、壮医药文化自身存在的一些问题有待进一步解决

文字是文化得以稳定持续传承的载体，一旦离开了文字，许多传承会发生偏离或断裂。新中国成立以前，壮族历史上没有统一规范的文字，壮医药文化靠口耳相传几千年，这其中难免发生偏离，许多偏方、技法，今天我们只能从汉史典籍中窥其一斑，而更多的已湮灭在历史的长河中。今天，我们从民间挖掘、整理的壮医药文化，一方面是真伪难辨，因为许多诊疗方法和药方都还有待进一步研究验证；另一方面是已整理出来的壮医药，毕竟经验的积累还是占较大的比重，其基础理论与临床诊疗之间的作用机理仍是笼统、模糊的，不能以严格的逻辑来推理疾病的内在辩证发展规律。即使是技法丰富、适应证很广的壮医药线点灸、壮医针刺等疗法，仍然表现为一种直接实用的状态。无论是何种医学模式，要生存发展，首先要能够把积累的经验上升为理论，使之具有普遍的指导意义；其次是在理论的指导下采用一定的诊疗方法有效地防病治病。因此，进一步挖掘整理、完善壮医理论体系，使其更有效地指导临床实践，是相当长一段时间内的主要任务。

第二节　壮医药文化传承和发展应遵循的原则

一、尊重壮医药文化变迁的规律

每一种文化都是在历史的塑模下与现实结合的产物。壮医药文化的内涵结构，我们可以用图12-1来表示，最外围的是壮医药物质文化，主要包括诊疗和药物采制器皿等；处于中间的是壮医药组织制度文化，主要包括诊疗方法、用药规则以及一些医药卫生习俗；核心是壮医药理论体系。一个成熟的医药文化体系，应是在其核心理论的指导下，以该时代物质条件为基础，以符合时代伦理规范为方法手段的。其核心理论历经数代人的医疗经验积累，具有历史的意义。壮医药文化是一个开放的持续变迁的过程，随着时代的发展，人们对生命科学的认识不断深入，社会伦理观念不断变化以及物质条件的丰富繁荣，壮医药的药用器皿、诊疗行为以及相关的卫生习俗、核心理论等也随之不断变化。一般来说，处于外围的物质层面最易与外界发生反应并且随着外界改变而变化，处在核心位置的理论体系较难发生变化，中间层面的壮医药组织制度文化随着物质层面、时代伦理观念的改变而发生变化。

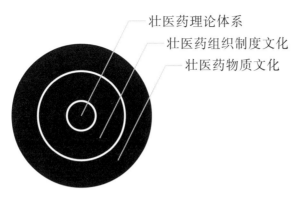

壮医药理论体系
壮医药组织制度文化
壮医药物质文化

图 12-1 壮医药文化的内涵结构图

因此，在壮医药文化传承和发展的过程中，我们要遵从文化发展的规律，在物质文化层面上，尽可能地利用现代社会的成果作为自我完善及发展的手段和条件。中间层面的诊疗方法、用药规则、药物采制方法以及一些医药卫生习俗，则要研究筛选，去伪存真，扬长避短；最核心的理论体系是壮医药的精华和特色所在，对壮医药而言具有普遍意义，是壮医药文化可持续发展的基础，要谨慎辩证，不能轻易动摇。

二、把握壮医药文化发展的方向

在现代科学技术的浪潮下，西方医学以强劲的势头席卷了整个世界，给传统医学发展带来了比历史上任何一次都更强大的冲击。一些观点对民族医药的存在和发展提出了质疑，包括中医药在内的许多民族医学经受了考验。在壮医药的传承和发展问题上，要注意把握方向，防止两种倾向：一是唯心主义思想。古代人们受生产力和认识水平的影响，不能客观地揭示病因病机，把疾病原因归结为超自然的东西，一旦生病就请巫师祭鬼神或驱邪治疗。古代的一些民族医学在历史上曾有过较高的成就，但是因为停留在经验水平层面，没有对病证的机理进行客观地挖掘和分析，依靠主观推断或归于超自然力量，从而走入唯心主义的歧途，最终被其他医学所代替。这种唯心主义思想在很长一段时间内阻碍了壮医药发展。把巫师祭鬼神或驱邪治疗归于唯心思想，今天已有普遍的认识，但是对于另一种形式的唯心主义往往容易忽略，那就是不能正确认识决定和影响疾病的因素，把一些过程或某一方面加以夸大，使之绝对化，造成理论和临床实践的分离。二是虚无主义。表现为否定民族文化传统和历史遗产，甚至认为壮医药文化是虚构的概念，根本否认壮医药文化2000多年的历史和存在，或者以壮医药某一阶段、某一方面的缺陷来否定它的全部，这实质上是西方医学至上主义的一种表现。因此，在壮医药的整理过程中，我们要以保持壮医药的精华和特色为前提，以尊重历史、尊重现实的态度，以严谨的思维，用多学科融合的手段，吸收现代科学技术成果，构建适合壮医药特点的研究方法体系，对壮医药基础理论进行现代诠释，厘清需要重新认识或加以摒弃的部分，构建一个符合时代要求的壮医药文化体系，坚决反对以现代化的名义把壮医药肢解成碎片后粘贴到西方医学体系上。

第三节　壮医药文化传承和发展的方法与途径

一、繁荣壮族传统优秀文化

壮族传统文化是几千年来壮族人民辛勤劳动和努力创造的结果，内容丰富，成就显著。壮族传统文化的优秀代表稻作文化、铜鼓文化、干栏文化、医药文化等，对人类的进步和文明的传播曾产生过巨大的作用。壮医药文化根植于壮族传统文化，是壮族人民日常生活的重要组成部分。随着 21 世纪我国现代化进程的不断加快，壮族人民的生活方式也在悄然发生着变化，壮族传统文化在人们的生活中存在着弱化的倾向，壮医药文化生存的空间受到挤压。优秀壮族传统文化繁荣发展，不仅是民族团结、民族认同的问题，而且也是壮医药文化生存和发展的问题。繁荣发展壮族传统优秀文化，与现代化不是相对立的。现代化是当前人类社会发展的一个共同经历，是发展中国家为了共享人类社会已获得的科学技术成果而经历的一次大的文化变迁而已，其目的是利用现代科学技术提高人们的生活质量，因此现代化是人类社会发展的途径而不是目的。人类生存的环境千差万别，不同的文化类型与不同的环境相适应，保留文化的多元性如同保留地球上物种的多样性一样，对人类而言是十分有必要的。因此，对于壮族人民优秀的精神文化内核，如勤俭和睦、善良宽容、崇尚自然、团结互助、热爱生活的理念，以及体现这些文化内核的习俗、制度、节庆应加以宣传推广，重新构成当代壮族人民的理想追求和社会规范。重视对少数民族文化遗产载体的保护，特别是对于蕴含丰富养生保健内涵的壮族文化特质，如喝油茶、佩戴香囊、端午节洗药浴逛药市等应加以宣传，对刮痧、拔罐等养生保健方法大力推广，使其成为壮族人民保健养生的重要手段。对一些潜在经济价值较大的壮医药文化项目，可通过发展文化产业，将文化优势转化为产业优势。

二、挖掘整理壮医药文化

壮医药文化是否能够较好地传承发展，关键在于它是否能有效地指导人们的医疗实践，为人们的防病治病提供能够推而广之、行之有效的解决方案。因此，在临床实践中进一步证明其疗效，并提高壮医药在医疗卫生体系中的服务能力是壮医药传承和发展的关键。壮医药是我国第一个缺乏文字记载，通过整理形成比较完善的民族医学体系，目前对壮医药的研究尚处于完善和充实阶段。许多诊疗技法、偏方验方有待于我们进一步运用现代科学手段对其进行定性、定量研究，使壮医理论更系统化，临床诊疗更客观化，壮药的生产和使用更加标准化，从而扫除壮医药与现代医疗体系相接轨的障碍，提高壮医药的服务能力。比如，壮医里面最有特色的痧证治疗法。壮族民间有"万病从痧起"之说，民间壮医对痧证的分类十分复杂，达上百种之多。壮医痧证主要从民间口碑中整理，由于言语不通及各家之见，存在着对其概念认识不统一，病证分类不规范，病名概念和内涵模糊，病证特征不明确等问题，阻碍了壮医药的传承和发展。对于临床上常见的热痧、寒痧、蚂蟥痧、红毛痧、标蛇痧等，应对病名的概念和内涵、临床表现和特征、病因病机、辨治规律等进行规范化研究，同时建立痧证临床信息采集资料库，在此基础上不断完善痧证的诊断方法、治则治法，从而建立壮医常见痧证诊断标准，拟定常见痧证规范化诊疗方案。当然，壮医药的规范化研究也不是绝对化的，对于尚未能进入规范化研究或目前尚不能证明其疗效的民间诊疗技能和偏方验方，我们也要谨慎对待，毕竟壮医药文化是经历代经验积累，一点一滴传下来的，而我们运用现代技术对它进行规范化研究才刚刚起步，更何况医学远比科学技术复杂，现阶段我们应该用科学技术手段来解释、完善壮医药文化，而不是用科学技术手段来约束、肢解壮医药文化。随着未来科学技术的发展以及人们对生命科学的认识不断深入，对壮医药文化可能会有新的研究方法、新的发现和新的认识。

三、发展壮医药文化教育

发展壮医药文化教育应该从以下三个方面开展工作：

1. 提高壮医药文化教育的层次

由于壮族在历史上没有统一的文字，壮医药一直在民间口耳相传，直至20世纪80年代以后，广西中医药大学将壮医药科研成果纳入中医学专业课程体系，从学术讲座、辅修课等教育形式起步，经过30多年的不断总结和提升，现已开展了壮医学本科和硕士研究生层次教育。但当前的教育层次仍然不能满足壮医药事业发展的需要，只有使壮医药教育达到博士生层次，才能更有利于进一步提升壮医药理论研究、临床应用推广、药物研究开发水平，从而使植根于民间的壮医药理论更具完整性、系统性和科学性。

2. 扩大壮医药教育的范围

壮医药教育应不仅局限于院校教育，而且还应包括民间壮医师队伍的建设和医疗卫生机构中的壮医药文化建设。壮医药民间医师是壮医药文化的重要载体，也是壮医药文化繁荣发展的基因。壮医药教育应把民间医师教育纳入壮医药人才队伍管理，不断提高他们的业务水平和业务能力，鼓励民间壮医师以带徒授业等方式，将壮医药文化代代相传。对于成熟的壮医药诊疗技术，应当作为适宜技术在各级医疗机构积极推广。

3. 创新壮医药教育的形式

壮医药教育来源于民间,已经整理进入教材、进入课堂的壮医药文化知识毕竟有限,目前高等学校集中化的培养方式也有一定局限性。因此,壮医药教育更应该侧重于实践教学和田野调查。在师资队伍的建设上,对于确有专长的民间医师应聘请为学校兼职教师,为他们配备高学历徒弟,开展名老壮医药专家学术思想及临床经验的传承研究,加强个人行医经验的师承。同时,高校应招收一定比例的通晓壮族语言或有壮族文化背景的学生,培养本土化人才,有利于民间壮医药的挖掘整理。

参考文献:

[1] 覃主元. 对壮族传统文化的几点反思 [J],经济与社会发展,2013 (12):144-146.

[2] 付广华. 论新桂系政权的民族同化政策 [J],桂海论丛,2008,24 (5):74-78.

[3] 庞宇舟,王春玲. 壮医药文化概述 [J]. 中国中医基础医学杂志,2009,15 (10):800-802.

1 Introduction

1.1 Interpretation of Zhuang medical culture

1.1.1 Definition of culture

The word "culture" should be one of the most frequently used words in the world today. It comes from the Latin word "colere", originally used to describe the tilling and improvement of land. Later, it acquired multiple meanings including processing, accomplishment, education, and courtesy. In the seventeenth century, the German jurist Pufendorf proposed, "Culture is the sum of what is created in human activities and what exists depending on the social life of humans." In the mid-nineteenth century, when the first cultural craze arose, British anthropologist Tylor was recognized as the founder of contemporary culturology. He defined culture in his famous work *Primitive Culture*, "Culture or civilization is that complex whole which includes knowledge, belief, art, morals, law, custom, and any other capabilities and habits acquired by man as a member of society."

In the twentieth century, the definitions of culture in different nations became diversified. *La Grande Encyclopédie* says, "culture is the sum of phenomena of civilization peculiar to social communities", and "Culture is a complex whole which includes knowledge, belief, art, morals, law, custom, and any other norms and habits shared by man as a member of society." *Meyer Encyclopedia*, published in German in 1971, says, "Culture is the material and ideological wealth created by human societies in the conquest of nature and self-development." *Great Soviet Encyclopedia*, published in 1973, defines culture in a broad sense as "it is the development level of socie-ties and human beings in the history, manifesting as types and forms of human life and activities as well as material and spiritual wealth created by human beings", and in a narrow sense as "simply the field of human spiritual life".

Famous Chinese scholar Liang Shuming explained in his book *Highlights of Chinese Culture*, "The core of culture is all-embracing, not excluding economy and politics." So, the meaning of culture is broad in nature. At present, there are two popular definitions of culture in China. One is explained by *Cihai* that culture refers to, in the broad sense, the sum of the acquired material and spiritual productive forces and created material and spiritual wealth in the historic course of social practice, and in the narrow sense, it refers to spiritual productive forces and spiritual products including all forms of social consciousness, such as natural science, technical science and social ideology. The other is explained by *Modern Chinese Dictionary* that culture is "the sum of the created material and spiritual wealth in the historic course of social practice, particularly spiritual wealth, e.g., literature, art, education, and science".

1.1.2 Concepts of Zhuang medical culture

The great medical scientist Pavlov once said, "There was human; and now there are medical activities." Medicine is an inherent need of human beings, in which every nation has their own creation and accumulation through their history. Zhuang is an ethnic minority with a long history and splendid culture, derived from Xi'ou and Luoyue tribes in ancient Baiyue in South China. According to archeological discovery, there were ancient human activities in the Zhuang region as early as the Old Stone Age. In ancient times, conditions for life were harsh in the Zhuang region. According to the record of *Strange Stories in Lingnan* by Liu Xun in the Tang Dynasty, "Peaks rise one after another in Lingnan, where the terrain is so tough that miasma emerges and converges among the misty hills. People who touch miasma tend to be sick, with abdominal distended." In the process of struggling against diseases, Zhuang ancestors have accumulated rich medical knowledge and experience, and a unique system of Zhuang medical culture has been formed.

The Zhuang medical culture is: the sum of medicine-related spiritual, institutional and material cultures in the traditional Zhuang culture, as well as the manifestations of Zhuang ancestors' physiological and pathological views, etiological and pathogenetic theories, methods of diagnosis and treatment, and relevant material and non-material (e.g., psychological orientation, symbols, folklore, medicine and utensils). And it is the combined result of Zhuang medicine and various Zhuang cultures.

On the one hand, Zhuang medical culture, the medical culture created by the Zhuang nationality through their history, essentially belongs to the category of medicine, making indelible contributions to the survival and reproduction of Zhuang by observing and tracking the phenomena of human life, reflecting on the relationship

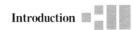

between humans and nature and summarizing it. On the other hand, there are several human dimensions in it as it contains ethnic wisdom, spiritual value, ways of thinking and other intangible content. In short, Zhuang medical culture is natural, humanistic, material, non-material and dual as non-material culture dwells in material one in an inseparable way.

As one kind of material and spiritual wealth created by the Zhuang nationality, Zhuang medical culture is undoubtedly an integral part of human culture, especially Zhuang culture.

1. 1. 3 Basic types of Zhuang medical culture

1. 1. 3. 1 **Spiritual culture**

In Zhuang medicine, its spiritual culture reflects its philosophical foundation, physiological and pathological views and therapeutic ideas, the core part of which is its theoretical system.

The spiritual culture of Zhuang medicine falls into the category of materialistic dialectics as a whole.

First of all, in terms of the understanding of Zhuang medicine towards nature and human, Zhuang ancestors believed the universe, made of "the three realms" — heaven, earth and waters — was objective and material, was not the imaginary consciousness. Accordingly, the human body is divided into three parts that are closely linked — human qi, heaven qi and earth qi. "Humans cannot act in defiance of heaven and earth". The human life cycle is nourished and constrained by the ever-changing heaven and earth qi, to which humans, as the wisest of all creatures, can proactively adapt.

Secondly, in terms of the physiological and pathological understanding of human body, it is deemed by Zhuang medicine that internal organs, qi, blood, bones and flesh are the main physical bases of the human body. All the relatively independent entities within the cranium, thoracic cavity and abdominal cavity are called zang and fu organs, and no clear distinction is made between "zang" and "fu". In the Zhuang language, the encephalic content is called "uk", which means coordination, thinking and control of mental activities. For example, in Zhuang medicine the psychiatric symptom of psychosis is called "uk luenh" or "ukgyaeuj luenh", which means dysfunction of general headquarters. The heart is called "simdaeuz", which means head of zang and fu organs. The lung is referred to as "bwt", the liver as "daep", the gallbladder as "mbei", the kidney as "mak", the pancreas as "mamx", the spleen as "lenzded", the stomach as "dungx", the intestines as "saej", the bladder as "rongznyouh", and the uterus as "saejva". All the internal organs play their own role in jointly maintaining the body's normal physiological state. When they are damaged or do not function properly for other reasons, diseases will be caused. Bones (referred to as "ndok" in the Zhuang language) and flesh ("noh" in Zhuang language), constituting the body's frame and form, protect organs within the body from exterior injury normally. Also, bones and flesh are locomotive organs. It is claimed by Zhuang medicine that the blood ("lwed" in Zhuang language) is an extremely important substance that nourishes the whole body including bones, flesh and zang and fu organs, and that is generated by qi of heaven and earth and depends on it to circulate. Zhuang medicine attaches great importance to qi ("heiq" in Zhuang language). Qi is power and function, as well as the manifestation of the force body's life energy. Qi is invisible, but it can be felt.

The Zhuang nationality, one of the first Chinese ethnic nations to grow rice, knows that grain crops grow naturally with the blessing of heaven and earth qi, and that grain crops nourish the body with heaven and earth qi within them. The tract leading to the inside body and enabling digestive absorption is called "Gudao" ("diuzgwnngaiz" in Zhuang language), and it mainly refers to the esophagus, the stomach and the intestines. The body's "Shuidao" is the tract where water, the source of life, comes into and out of the body, and it allows the most direct and closest connection between the body and nature. Gudao and Shuidao are congenetic but differentiated. After the essence of water and food is absorbed, Gudao allows defecation and Shuidao allows perspiration and urination. "Qidao" is the tract that enables the exchange between the body and natural qi, and the mouth and nose are inlets and outlets. When the three tracts are unblocked and well-regulated, human qi with heaven and earth qi can remain synchronous, coordinated and balanced, namely we can stay healthy. However, if they are blocked or not well-regulated, the asynchrony of triple initial qi will cause diseases.

In Zhuang medicine, "Longlu" and "Huolu" are two extremely important closed-ended tracts inside the body, which are not directly connected to nature but able to maintain the body's vitality and reflect the dynamic of diseases. In Zhuang tradition, it is believed that dragon (Long in Chinese) can control water. Longlu is the tract of blood inside the body (so some Zhuang physicians call it blood vessel or dragon vessel), which is able to deliver nutrition into internal organs, bones and flesh. Longlu circulates in all of the body through its trunk and network, with the heart as its pivot. Fire (Huo), as a trigger, is quick in nature (fire usually means quick in Chinese words) and scorching hot. In Zhuang medicine, it is believed that Huolu is a sensing tract inside the body, which means "information channel" in modern languages. Its pivot is in "ukgyaeuj" (referring to brain in Zhuang language). Like Longlu, Huolu circulates in all of the body through its trunk and network. So the normal body is able to sense information and stimuli from outside in a remarkably short period of time, and send them to the pivot "ukgyaeuj" for processing and rapid response. That is how the body adapts to external changes and how the equilibrium state — "synchrony of triple initial qi" is achieved physiologically.

The Zhuang region is located in the subtropics, characterized by thick mountain forest and damp and hot climate. The decaying animals and plants produce miasmic toxin, and there are also many wild poisonous animals, plants and other poisonous substances, e. g., poisonous herbs, poisonous trees, poisonous insects, poisonous snakes, poisonous water and poisonous minerals. The Zhuang ancestors have particularly direct and impressive feelings about toxin, as there are many instances and lessons about diseases and death caused by poisoning. After the pathogenic toxin or poisonous substances enter the body, whether you are susceptible to diseases depends on your body's resistance to toxin and capability of detoxification, namely the strength of healthy qi within your body. In addition, Zhuang medicine believes that deficiency is one of the two major pathogenic factors. It refers to the deficiency of healthy qi or qi-blood. It is the cause of diseases as well as the reflection of pathosis. Toxin and deficiency turn the body from normal state into diseased state.

Finally, in terms of treatment ideas in Zhuang medicine, objective idealism is reflected. From primitive society to feudal society, the Zhuang ancestors failed to give reasonable explanations of certain diseases and attributed them to haunting ghosts and gods and curses. They believed sorcery can dispel pathogenic and noxious factors. With an increasing understanding of the body's physiology, pathology, etiology and pathogenesis, Zhuang medicine has gradually formed the therapeutic principle of "regulating qi, removing toxin and rectifying deficiency", which is a guide to effective clinical treatment.

1. 1. 3. 2 Institutional culture

The institutional culture of Zhuang medicine mainly includes methods for diagnosis and treatment, rules of drug usage and healthcare customs.

The methods for diagnosis and treatment are diverse and distinctive. It holds that the body is a well-balanced life entity. Apart from aberrant foci of infection, there is exosyndrome on the body surface when lesions occur in any part of the body. So diseases can be diagnosed through the observation of body surface or simple tests. Its diagnostic methods can be divided into five categories and dozens of diagnostic techniques. The five categories are known as (1) inspection, (2) listening and smelling, (3) enquiry, (4) palpation, and (5) probing. Amongst the diagnostic techniques are: (1) inspection of the eyes, (2) feeling of pulse, (3) inspection of nail, (4) inspection of finger, (5) abdominal palpation, (6) illness detection with Yeyutou (*Colocasia antiquorum* Schott), (7) illness detection with Shihuishui (*Aqua Calcis*). Also, it has dozens of therapeutic methods including herbal medicine for oral administration, irrigation, fumigating and, steaming, peste application, aromatic pendant, scrapping with animal bone, horn treatment, moxibustion and needle-pricking.

The Zhuang region is situated in the subtropical zone, characterized by temperate climate, plentiful rainfall, lush and evergreen vegetation. It is rich in drug resources. Local materials are preferred in Zhuang medicine, and the custom of using fresh herbs has been gradually developed. Many fresh herbs can be taken internally and applied externally, such as Xianrenzhang [*Opuntia stricta* (Haw.) Haw. var. *dillenii* (Ker-Gawl.) Benson], Pugongying (*Taraxacum mongolicum* Hand.-Mazz.), Shengdi [*Rehmannia glutinosa* (Gaetn.) Libosch. ex Fisch. et Mey.], Lugen (*Rhizoma Phragmitis*), Shihu (*Dendrobium nobile* Lindl.), Huoxiang [*Agastache rugosa* (Fisch. et Mey.) O. Ktze.]. From the long-term clinical practice of Zhuang medicine, knowledge of the actions of medicinal herbs has accumulated, and is expressed in a widespread pithy formula — "Pungent flavor can promote circulation of qi and blood, release exterior, treat trauma, dispel wind-dampness and expel cold. Sour flavor can astringe and invigorate the kidney to preserve essence, relieve diarrhoea, secure semen and treat excessive sweat due to deficiency. Bitter flavor and cold nature can dispel dampness, purge, treat excess heat and constipation. Numbness can ease pain, expel carbuncle and boil, and treat tongue injury and chronic phlegm. Astringent flavor has astringent, antimicrobial and hemostatic actions, and it can treat burns and reduce inflammation. Salty flavor can treat scrofula and abdominal mass, promote purgation, and soften hard mass. Sweet flavor can harmonize the middle, nourish the body, regulate actions of many other medicines, and modify the taste. Bland flavor can dispel dampness, excrete water, tranquilize mind, relieve dysphoria, and help sleep." In

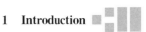

Zhuang medicine, knowledge of the relationship between the appearance and function of medicine is organized in a formula — "Hairy herbs can disperse wind, and sap can draw out pus. Hollow herbs can excrete water, and square stems have dispersing action. Most thorny herbs can alleviate edema, and vines can treat joint diseases. Leaves showing bilateral symmetry in being divided via a stem can treat trauma, dispel wind-dampness and relieve pain. Herbs with hairy leaves and stalks can stop bleeding and treat burns. Most flowers have an action of dispersing, and most seeds are sinking and lowering. Herbs with square stalks and white flowers are cold in nature. Herbs with round stalks and red flowers are mostly pungent in flavor and warm in nature." Drugs are classified as male, female, principal, auxiliary and messenger ones. The therapeutic effect of drugs can be improved by combining them as needed.

Zhuang have colorful customs of medicine and healthcare. In terms of hygiene, Zhuang people prefer having the hair clipped short, dressing in blue black, living in ganlan houses (house in stilt style). In terms of healthcare, they wear herbal sachets, go to the drug fairs, and hang Ai (*Artemisiae argyi*) on the door. In diet and health preservation, they attach importance to the diet for seasonal occasions. For example, they pick Baitouweng (*Radix pulsatilla*) and Aiye (*Folium Artemisiae argyi*) and use them with rice to make zongzi at the end of the first lunar month; they pick Jinyinhua (*Flos Lonicerae*), Aiye (*Folium Artemisiae argyi*) and other herbs to make ciba cakes on the third day of the third lunar month; they cook and eat black rice to dispel plague at the Buddha's Birthday Festival on the eighth day of the fourth lunar month; they drink Changpu (*Acorus calamus* L.) wine and Xionghuang (realgar) wine to dispel plague on the fifth day of the fifth lunar month. They are good at making medicated diet, for example, Longhudou (the main ingredients are snake and cat), Longfenghui (the main ingredients are snake and chicken) and Sanshe wine (sanshe consists of cobra, krait and Chinese rat snake).

1.1.3.3 Material culture

In Zhuang medicine, material or tangible culture means tangible medicine-related things, which mainly include tools for diagnosis and treatment, drugs and utensils for collecting and processing drugs.

Without standard written characters throughout their history, the Zhuang nationality has relied on word of mouth to disseminate medical knowledge, which has led to variable understanding and interpretation in different era. We can hardly deduce the journey of Zhuang medical culture precisely from current myths, folktales and customs. However, its material culture clearly represents the situation of medicine and healthcare in the ancient Zhuang region. The bronze needles, unearthed in an ancient tomb in Matou Township, Wuming District, Nanning City, Guangxi, can date back to the period between Western Zhou Dynasty and Spring and Autumn Period. The Tiedongqing (*Ilex rotunda* Thunb.) and silver needles, found in an ancient tomb in Guigang City, Guangxi, can date back to the Western Han Dynasty. They show that there was a high level of healthcare and treatment in the Zhuang region. There are various Zhuang medical tools, a great part of which are still used until this day. They include needle, medicated thread, porcelain bowl, bone bow, drug hammer, ox horn and bamboo jar. Also, the Zhuang region is home to many rare medicinal materials which have long been known and applied extensively by the Zhuang people. They include Tianqi or Sanqi [*Panax pseudoginseng* Wall. var. *notoginseng* (Burkill) Hoo et Tseng], Rougui (*Cinnamomum cassia* Presl), Bajiaohuixiang (*Illicium verum* Hook. f.), Yiyiren (*Semen Coicis*), Luohanguo [*Siraitia grosvenorii* (Swingle)], Zhenzhu (*Margarita*). According to the *Compendium of Materia Medica* by Li Shizhen in the Ming Dynasty, "Tianqi or Sanqi [*Panax pseudoginseng* Wall. var. *notoginseng* (Burkill) Hoo et Tseng], native to remote mountains of Nandan County and other counties in Guangxi, is an important drug for treating slash or stab wound." They all have the attributes of material objects and belong to the primary forms of material culture in Zhuang medicine, which has been enriched by the popularization and development of science and technology since the establishment of the People's Republic of China. Also, its connotation has been quietly influenced by modern pharmaceutical machinery and wonderful and scientific medical instruments.

1. 2　Journey of Zhuang medical culture

Zhuang medical culture has been formed in an evolutionary process, which can be analyzed both internally and externally. In terms of internal factors, it has been enriched and developed, from simple to complex, with the productivity growth of Zhuang, social progress and improvement of Zhuang medicine. It has changed steadily and continuously according to its own rules. In terms of external factors, part of its changes is caused by the shock and infiltration of different forms of medical cultures from other ethnic. That change is limited and evolved according to the level of its material technologies or non-core theories. That is the foundation on which it can maintain its cha-racteristics and continue to exist. Judging from its vertical evolution, it can be divided into several phases— infancy (from ancient times to the Pre-Qin Period), beginning (from the Qin Dynasty to the Sui Dynasty), enrichment (from the Tang Dynasty to the period of Republic of China), and integrated development (since the founding of the People's Republic of China).

1. 2. 1 Infancy (from ancient times to the Pre-Qin Period)

The emergence of medical culture accompanied that of production culture. About 50,000 to 20,000 years ago, there were traces of human activities in the Zhuang region. Archeologists have discovered more than 100 paleolithic sites in areas inhabited by the Zhuang nationality. 75 sites are located in the river terrace on both sides of Youjiang River within 4 cities (counties) — Baise, Tianyang, Tiandong and Pingguo. Over 1,100 chipped stone tools have been collected in all shapes and sizes. It shows that as early as the Paleolithic Age, Zhuang ancestors had learned to choose the appropriate broken stones, shape them, produce rough but practical blades and sharp tools, and use them to chop, hit and dig. When using such tools, they found they could relieve the pain or cure some disease by using the tools to hit certain parts of their body. While they were working or fighting against wild beasts, they were often wounded by broken stones and bled, which also gave some relief to the pain. Over the years such life experiences were repeated, and then people paid attention to them. Now it has been handed down to us and become acupuncture therapy through repeated practice and lessons.

Throughout the Neolithic Age, Zhuang ancestors' economic life changed with continuous improvement in productivity, stronger capability of fighting against nature and wild beasts, and secure source of income. Compared with the Paleolithic culture, the Neolithic culture had improved significantly, and medicine and health had also been developed greatly. The Zhuang ancestors invented ganlan houses (house in stilt style), where humans and animals lived apart. It was a really important hygiene practice for their survival in a harsh environment. Also, they were aware of the hygienic need to have people and animals live apart. They invented polishing technology for stone implements and earthenware. A great number of colorful polished stone artifacts have been unearthed in Zengpiyan in Guilin, Liyuzui in Liuzhou, Baozitou in Nanning and other sites, and these unearthed items of pottery (in pieces) are now the earliest discovered in China. People were able to cook with pottery, so that better absorption of food could improve their health. Meanwhile, pottery needle therapy emerged in Zhuang medicine with the rise of ceramic culture in the Zhuang region. This therapy is still popular because it is effective in treatment and easy to use.

From the end of the Zhou Dynasty to the Spring and Autumn Period, Zhuang people entered the Metal Age. Metal smelting technique improved their cultural life as well as tools for acupuncture treatment. Two exquisite bronze needles have been unearthed in an ancient tomb in Matou Township, Wuming District, Nanning City, Guangxi, which can be dated back to the Western Zhou Dynasty and Spring and Autumn Period. According to research, these were acupuncture tools used by the Zhuang ancestors, indicating that the ancient Zhuang ancestors' medical achievements went hand in hand with social development.

During the Pre-Qin Period, the Zhuang society still existed as low-productivity tribal alliances. Mother Nature's secrets are boundless, and she is ever-changing. Zhuang ancestors failed to explain natural phenomena (e.g., earthquake, flood and volcanic eruption) and even the common ones (e.g., sunrise, sunset, wind, rain, thunder and lightning). In particular, they felt mystified by night dreams, birth, death, old and disease. Therefore, based on boundless imagination, they assumed that there must be supernatural powers and mysterious realms dominating nature and society. Hence sorcery culture came into being, and this had a significant impact on Zhuang medicine. For example, murals on the Huashan Mountains on both sides of Zuojiang River represent Zhuang ancestors' worship of the sun, moon and stars. Some scholars believe that in addition to dance movements, there may be depictions of diagnosis and treatment in those murals, where we can see people performing witchcraft, holding instruments and being subjected to witchcraft. Considering the scenes of sacrifice in those cliff paintings and the features of Zhuang ancestors' sorcery culture, we can say there is evidence of treating diseases by witchcraft medicine in those cliff paintings. In terms of the influence of sorcery culture on Zhuang medicine, they were one and the same in the beginning, then they coexisted, and finally Zhuang medicine prevailed.

1.2.2　Beginning（from the Qin Dynasty to the Sui Dynasty）

Because of historical and geographical circumstances and other reasons, social development was slow in the Zhuang region. During the Shang and Zhou periods, the Central Plains had entered slave society, while the Zhuang region in Lingnan remained a backwater and was in the late period of primitive society and had the form of tribal alliance or military democracy. It was not until the Qin Shihuang (the first emperor of Qin) unified China in 221 B. C. that the Zhuang region started to be governed directly by a centralized feudal dynasty and started rapid development of the economy and society.

From the Qin Dynasty to Sui Dynasty, the Zhuang ancestors began to be well aware of hygiene and environmental protection with the development and progress of productivity. The unearthed cultural relics, especially the sanitary appliances, reflected that they had developed good hygiene habits as early as 2000 years ago. For example, the bronze phoenix lamp for smoke abatement (unearthed in the late Western Han Dynasty tomb in Wangniuling, Hepu, Guangxi), ceramic model of toilet (in the Eastern Han Dynasty tomb in Zhongshan, Guangxi), ceramic chamber pot (in the Eastern Han Dynasty tomb No. 11 in Xincun, Guigang City, Guangxi), gilded bronze earpick (in the Western Han Dynasty tomb in Luobowan, Guigang City, Guangxi), ceramic spittoon (in the Han Dynasty tomb in Xingping, Lipu County, Guangxi). The awareness of hygiene was extremely valuable given the slow social development, laggard productivity, and poor medical and sanitary conditions.

During this period, the Zhuang ancestors had a certain understanding of how diseases damaged human health. *Biography of Ma Yuan*, *Book of the Later Han* says, "in an expedition to Jiaozhi, many soldiers suffered from miasmic malaria", and "about half the military officers died of miasmic malaria". In *General Treatise on the Causes and Symptoms of Diseases*, Chao Yuanfang in the Sui Dynasty pointed out, "Warmness gives birth to miasma", and "Miasma emerges from the moisture around mountain streams". But people still had a vague understanding of diseases and were not able to distinguish types of diseases. So pathogenic factors were collectively named as "miasma" and names of diseases as "miasmic malaria". In *Handbook of Prescriptions for Emergencies*, Ge Hong in the Jin Dynasty recorded the Zhuang ancestors' experience in preventing and treating beriberi and chigger disease (tsutsugamushi disease), and repeatedly mentioned toxin and their methods of detoxification.

During the same period, new drugs were increasing and old drugs had additional usage in the Zhuang region. In *Classic of Mountains and Seas* and *Classic of Herbal Medicine*, there are many records about drugs in the Zhuang region and the Zhuang ancestors' experience of treatment with medicine during the Pre-Qin Period. There are more records about drugs in Zhuang medicine during the Qin, Han, Wei, Jin dynasties and the Northern and Southern Dynasties. For example, *Nanfang Caomu Zhuang* (*Plants of the Southern Regions*), attributed to the scholar Ji Han in the Jin Dynasty, has recorded Jilicao, Water Spinach, Doukouhua (*Amomum kravanh* Pierre ex Gagnep.) and other drugs in Zhuang medicine. Another classic *General Treatise on the Causes and Symptoms of Diseases*, attributed to the scholar Ge Hong in the Jin Dynasty, has recorded the Zhuang ancestors' experience of drug usage in preventing and treating miasma, parasitic tympanites and toxin. Plenty of seeds and fruit were unearthed in 1976 in the Han Dynasty tomb No. 1 in Luobowan, Guigang City, Guangxi. It has been identified that many of them are from medicinal plants, indicating that botanical drugs had been widely used to prevent and treat diseases and the foundation of pharmacotherapy had been laid in the Zhuang region at that time.

Also, Han culture had a significant impact on the Zhuang region from the Qin Dynasty to Sui Dynasty. Confucianism was widely promoted with the establishment of city and county schools. With the continuous in-depth exchanges between the Zhuang nationality and the Han nationality in the Central Plains, the Han people's writings had recorded and disseminated the society, politics, culture, customs, medicine and other aspects of the Zhuang region. There are increasing documentary records of Zhuang medicine after *Classic of Mountains and Seas* and *Classic of Herbal Medicine*.

1.2.3　Enrichment (from the Tang Dynasty to the Republic of China)

From the Tang Dynasty to the Republic of China, it was the golden age of Zhuang medical culture, which was rich and prosperous with the economic, political and cultural development of the Zhuang region.

The Tang Dynasty and Song Dynasty have witnessed the thriving feudal economy in China. With the great economic development of the Zhuang region, the knowledge of Zhuang medicine was becoming systematic, and its theory was budding. It had good success in preventing and treating common diseases, such as miasmic malaria, toxin, parasitic tympanites, sha (filthy-attack diseases caused by spotted qi), wind syndrome and dampness. In the Tang Dynasty, the writer and politician, Liu Zongyuan was the City Governor of Liuzhou. He personally collected proven Zhuang prescriptions and applied them to himself. Then he wrote *Liuzhou Prescriptions for Three Deadly Diseases* that recorded treatment of furunculosis, beriberi and cholera. In the Song Dynasty, Fan Chengda pointed out in *Guihai Yuheng Zhi* (*Record of an Offi-*

cial Posting in the Gui Region），"Except Guilin, there is miasma everywhere in Guangdong and Guangxi. Zones in the south of Guilin are all miasmatic." And "Zuojiang and Youjiang basins are harsh, and there is miasma all the year around", "Moisture comes from water in mountainous and grassland regions, and is so excessive that it forms miasma which seems to affect people with malaria". It clearly points out that the symptoms of miasmatic disease are similar to that of malaria. In *Lingwai Daida* (*Answer on Outer of the Five Ridges*), Zhou Qufei in the Song Dynasty has not only elaborated on the Zhuang therapeutic methods for miasmic disease, but also pointed out its etiology and pathogenesis, "In hot and humid climate, Yang Qi leaks out of the body, and this does not stop even in the winter. Both grass and waters bear filthy qi, which haunts people. People who live in such environment suffer from insecurity of original qi, which evolves into miasmatic disease." Those documentary records were not directly written by practitioners of Zhuang medicine, but they are referential and reflect those practitioners' understanding of miasmatic disease at that time, because their authors, as local officials in the Zhuang region for many years, knew local customs and practices. Meanwhile, Zhuang medicine formulas and pharmacy emerged. The *Tang Materia Medica*, attributed to 22 people including Su Jing in the second year of Emperor Xianqing of Tang (in 657), had been completed through two years of efforts and issued by the imperial court as a pharmacopeia. It is the first national pharmacopeia in the world, recording 850 types of drugs including part of those in the Zhuang region, such as Ranshedan (boa gallbladder), Huashi (talc), velamen of Diaozhang (*Lindera erythrocarpa* Makino), Fuling [*Poria cocos* (Schw.) Wolf.], Gui (*Cinnamomum cassia* Presl), garlic (*Allium sativum*), betel nuts (*Areca catechu* L.), Baihuateng (*Clematis maximowicziana* Franch. Et Sav.), Shacaoke (*Cyperaceae*), Sufangmu (*Caesalpinia sappan* L.), and Langbazi (*Wisteria sinensis*). *Bencao Shiyi* (*A Supplement to the Compendium of Materia Medica*) also includes famous Chenjia Baiyao and Ganjia Baiyao from the Zhuang region.

During the Yuan, Ming and Qing dynasties, the Zhuang region entered the era of the Tusi (native chieftain) system, and Zhuang medicine had seen fast development in the long journey. In the Tusi system, official medical organizations were established, and there were a number of full-time officials and non-governmental medical workers, which was recorded clearly in the annals of xian (counties), zhou (secondary prefectures) and fu (supreme prefectures) in Guangxi since the Ming Dynasty. In the tenth year of Emperor Jiajing of Ming (in 1531), according to incomplete statistics, Tusi established medical academies in each of the more than 40 xian, zhou and fu of Guangxi where the Zhuang nationality lived, such as Qingyuan, Si'en, Tianhe, Wuyuan, Yongchun and Nanning. In particular, the positions of medical officials in those medical academies were assumed by native doctors, and this promoted the development of Zhuang medicine, indicating the importance placed on native traditional medicine by Tuguan (native civilian commanders).

During the Ming and Qing dynasties, Zhuang medicine had a deep understanding of the body's etiology and pathogenesis, as well as local common diseases. According to the syndrome, etiology and pathogenesis, they were classified as sha (filthy-attack diseases caused by spotted qi), miasmic malaria, parasitic tympanites, toxin, wind syndrome and dampness. It not only accumulated various diagnostic methods (e.g., observation of the eyes, feeling of pulse, inspection of nail, inspection of finger, abdominal palpation), therapeutic methods (e.g., herbal medicine for oral administration, irrigation, fumigating and steaming, paste application, wearing herbal sachets, scrapping with animal bone, horn treatment, moxibustion and needle-pricking), but also created a great number of proven prescriptions and secret recipes. In the late Qing Dynasty and the period of the Republic of China, an integral but preliminary system of Zhuang medicine had formed after a long historical development, for which the emergence of medical works and famous doctors laid the foundation.

In the long-term evolution from the Tang Dynasty and Song Dynasty to the Republic of China, increasingly importance was attached to Zhuang medicine and relevant cultures were also increasingly prosperous with the accumulation and application of medical knowledge. Notably, myths and legends about the origin of Zhuang medicine were around in the Zhuang region, such as "the miracle-working doctor Sanjiegong (literally the Lord of the Three Realms) " and "Yeqi's fight against the God of Plague". Famous and miracle-working doctors and the King of Medicine were worshipped and commemorated. Take annals in the Qing Dynasty for example, *Ancestral Shrine*, *Volume 1*, *Annals of Ningming Zhou* records, "Yiling Temple is near to the city wall outside the east gate." *Annals of Ritual Offering*, *Volume 43*, *Annals of Yongning Xian* says, "Yaowang (the King of Medicine) Temple is on the North Gate Street, on the left side of Dongyue Temple." The book *Volume 3*, *Annals of Liuzhou Xian* records, "Yaowang (the King of Medicine) Temple is inside the west gate." Before the Qing Dynasty, there were basically no Western-style doctors and few doctors of traditional Chinese medicine in the Zhuang region. Those nameless mir-

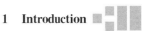

acle-working doctors and the King of Medicine, commemorated in the temples, were largely famous folk doctors, namely Zhuang doctors in the Zhuang region. They were held in high esteem by people because they were able to treat patients' diseases and relieve their pain with excellent medical skills and noble medical ethics. For another example, currently there is still one Sanjie Temple buit in the Qing Dynasty near the Tusi yamen (administrative office of a local bureaucrat in imperial China) in Xincheng. Sanjie was a miracle-working doctor who was proficient in internal medicine, surgery, ophthalmology and otorhinolaryngology and other departments. He was so famous that people built a temple which was consecrated to the memory of him. Sanjie Temple was allowed to be built close to Tusi yamen, which revealed the lofty image of that miracle-working doctors in the eyes of Zhuang people. This phase has seen the formation of the custom of drug fairs. Vegetation and drug resources are plentiful among the heavily forested mountains of the Zhuang region. On the fifth day of the fifth lunar month in each year, Zhuang villagers go to the drug fairs in the market town, where they either sell a variety of medicinal materials picked by themselves, or browse, smell and buy medicine. In Zhuang folklore, lush herbs exhibit strong efficacy and the best therapeutic effect on the fifth day of the fifth lunar month. When people go to the drug fairs on that day, they can absorb the qi of medicine, prevent diseases, and consequently fall ill as rarely as possible throughout the year. Over time, going to the drug fairs became a Zhuang custom. Zhuang people go to the drug fairs on that day to absorb the qi of medicine with all their family even though they have no medicine for sale. That custom of mass prevention and treatment still survives now in the Zhuang region.

1.2.4 Integrated development (since the founding of the People's Republic of China)

Zhuang medical culture has a long history and rich content. However, it was not until the founding of the People's Republic of China that it received the necessary attention from the government because of the prejudice and discrimination against ethnic minorities in the society. Since the founding of the People's Republic of China, Chinese government has attached importance to support the investigation, organization and research of Zhuang medical culture, guided by the party's ethnic minority and TCM policies. Based on the relevant non-governmental research and articles on Chinese herbal medicine between the 1950s and 1970s, there has been comprehensive, systematic and large-scale study and organization of Zhuang medical culture particularly since the National Working Conference on Ethnic Medicine in 1984.

According to local chronicles, there were medical facilities in Tusi yamen before the founding of the People's Republic of China. However, all of them vanished with the founding of the People's Republic of China. For the inheritance and promotion of Zhuang medicine, Guangxi College of Chinese Medicine current Guangxi University of Chinese Medicine, established the Laboratory of Zhuang Medicine in 1984, where Professor Ban Xiuwen, as one of the first TCM Masters, was appointed as director. Also, in 1985, the laboratory enrolled the first postgraduates of History of Zhuang Medicine in China's medical history. In April 1985, China's first outpatient department of Zhuang medicine was opened in the headquarters of Guangxi University of Chinese Medicine after receiving the approval of Health Department of Guangxi Zhuang Autonomous Region. Many famous experts of Zhuang medicine were recruited to that outpatient department, for example, Long Yuqian (expert of Zhuang medicated thread moxibustion), Luo Jia'an (expert of Zhuang needle-pricking therapy) and Guo Tingzhang (expert of miscellaneous diseases).

In 1985, China's first provincial-level scientific research institution for ethnic medicine, Guangxi Institute for Ethnic Medicine, was established in Nanning after being granted the approval of People's Government of Guangxi Zhuang Autonomous Region and State Scientific and Technological Commission. In February 1993, China Academy of Chinese Medical Sciences decided to take Guangxi Institute for Ethnic Medicine as its research base for ethnic medicine, and endowed the institute with the title "Guangxi Institute for Ethnic Medicine under China Academy of Chinese Medical Sciences".

In the second half of 1986, Health Department of Guangxi Zhuang Autonomous Region set up a leading group for general investigation and organization of ancient books on ethnic medicine. More than 200 personnel in Guangxi were transferred to make up a professional investigation team. And the investigation members spent six years collecting and arranging a large quantity of Zhuang medical literatures distributed in local chronicles, books of natural history, historical records (including official and unofficial history), works of traditional Chinese history and other relevant materials (e.g., about ethnic minorities, folklore and archeology), registering thousands of folk practitioners of Zhuang medicine, and compiling and collecting a great many of private proven prescriptions, secret prescriptions and drug samples.

After working tirelessly and painstakingly on detailed literature collection, extensive and in-depth field study, and analysis of hundreds of types of local chronicles and other relevant Chinese materials, scientific researchers aggregated many written materials recording Zhuang medicine, collected thousands of proven prescriptions and secret prescriptions of Zhuang medicine, investigated and sorted out a variety of unique and effective methods of diagnosis and treatment applied by practitioners of Zhuang medicine, acquired cultural relics and manuscripts about Zhuang medicine, and registered more than 3,000 highly-skilled famous Zhuang doctors. From these, a great number of papers and monographs on Zhuang medicine were published. Among those articles are *Investigation Report on the Folk Medicine of Zhuang in Jingxi County*, *Preliminary Discussion on the Medical History of the Zhuang Nationality*, *Primary Investigation on the Origin of Zhuang Medicine*, *Study on the Zhuang Ancestors' Usage of Microneedle*, *Physical Geography of Guangxi and Zhuang Medicine*, *Ethnic Medicine of Guangxi under the Native Chieftain System*, *Brief Introduction to the Theoretical System of Zhuang Medicine*, *Discussion on the Specific Application of Theory of "Sandao Lianglu" in Zhuang Medicine*. Published monographs include: *Investigation and Organization of Zhuang Medicine*, *Compilation of Proven Prescriptions of Ethnic Medicine in Guangxi*, *Compilation of Selected Zhuang Medicine*, *New Zhuang Medicinal Resources in Guangxi*, *Medical History of the Zhuang Nationality* and *Zhuang Medicine in China*. In Guangxi University of Chinese Medicine and Guangxi Institute for Ethnic Medicine, researchers have used traditional and modern methods to investigate, organize and study Zhuang medicated thread moxibustion and Zhuang cupping. With significant achievements, they applied and rolled out moxibustion and cupping into clinical practice step by step. In May 1995, researchers of Guangxi Institute for Ethnic Medicine presented a report on *Preliminary Discussion on the Basic Theories of Zhuang Medicine*, at the National Academic Seminar for Ethnic Medicine in Nanning approved by State Administration of Traditional Chinese Medicine. The theoretical system of Zhuang medicine, including "synchrony of triple initial qi" "Sandao lianglu" and "pathogenicity of toxin and deficiency", was elaborated and discussed comprehensively and systematically in the report which was based on years of investigation. It was a sign that the investigation, organization and study of Zhuang medicine had overall been raised to a new level.

With over 30 years of efforts, there have been remarkable results of Zhuang medicine in many aspects, for example investigation and organization of ancient books, establishment of theoretical system, study on methods of diagnosis and treatment, research of medicine, and clinical application and roll-out. Meanwhile, the ancient Zhuang medical culture has been enriched and is evolving, as a result of the integrated process of utilizing historical accumulation and absorbing the essence of advanced cultures through the development of research into the relationship between Zhuang culture and Zhuang medicine, the value, development and utilization of Zhuang medical culture and other respects.

References:

[1] Liang Tingwang. An Introduction to Zhuang Culture [M]. Nanning: Guangxi Education Press, 2000.

[2] Guo Jianqing. An Introduction to Chinese Culture (2nd Edition) [M]. Shanghai: Shanghai Jiao Tong University Press, 2005.

[3] Huang Hanru, Huang Jingxian, Yin Zhaohong. Medical History of the Zhuang Nationality [M]. Nanning: Guangxi Science and Technology Press, 1998.

[4] Pang Yuzhou. Preliminary Discussion on the Concept and Connotation of Zhuang Medical Culture [J]. Chinese Journal of Ethnomedicine and Ethnopharmacy, 2007, 89 (6): 322 – 324.

[5] Pang Yuzhou, Wang Chunling. An Introduction to Zhuang Medical Culture [J]. Chinese Journal of Basic Medicine in Traditional Chinese Medicine, 2009, 15 (10): 800 – 802.

2　Features and Manifestations of Zhuang Medical Culture

2.1　Features of Zhuang medical culture

2.1.1　Long and glorious history

Zhuang medicine has a long and glorious history. As a native minority of the Zhuang region since ancient times, Zhuang ancestors lived in high mountains and lofty hills with plentiful rivers, vegetation and rainfall, frequently encountered miasmic malaria, and elusive poisonous insects and wild beasts. In the harsh natural environment and life conditions, they were forced to create primitive medical skills. As far as origin is concerned, medicine of Zhuang and other Chinese nationalities emerged simultaneously or successively.

Zhuang medical culture has been growing from nothing since ancient times. The Pre-Qin era witnessed its infancy; the period from Qin Dynasty to Sui Dynasty saw its practice and accumulation; the period from the Tang Dynasty and Song Dynasty to the era Republic of China demonstrated its formation and development; the time after the founding of the People's Republic of China witnessed its investigation, organization and improvement. Now it has been enriched and systematic throughout the long and splendid journey.

In different periods of history, it has had unique material and spiritual features, which have enriched the content of Zhuang culture and has been marked by traditional Zhuang culture.

2.1.2　Strong regional features

The social and historical development of Zhuang, as an integral part of the Chinese nation, is basically in tandem with that of the Han nationality in the Central Plains. However, because of the special geographical, political, economic and cultural circumstances, Zhuang has unique features in its social and historical development, which has had a great impact on the formation and development of Zhuang culture.

Zhuang has unique cultures. Take rice-farming as an example. With rice as the staple food for generations, Zhuang is one of the first nations to grow rice in the world and one of the first ethnic groups to create a rice planting civilization in China. In recent years, domestic and foreign scholars consider that Asian cultivated rice originated in the vast half-moon area from Hangzhou Bay in China to Assam in India, based on records and research on wild rice found in archeological materials and history books. Zhuang live in Lingnan with warm climate, plentiful rainfall, fertile land, rich water sources, which are all good for rice crop. Zhuang ancestors planted rice as early as 4000 years ago, as evidenced by millstones and stoneware in Shell Mound sites on Mount Yapu, Mount Malanju and Mount Beijiao in Fangchenggang City, Guangxi. In their long history of rice-farming, Zhuang discovered many solutions to issues in both grain production and development, and rice-farming culture, and these had an influence on its lifestyle and customs. To be more precise, rice-farming culture had a profound and lasting influence on the production, life, etiquette, national character and deep thought of Zhuang people.

As an important symbol of Zhuang culture, rice-farming culture is the base of Zhuang culture. It not only had a profound impact on Zhuang culture, but also endowed Zhuang medical culture with strong regional features. Rice takes root in the land, grows with the grace of heaven, and benefits human beings. Rice-farming culture brought Zhuang ancestors an early recognition of yin and yang, and gave rise to concepts of yin and yang. According to the record of *Volume 17*, *Guangxi Local Records* in the Ming Dynasty, Zhuang people sincerely believed in yin and yang. Paddy field is called "naz" in Zhuang language, so rice-farming culture is also referred to as "naz" culture. The "naz" is divided into at least three horizontal and two vertical rows, which gave a basic framework to the theory of "Sandao lianglu" (three paths and two roads) in Zhuang medicine. In daily life, Zhuang ancestors noticed that rice grows naturally with the blessing of heaven and earth qi, and that rice nourishes the body with heaven and earth qi within them. Humans live on "cereals", which are a necessary part of meals. Therefore the tract taking cereals inside the body and enabling digestion and absorption is called "Gudao" ("diuzgwnngaiz" in Zhuang language, literally cereal tract). Rice needs to be nourished by qi and water from heaven and earth, and the human body needs to exchange qi and water with heaven and earth through tracts, which are called "Qidao" ("diuzlohheiq" in Zhuang language) and

"Shuidao" ("diuzlohraemx" in Zhuang language). Rice-farming culture cannot do without water and fire. Zhuang ancestors worshipped dragon (long in Chinese) and believed it could control water. The human body also has a tract for blood circulation, which is therefore called "Longlu" ("lohlungz" in Zhuang language) in Zhuang medicine. Fire (huo in Chinese), as a trigger, is quick in nature (fire usually means quick in Chinese words). The human body has the tract for information sensing, which is like fire in nature and that is called "Huolu" ("lohfeiz" in Zhuang language) in Zhuang medicine. The theory of "Sandao lianglu" in Zhuang medicine is derived from Zhuang ancestors' basic understanding of humanity and nature and accumulation of practical experience.

Not only rice-farming culture has endowed Zhuang medical theories with strong regional features, other Zhuang cultures such as Zhuang customs, ballads, festivals, food, dwelling and sports also provide medical and sanitary values with strong regional ethnic characteristics. For example, in Zhuang food culture, it is a custom for Zhuang people in northwest Guangxi to have sheep offal soup and fresh sheep blood. It is hard for strangers to swallow them, but they are rare healthy delicacies for local Zhuang people as sheep offal soup can clear heat and nourish the stomach, and fresh sheep blood can tonify deficiency and make the body strong.

2.1.3 Rich medical connotation

2.1.3.1 The plain man-nature theory

Zhuang ancestors formed the unique man-nature theory over the long-term medical practice. Zhuang medicine divides the space of the natural world into three parts—the upper, middle and lower part as "heaven, earth and human", and the qi of the three parts is synchronized. The human body is also divided into three parts — the upper part as heaven ("gyaeuj" in Zhuang language), the lower part as earth ("dungx" in Zhuang language) and the middle part as human ("ndang" in Zhuang language). The qi of the three parts of the human body is also synchronized. Physiologically, humans can keep healthy only when the heaven, earth and human parts of the body, and the natural world interact with each other, move synchronously, and emerge naturally; pathologically, all kinds of diseases and ailments will break out if the heaven, earth and human qi do not move in synchrony. Actually, both the man-nature theory in Zhuang medicine and the unity of man and nature in TCM belong to the category of "holism", while Zhuang medicine focuses more on the equilibrium among human, nature and all parts of the body, and regards "asynchrony of heaven, earth and human qi" as an important aspect of pathogenesis.

2. 1. 3. 2 Unique physiological and pathological theories

(1) Theory of "yin-yang basis". It is believed in Zhuang medicine that all things fall into the categories of yin and yang and that all changes are due to yin and yang, which is the theory of "yin-yang basis". Yin and yang are widely used by Zhuang ancestors in production and life to explain the relationship between nature and humans as well as the body's physiology and pathology. For example, in the natural world, heaven is yang, and earth is yin; daytime is yang, and night is yin; fire is yang, and water is yin. In the human body, the back is yang, and the abdomen is yin; the exterior is yang, and the interior is yin. And in terms of diseases, there are yin syndromes and yang syndromes. Therefore, it is believed in Zhuang medicine that all changes in the natural world are the results of yin and yang changes, so are all physiological and pathological changes in the human body, and so are the changes of states of illnesses. In *Illustrations of Acupuncture for Sha Diseases*, attributed to famous Zhuang doctor Luo Jia'an, exuberant yin and declined yang, exuberant yang and declined yin and exuberant yin and yang are used as the general principles of pattern identification in classifying sha diseases.

(2) Theory of synchrony of triple qi. Synchrony of triple qi means only when the triple qi (heaven, earth and human qi) moves harmoniously and steadily can the human body maintain the best state of being. "Heaven" is referred to as heaven qi, "earth" as earth qi, and these two make up the qi of the natural world. "Triple qi" means heaven, earth and human qi, and synchrony means maintenance of harmony and balance. Synchrony of triple qi means the harmony and balance among heaven, earth and human. The connotation of "synchrony of triple qi" includes: human beings, growing with the blessing of heaven and earth qi, are the wisest of all creatures; the human life cycle is nourished and constrained by the ever-changing heaven and earth qi, and human qi and heaven and earth qi are interlinked; heaven and earth qi has created "rules" for human survival and health; humans are a finite microcosm; the unity of the body's structure and function, and the harmony of congenital qi and acquired qi, enable the body to adapt, defend and consequently maintain health with the synchrony of triple qi. The synchrony of triple qi has formed the physiological and pathological views of Zhuang medicine and becomes one of its important theoretical foundations for diagnoses and treatment.

(3) Theory of "Sandao lianglu". Sandao means Gudao, Qidao and Shuidao. They are tracts for the generation, storage and circulation of nutriments maintaining vital activities within the body, and are also tracts for the excretion and distribution of waste matter. Lianglu means Longlu and Huolu. They are two extremely important close-ended tracts inside the body, which are not directly connected to nature, but are able to maintain the body's vitality and reflect the dynamic of diseases. In "Sandao lianglu", Gudao is the tract for the digestion and absorption of food, the distribution of nutriments, and the excretion of waste matter; Qidao is the place for the generation, distribution and storage of human qi; Shuidao is the place for the generation, storage, distribution and circulation of body water; Longlu is the place for restricted blood circulation with the heart ("simdaeuz" in Zhuang language) as its pivot, and its main function is to supply the internal organs, bones, flesh, the five sense organs and orifices with nutriments; and Huolu is the tract for information sensing, so as to maintain a balance between the environments inside and outside the body, and to regulate physiological equilibrium. "Sandao lianglu" perform their own functions cooperatively. Physiologically, they are interlinked with each other and work in coordination. Pathologically, they influence each other through transmission and change.

(4) Understanding of zang and fu organs, qi, blood, bone, flesh and brain. In Zhuang medicine, it is believed that zang and fu organs, qi, blood, bone and flesh are the material bases of the body. Relatively independent entities within the cranium, thoracic cavity and abdominal cavity are called zang and fu organs. Zang and fu organs have different physiological functions, roles and objects to govern in the life process. Qi ("heiq" in Zhuang language) is power and function, as well as the manifestation of the body's life force. Blood ("lwed" in Zhuang language) is an extremely important substance that nourishes the whole body including bones, flesh and zang and fu organs. The locomotive organs — bones ("ndok" in Zhuang language) and flesh ("noh" in Zhuang language), constituting the body's frame and form, normally protect organs within the body from exterior injury. The body's Gudao, Qidao, Shuidao, Longlu and Huolu work within them. The injury of bones and flesh can potentially lead to the damage of important tracts within the body, and other diseases. In Zhuang medicine, it is believed that mental activities, linguistic competence and thinking capacity are the functions of the brain ("ukgyaeuj" in Zhuang language). "Ukgyaeuj", governing spiritual thinking, is the place for marrow aggregation, where the essence and mind get together. In Zhuang medicine, the psychiatric symptoms of psychosis are

called "ukgyaeuj luenh".

2. 1. 3. 3　Distinctive etiological and pathogenetic theories

It is believed in Zhuang medicine that toxin and deficiency are important etiology and pathogenesis that damage the human body and cause diseases. "Pathogenicity of toxin and deficiency" is the major etiological and pathogenetic theory of Zhuang medicine. In the broad sense, toxic factors are used as an umbrella term for all pathogenic factors. However, in the narrow sense, they refer to the pathogenic substances showing toxic effects on the human body. A wide range of toxic factors generally have similar pathogenesis. Some of them may cause flesh wound or affect the functions of zang and fu organs and "Sandao lianglu". Some of them show acute toxicity, and people who suffer from them will immediately fall ill and even die. Some show chronic toxicity and their adverse effects occur slowly. Toxic factors cause diseases by damaging healthy qi, functions of zang and fu organs or the body. There are a variety of typical clinical symptoms and signs due to the different properties of different toxic factors.

Deficiency, a cause of diseases, is also a pathological result and morbid manifestation. Zhuang medicine pays extra attention to the important role of "deficiency" in etiology and pathogenesis. As a cause of disease, deficiency can lead to the hypofunction of zang and fu organs, and a decline in the ability to defend against external pathogenic factors, and then deficiency and toxin coexist, they pathologically manifest a vicious circle through their interaction. If healthy qi is insufficient, the body's adaptive and regulating abilities will decrease, and the body comes prone to react violently to external emotional stimulation, which will cause emotional diseases. As a pathological result, deficiency can cause not only diseases but also death. Deficiency of healthy qi causes diseases as "pathogenic qi" grows inside the body. To be more precise, the body will be less able to regulate the functions and activities of zang and fu organs, the five sense organs and orifices, and these disorders will generate pathological products and cause diseases. People will possibly die when they lose the ability to regulate the body because of the severe deficiency of healthy qi.

In Zhuang medicine, it is believed that toxin and deficiency, as major causes of diseases, turn the body from normal state into diseased state. The body can recover to the normal state with illnesses cured if it receives appropriate treatment or defeats pathogenic toxin and deficiency through its self-defense and self-healing capabilities. Otherwise, the asynchrony of triple initial qi will cause qi collapse, qi exhaustion and death.

2. 1. 3. 4 Distinctive methods for disease diagnosis and identifying

Zhuang medicine attaches great importance to the eyes ("lwgda" in Zhuang language), and it is believed that the eyes are the body's windows endowed by nature; eyes are light bringers and the essence of heaven, earth and human qi. The eyes, in which the essence of zang and fu organs concentrates, are all-embracing and insightful, reflecting various diseases. In Zhuang medicine, inspection of the eyes is of great importance in disease diagnosis because we have eyes on the head ("ukgyaeuj" in Zhuang language) and they are directly controlled by the head. In Zhuang medicine, inspection of the eyes means diagnosing diseases throughout the body by observing subtle vascular changes in patients' eyes, such as the distribution, trend, size, color, tortuosity and spot of blood vessel. That is so-called "yi mu liao ran" (a Chinese idiom meaning "obvious at a glance"). We can make a definite diagnosis, predict prognosis and confirm death by the inspection of the eyes. For example, we can obtain relatively accurate information about the functions of zang and fu organs, "Sandao lianglu" and "ukgyaeuj" by inspecting the eyes. Zhuang medicine values inspection of the eyes but also recognizes other diagnostic methods, many of which are characteristic, for example inquiry, listening and smelling examination, feeling of pulse, inspection of nail, inspection of finger and abdominal palpation.

Zhuang medicine focuses on disease differentiation. There are hundreds of names of syndrome collected through documentary records and field investigation, and many of them are strongly influenced by regional local minorities in Lingnan. Internal medical diseases can be summarized as follows: sha (filthy-attack diseases caused by spotted qi), miasmic malaria, parasitic tympanites, toxin, wind syndrome and dampness. Disease differentiation in Zhuang medicine is similar to that in Western medicine, therefore specific diseases are treated with specific prescriptions and medications in Zhuang medicine, and therapeutic principles and prescription selection are mainly determined by disease differentiation.

2. 1. 3. 5 Therapeutic principles as effective guides to practice

According to the understanding of the body's physiology, pathology, etiology and pathogenesis, Zhuang medicine has formed the therapeutic principle of "regulating qi, removing toxin and rectifying deficiency", which is an effective guide to clinical practice.

Regulating qi means making human qi work well and synchronizing it with heaven and earth qi by regulating, stimulating or unblocking qi by specific therapeutic methods （mostly non-pharmaceutical therapies, such as acupuncture, pricking blood, cupping, dancing and Qigong— literally "life energy cultivation"). The clinical manifestations of Qi diseases are pain and other functional diseases, which can be cured with acupuncture, pricking blood, cupping and qi regulation through medicine.

Removing toxin means synchronizing triple initial qi and curing diseases by reducing toxic factors coming into the body, promoting the excretion of poisonous substances or dissolving toxin within the body through medicine for internal and external use. The clinical manifestations of toxic diseases are acute inflammation and pathologic and functional changes of organs, for example inflammation, thermalgia, ulceration, tumor, sore and furuncle, jaundice and blood disease. Some toxic materials can be dissolved within the body or eliminated via "Sandao" through treatment with and without medicine. Human body can restore healthy qi and recover by removing toxin.

Tonifying deficiency means supplementing insufficient qi and blood and regulating unbalanced triple initial qi within the body through orally administered medicine or dietotherapy, so that the body's triple initial qi can work well and human qi can be kept harmonious with heaven qi and human qi. The clinical manifestations of deficiency are common in chronic and senile diseases, and during the recovery phase after removing pathogenic toxin. Tonifying deficiency should be a top priority for these diseases. In Zhuang medicine, great importance is attached to dietotherapy and animal medicine. It is believed that human should let nature take its course, and dietotherapy is a common and natural way to tonify deficiency. Human beings are miracles and like attracts like. So it is believed in Zhuang medicine that the most effective way to tonify deficiency is to use animal medicine, as animals have flesh, blood and emotions like human beings.

2. 1. 3. 6 Rich medicinal knowledge, practice of drug usage and creative combination of medicines

In Zhuang medicine, it is believed that the therapeutic effects of Zhuang medicines are brought into play by regulating abnormal exuberance of yin or yang, asynchronized triple initial qi, obstructed "Sandao lianglu" and other pathological conditions through natures and flavors of medicines. There are animal, herbal and mineral medicine. According to their action, medicines can be categorized as toxic, detoxicating, heat-clearing, tonifying, antirheumatic and vermifugal medicines, drugs for miasmic malaria, trauma and sha diseases, and so on. There are a great variety of medicines and poisonous animals and plants in the Zhuang region. In the long-term practice, Zhuang people have bravely used local toxic medicines to treat diseases, have accumulated rich experience, and have formed unique theory of toxic medicine application. Also, detoxicating drugs are used skillfully in Zhuang medicine. It is believed that pathogenic toxin can be eliminated through corresponding detoxicating drugs, namely "everything has its vanquisher".

There is plentiful lush and evergreen vegetation in the Zhuang region, so the custom of using fresh herbs has been developed in Zhuang medicine. In the long-term medication practice, it was found in Zhuang medicine that the combination of one drug with other drugs can produce better therapeutic effect. Through generations of accumulation, ingenious methods for combination of medicines and prescription have been gradually developed. Zhuang medicine considers that there are only two syndromes — yin syndrome and yang syndrome. In Zhuang prescriptions, male drugs are for yin syndrome and female drugs are for yang syndrome. It is required by Zhuang medicine that combination of medicines be simple, convenient, inexpensive and proven. A prescription comprises principal, auxiliary, messenger and detoxicating drugs, which are compatible and combined in order of importance with specific actions. Generally one prescription consists of four or five drugs, but rarely more than ten.

2. 1. 3. 7　Special contribution to the formation and development of acupuncture

In the Neolithic Age, pottery needle therapy emerged with the development of ceramic culture in the Zhuang region. In the Warring States Period, it became popular and had a positive effect on the formation of "nine needles" in TCM. According to research on existing pottery needle in Zhuang medicine, it is similar to the first of nine needles — shear needle (chan zhen in Chinese). Even now it is still widely used by Zhuang people. Two exquisite bronze needles were unearthed in the Western Zhou Dynasty tomb in Matou Township, Wuming District, Nanning City. According to research, they are acupuncture apparatus used by Zhuang ancestors. As it is written in *Huangdi Neijing* (*Inner Canon of the Yellow Emperor*), "So, the therapy with nine kinds of needle also comes from the south." It suggests that the Zhuang region is one of the birthplaces of acupuncture therapy and nine needles. For two thousand years, Zhuang ancestors had high needle making techniques, and overall, their acupuncture therapy and medical level were advanced for the time.

2.1.4 Colorful medical customs

2.1.4.1 Hygiene practice

(1) Close-cropped hair. According to *Xiaoyaoyou*, *Inner Chapters*, *Zhuangzi*, "A man in the State of Song purchased hats and sold them in the State of Yue. But hats were useless for Yue people because they liked cutting the hair and tattooing the body". That means Yue people had the hair clipped short and they were free from Shufa and Jiaguan (tying the hair and wearing a hat). In *Treatise on Geography*, *Book of Han*, it is recorded that it was a custom for Yue people, from Wuyue to Nine Prefectures of Lingnan, to "have the hair clipped short". From the cliff painting portraits of the Huashan Mountains in Ningming, Guangxi, it can be seen that Zhuang ancestors — Luoyue people — had the hair clipped short. Whatever the reason for doing this was, it was still a good sanitary practice to cut the hair, considering that short hair dried fast and promoted cooling of the human body in the damp and hot climate of Luoyue region.

(2) Dressing in blue black. Zhuang developed the habits of cotton planting and spinning. "Jiaji" is the cloth woven with the homespun yarn made of home-grown cotton. Indigo is a dye preferred by ancient and modern Zhuang people. They get their traditional costumes dyed black or blue, with black as the dominant hue. Even now that dominant hue still can be seen in Zhuang groups in Napo County, Longzhou County and other places, for example Black-clothes Zhuang inhabiting Napo County in Baise City, and Zhuang people calling themselves "Budai" in Jinlong, Longzhou County, Chongzuo City. It is recorded that indigo is a dye refined from leaves of plants such as Songlan or Caodaqing (*Isatis indigotica* Fortune), or Mulan (*Indigofera tinctoria* Linn.), or Malan [*Baphicacanthus cusia* (Nees) Bremek.], or Liaolan (*Polygonum tinctorium* Ait.), family Cruciferae, Leguminosae, Acanthaceae or Polygonaceae. Indigo can clear heat and remove toxin. Therefore, blue and black Zhuang costumes fit the climate and environment in the Zhuang region as they have the actions of removing toxin and repelling mosquitoes and other insects.

(3) Living in ganlan houses. Based on the geographical environment and climate conditions in the Zhuang region, Zhuang people invented ganlan houses very early. The ganlan houses are characterized by two floors, with the upper layer for human habitation and the lower layer for storing farm implements or rearing livestock. *Liaoren Chapter*, *Book of Wei* says, "Liao possibly belongs to an ethnic group of Nan-

man (Southern Barbarians)... They pile up wood against trees and live aloft in the so-called ganlan." High off the ground, ganlan houses can avoid tigers, wolves, snakes, insects, toxic factors and miasma. To seperate humans from livestock, ganlan houses are also a hygiene practice. Many Zhuang-inhabited areas carry on that residential custom.

2.1.4.2 Customs of sorcery and ancestor worship

(1) Sorcery. Sorcery was a key activity of primitive religions. During the Pre-Qin Period, Luoyue people worshipped sorcery, ghosts and gods. Zhuang ancestors' belief in ghosts and gods gave rise to sorcery culture. In ancient times, Zhuang sorcerers were divided by gender — female sorcerers and male sorcerers. When there was sickness or disaster in the host family, the host would invite female sorcerers to ask immortals about the causes of the sickness or disaster. Then the host would pick an auspicious day to invite male sorcerers to carry out religious rites, where animals were killed for worship, immortals were urged to depart, people prayed for the ending of the disaster, and male sorcerers brandished swords, heated up a pot with oil, and drove away evil spirits. In modern times, witchery remains in the Zhuang region. In terms of the influence of sorcery culture on Zhuang medicine, they were one and the same in the beginning, then they coexisted, and finally Zhuang medicine prevailed.

(2) Tattoos. Tattooing is a custom of Zhuang ancestors as early as the prehistoric society. As it is written in *Taiping Huanyu Ji* (*Universal Geography of the Taiping*) in the Song Dynasty, "people preferred forehead, face and body tattoos and tooth extraction" in zhous (prefectures) along the Zuojiang River and Youjiang River in Yongzhou. The custom of tattooing can be traced back to the totem images or signs of clans and tribes, and had the purpose of asking a blessing from the Totem God. Those totems can "avoid the harm of flood dragon" , and enable identification and distinction in communication and intermarriage. Tattooing provided a boost to the formation and development of shallow needling therapy in Zhuang medicine. Shallow needling was used for tattooing. And more importantly, tattooing was a religious activity, which motivated Zhuang people to follow.

(3) Bone-collecting reburial. "Secondary burial (bone-collecting reburial) " is still popular in the Zhuang region. In the third year after the death of family members, the offspring collect their bones, put them into a pottery urn ("guenq" in Zhuang language), and select another cemetery hill with good Fengshui for reburial. Bone-collecting reburial demonstrates Zhuang's ancestor worship and recognition of Fengshui of

cemetery hills. It also promoted the correct understanding of human skeleton in Zhuang medicine.

2. 1. 4. 3　Customs of disease prevention and healthcare

（1）Focus on prevention. Zhuang region is characterized by high mountains, thick forests, plentiful rainfall and severe heat. Zhuang people hold ginger in the mouth to repel foulness when they go out in the morning in the miasma, mist and dew. They shower with ginger and shallot decoction and drink it before it cools down to dispel cold and dampness after getting wet from rainstorms when farming. They use alum to settle water before drinking it, and eat fresh garlic to stop the growth of parasites and toxin inside the body in the rainy and hot summer. In plague season, they repel foulness and remove toxin by taking a shower with herb decoction after going back home. The old and infirm sleep on a mat covering things to repel foulness, remove toxin, relax sinew and activate collaterals. Growing children wear fragrant accessories for detoxification, on the chest or belly.

（2）Going to the drug fairs. There is a plentiful supply of evergreen vegetation and drug resources in the Zhuang region. On the fifth day of the fifth lunar month in each year, Zhuang village people go to the drug fairs in the market town, where they either sell a variety of medicinal materials they have picked, or browse, smell and buy medicine. In Zhuang folklore, lush herbs exhibit strong efficacy and the best therapeutic effect during this Dragon Boat Festival. When people go to the drug fairs on that day, they can absorb the qi of medicine, prevent diseases, and consequently fall ill as rarely as possible throughout the year. Over time, going to the drug fairs became a Zhuang custom, and the drug fairs of Jingxi City during the Dragon Boat Festival are most famous. Zhuang people go to the drug market to absorb the qi of medicine during the Dragon Boat Festival with all their family even though they have no medicine for sale. Drug fairs not only provide a great opportunity to exchange the know-ledge of medicinal materials and disease prevention and treatment, but also reflect Zhuang's emphasis on medicine.

（3）Hanging Ai （*Artemisiae argyi*） on the door. Hanging Ai and drinking Changpu （*Acorus calamus* L.） wine are key activities for Zhuang during the Dragon Boat Festival. *Annals of Jingxi Xian* records, "On the fifth day of the fifth lunar month, all families hang Ai and calamus leaves on the door, and drink Xionghuang （realgar） wine to dispel plague." Early on the morning of the fifth day of the fifth lunar month, Zhuang people pick Ai before the rooster crow. They shape Ai leaves and roots to resemble a human or tiger (commonly known as Ai tiger), and center them on the lintel. They also shape calamus leaves like swords and hang them under the roof. On that day, they also heat up water with Ai leaves, calamus and garlic in it. Then they shower with the water, and scatter it around the house. In fact, it is a good sanitary practice in the summer. The weather turns hot after the Dragon Boat Festival, and bacteria grow and multiply fast. Scattering water with Chinese medicinal herbs can effectively inhibit and kill bacteria and keep the environment clean. It is just like drinking calamus wine during the Dragon Boat Festival. Calamus, warm in nature, is able to resolve phlegm, dispel dampness, moisten lung and dispel wind-cold. It has an action of preventing external-contraction diseases in summer.

2. 1. 4. 4　Customs of plague and toxin prevention

(1) Wearing medicine accessories. Zhuang live in Lingnan, a subtropical zone. There are rolling hills, numerous rivers, thick forests and plentiful vegetation. Miasmic toxin emerges in the damp and hot air, together with rainy and humid climate. Miasmic toxin gives rise to "miasmic malaria", a common and frequently encountered disease in the Zhuang region at that time. *Biography of Ma Yuan*, *Book of the Later Han* says, "In an expedition to Jiaozhi, many soldiers suffered from miasmic malaria", and "About half the military officers died of miasmic malaria". It is thus clear that miasmic malaria does great damage. Zhuang ancestors accumulated characteristic methods for treating miasmic malaria. Every spring and summer, they bundled picked herbs and put them on the door or in the house to repel foulness and miasmic malaria. These common herbs were leaves of Changpu (*Acorus calamus* L.), Peilan (*Eupatorium fortunei* Turcz.), Ai (*Artemisiae argyi*), Qinghao (*Artemisia carvifolia*) and so on. Juveniles were asked to wear herbal sachets made from aromatic medicine, aiming at reinforcing healthy qi and repel miasmic malaria. Common fragrant herbs were Tanxiang (*Santalum album* L.), Cangzhu [*Atractylodes lancea* (Thunb.) DC.], Muxiang [*Sabina saltuaria* (Rehd. et Wils.) Cheng et W. T. Wang] and so on. In the season of miasmic malaria, all villagers — men and women, young and old — wore herbal sachets to repel pathogenic qi and miasmic malaria, so that people could prevent the disease or reduce the chances of getting in. Those customs of miasma prevention have been carried on till now.

(2) Nasal drinking. One method of nasal irrigation and aerosol inhalation has been handed down in the Zhuang region. Patients flush their nasal cavities with a decoction or inhale aerial fog produced by boiled herbs, so that some epidemic diseases

can be prevented. It was called "nasal drinking" in ancient times, and was handed down in Ancient Yue tribes, and recorded by many history books and annals. It can be found as early as *Yiwu Zhi* (*Record of Foreign Matters*) in the Han Dynasty, "Wu-hu is an alias of Nanman (Southern Barbarians). They live in a nest and drink through their noses." In *Lingwai Daida* (*Answer on Outer of the Five Ridges*), Zhou Qufei in the Song Dynasty elaborated on nasal drinking, "there is a custom of nasal drinking in the mountainous region where minorities dwelled in Yongzhou and villages in Qinzhou. Pour a small quantity of water in a ladle with an aperture, and add salt and several drops of Shanjiang [*Alpinia japonica* (Thunb.) Miq.] juice into it. Use a small tube, and insert it into the nose. Suck water into the head, and then it will flow into the throat ... Have a piece of preserved fish before nasal drinking, then you will not feel choked by water. Exhale after drinking water, and the head and dia-phragm will be cooled down, which is wonderful." The peculiar custom of healthcare contains scientific knowledge such as physical cooling and mucosal drug delivery, and it has certain therapeutic effects on nasal, laryngeal, and respiratory diseases.

(3) Chewing betel nuts. It is a prevailing custom to "serve guests with betel nuts instead of tea" in some Zhuang villages of Guangxi, such as Longzhou, Fangcheng-gang, Shangsi and Ningming. *Annals of Pingle Xian* says, "With miasma in the air, chewing betel nuts is just like enjoying a feast." Judging from the medicinal value of betel nuts, they can repel foulness, expel miasma, promote circulation of qi, excrete water, kill parasites and resolve accumulation. Prevention and treatment of miasmic malaria is one of the reasons why Zhuang chew betel nuts.

2.1.4.5　Customs of food and health preservation

(1) Diet for seasonal occasions. Zhuang have attached great importance to the diet for seasonal occasions since ancient times. For example, they pick Baitouweng (*Radix Pulsatilla*) and Aiye (*Folium Artemisiae argyi*) and use rice with them to make zongzi at the end of the first lunar month, and both Baitouweng and Aiye are common Zhuang medicines; they pick Jinyinhua (*Flos Lonicerae*), Aiye (*Folium Artemisiae argyi*) and other herbs to make ciba cakes on the third day of the third lunar month — it is said that it can ward off diseases and maintain health to have ciba cakes; they cook and eat black rice to dispel plague at the Buddha's Birthday Festival on the eighth day of the fourth lunar month; they drink Changpu (*Acorus calamus* L.) wine and Xionghuang (realgar) wine to dispel plague on the fifth day of the fifth lunar month. These customs stress both food nutrition and actions of medicine, in the spirit

of health preservation and healthcare in Zhuang medicine, and they are well received by Zhuang people.

(2) Medicated diet. In the long-term life practice, Zhuang developed many medicated diets containing food, medicine and spices, which can prevent and treat diseases, improve health and promote longevity. For example longhudou (made from snake and cat), longfenghui (made from snake and chicken), sanshe wine (made from cobra, krait and Chinese rat snake), fruit and sticky rice cake (made from milk, fruit and sticky rice), and huatuan cake (made from sticky rice, pumpkin flower, peanut, sesame and pork ribs). Fruit and sticky rice cake and huatuan cake are popular along the Youjiang River. In the Zhuang region, there are plentiful fresh herbs and animal medicine, which are frequently used to treat diseases. Zhuang believe animal medicine is effective as animals have flesh and blood as well as emotion. For example, the combination of goat meat, sparrow meat, fresh and tender Yimucao [*Leonurus artemisia* (Laur.) S. Y. Hu], black soybean can prevent and treat female sterility, snake soup and Wuyuan (Francois' leaf monkey) wine can prevent and treat intractable osteoarthrosis, and stewing lotus root with pork, old female duck, teal and partridge can prevent and treat exhaustion of yin and dry cough.

2.1.5 Obvious mark of cultural exchanges between Zhuang and Han

Zhuang minority belongs to the Chinese nation, and its culture was deeply influenced by Han culture. Unearthed cultural relics reveal that Han culture permeated Lingnan as early as the Pre-Qin Period. For example, the Shang Dynasty bronze wares in the Central Plains style unearthed in Mianling, Wuming, Guangxi; the Shang Dynasty bronze you with beast face Veins (wine vessel) unearthed in Xing'an Guilin; and the Shang Dynasty stone chimes in the Central Plains style unearthed in Dasi Town, Qinzhou. Those cultural relics reveal that the culture of the Central Plains influenced southern Guangxi as early as the Shang Dynasty, and that the cultural exchanges between Zhuang and Han can be dated back to the Pre-Qin Period. Zhuang absorbed the appropriate content of Han culture with the introduction of Chinese characters, establishment of schools, and dissemination of Confucianism, Taoism and other schools of thought. In the long historic course of social practice, Zhuang culture became superficially similar to Han culture, but maintained its own features in the deep structures such as thoughts and ideas.

The cultural exchanges between Zhuang and Han greatly influenced the formation and development of Zhuang medical culture. Some ancient books of the Pre-Qin Period recorded the medical practice of Zhuang ancestors in the early days. Existing materials suggest that the records of Zhuang medicine began in the Han Dynasty, and more and more records can be seen in the successive dynasties. It's recorded that medical scientists (e. g., Ge Hong in the Jin Dynasty), non-hereditary officers (e. g., Liu Zongyuan in the Tang Dynasty) and scholars disseminated TCM to the Zhuang region. In the first year of Emperor Xianping of Song Dynasty, Chen Yaosou, the transportation officer of Guangxi, compiled *Jiyanfang* (*Collected Prescription*) and asked stonemasons to carve it on the stones along the vital communication line of Guilin; Fan Min, the zhifu (prefect) of Yongzhou, issued a decree to ban excessive religious activities, used his own salary to purchase drugs for local people, and asked stonemasons to carve books of prescriptions on the hall walls of yamen. *Compendium of Materia Medica*, compiled by Li Shizhen in the Ming Dynasty, is a great work in medical science with rich and extensive content. It has recorded herbs used by Zhuang in the Lingnan region, among which Tianqi [*Panax pseudoginseng* Wall. var. *notoginseng* (Burkill) Hoo et Tseng] is the most prominent rare drug developed and applied by Zhuang people. In the long-term interaction and cultural exchanges between Zhuang and Han, vast quantities of actual data of Zhuang medicine have been presented in the forms of literature (written in Chinese characters) and cultural relics.

Zhuang inhabit subtropics with high average temperature and four distinct seasons. The sun and the moon move back and forth with the changing of night and day as well as the changing of seasons. Those natural phenomena gave rise to the yin and yang concept in the Zhuang nationality very early, and that concept is widely applied in their production and life under the cultural influence of the Han nationality in the Central Plains. The yin and yang concept was also applied to Zhuang medicine and gave rise to a fundamental philosophy — "yin-yang basis". It is an argument for explaining the complex relationship between nature and the body's etiology and pathogenesis.

2.2　Manifestations of Zhuang medical culture

As the combined result of Zhuang medicine and traditional Zhuang cultures, Zhuang medical culture is colorful and diverse. We can see part of it in both material and non-material forms, in seemingly unrelated things, such as medicated thread, bone bow, drug hammer and other therapeutic utensils. However, most of it is implied in other cultural groups in the form of myth, customs, folk songs, drug fairs and so on. More precisely, Zhuang medical culture can be categorized as cultures of material, myth, witch doctor, symbol, oral inheritance, custom, ballad, medicinal food, reproduction and sports.

2.2.1 Material culture

Material culture is the sum of all activities in material production and their products formed in the long-term human activities of transformation to the objective world. It has physical forms and it is perceptible, tangible and visible. Therapeutic tools and methods were gradually formed in the long journey of Zhuang medicine. There are many material cultural things including stone tablet, bone artifact, bone needle and pottery in the primitive society, bronze needle and silver needle in the Pre-Qin Period and Han Dynasty. Besides, those Zhuang medical tools (e. g. needle, medicated thread, ox horn, bamboo jar and drug hammer) and therapeutic methods (e.g. fumigating aud steaming, washing, paste applicatim, wearing herbal sacbets, scrapping with animal bone and egg rolling) are still widely used currently. *Ou Xifan's Five Zang Organ Painting* in the Northern Song Dynasty drew the human body's internal organs, it is the first recorded realistic anatomical drawing of the human body in Chinese medical history, as well as a landmark object atlas in the history of Zhuang medicine. Zhuang live in Lingnan, a subtropical zone with plentiful drug resources. Many Zhuang medicines were developed and applied early, and some of them became famous Chinese medicines. Among the 365 types of medicines recorded in *Classic of Herbal Medicine*, there are many specialties of the Zhuang region, such as Jungui (root of *Cinnamomum cassia* Presl), Mugui (bark of *Cinnamomum cassia* Presl), Yiyiren (*Semen Coicis*), cinnabar and stalactite. The Zhuang region is home to many rare medicinal materials, for example Tianqi [*Panax pseudoginseng* Wall. var. *notoginseng* (Burkill) Hoo et Tseng], Rougui (*Cinnamomum cassia* Presl), Bajiaohuixiang (*Illicium verum* Hook. f.), Yiyiren (*Semen coicis*), Luohanguo [*Siraitia grosvenorii* (Swingle)], Zhenzhu (*Margarita*) and Gejie (*Gecko*). In particular, Tianqi is a famous Zhuang medicine produced chiefly in Tianyang, Tiandong, Napo, Debao, Jingxi areas in Baise City of Guangxi, and it is one of the important contributions of Zhuang to both Chinese and global traditional medicine. The above-mentioned Zhuang medical tools therapeutic methods and medicinal materials all have the attributes of material objects and belong to the primary forms of material culture in Zhuang medicine.

2.2.2　Culture of myth

Myths, as cultural treasures of all nations, are ancient people's imagination and fantasies of the origins of the world, natural phenomena and social conditions. We can see the early culture of a nation from deep inside its myths and legends, which underlie the national spirit and turn into collective unconsciousness, and have a profound influence on the overall cultural development in the course of history. The legend of the miracle-working doctor Sanjiegong (literally the Lord of the Three Realms) is popular in the Zhuang region, and it represents the medicine-related myth culture of the Zhuang nationality. It is said that the legendary Sanjiegong is the reincarnation of a fairy child. He met an immortal in the mountain, who gave him a colorful ribbon, a fairy wand, a fairy peach and a magic weapon — a book with golden text. He ate the fairy peach and became a miracle-working doctor who worked amongst the poor. He wrapped the wounded part of a patient's body with the colorful ribbon, and tapped the wounded part three times with the fairy wand, then fracture or crippled patients could run, those with edema could recuperate, and those with years of blindness could see again. During the prevalence of plague, Sanjiegong distributed Quwenling formulations to fellow villagers without asking for money. As the medicine took effect, villagers were cured and they deeply respected him. Many "Sanjie Temples" were built in the Zhuang region in memory of this miracle-working doctor. People went there to pray for his blessings as well as the removal of ill fortune and illness. Even now there is still one Sanjie Temple built in the Qing Dynasty, with continuously burning incense, near the site of Tusi yamen (administrative office of a local bureaucrat in imperial China) in Xincheng County, Guangxi. The legend of the miracle-working doctor Sanjiegong gives a vivid description of Zhuang's pursuit of the true, the good and the beautiful, and has become an important carrier for the expression of Zhuang's thoughts of disease prevention and treatment.

2.2.3　Culture of witch doctor

In human culture, sorcery is the earliest attempt to conquer nature. The phenomenon of witch doctor, originated in ancient times, is a component of human culture, and it plays an important role in spawning and developing traditional medicine. Witch doctor and priest-doctor are the occupations that almost all nations in the world had in the early days. The culture of witch doctor has existed in the Zhuang region since ancient times. Zhuang ancestors could not understand natural phenomena, and they imagined that there could be mighty and mysterious gods behind those natural phenomena. From the knowledge of animism, they deduced that there were mysterious relationships between humans, human behavior and nature. Many documentary records show that Zhuang ancestors attached great importance to sorcery. In the Han Dynasty, the fashion of Yue sorcery caused a sensation throughout the capital. Kuang Lu in the Ming Dynasty wrote in *Chiya*, "In the second year of Emperor Yuanfeng of Han (in 109 BC), Yue sorcerers came after Yue was pacified. They were asked to worship gods and ghosts and practiced divination with chicken bones in worship activities, where there was a sea of necromancers and Confucians. When the emperor tried to solve national affairs, he preferred foreign rituals to traditional turtle-shell divination. Courtiers did not dare to express open admonition. So foreign rituals were well worth seeing." It is thus clear that the sorcery culture of Zhuang had a far-reaching influence. In the Qing Dynasty, there was still a fashion of sorcery in part of the Zhuang region in South China, where there remains the custom of sorcery right up to the modern age. Even now, some urban and rural people in Guangxi still use a spell to treat the night crying of children. They write on the incantation, "Dear gods of heaven and earth, there is a King of Night Cry in my house. Dear bypassers, please read out my words, then my little baby can sleep for the whole night." Then they throw the charm at the junction or paste it on the roadside tree trunk, telegraph pole or wall, and they believe that their baby will stop the night crying as soon as the bypassers read it out. It is an illustration of the culture of witch doctor. We can see details of how witch doctors treated diseases in *Miscellaneous Review*, *Lingbiao Jiman* (*Records of the Barbarians of Lingnan*) by Liu Xifan, "The barbarians use herbs to treat trauma, carbuncle and all other diseases requiring surgery. It is often effective, but they also treat those diseases through superstitious activities." He witnessed the treatment and wrote, "I have seen a patient with carbuncle invite a Zhuang fellow to treat him. When the Zhuang fellow came, he asked the patient's family to place in the hall a rooster, a ten-cent silver coin, water and rice. The performer put the ten-cent silver coin into a bag, took off his straw sandals, placed them on the ground, got some water and cast a spell. Then he sprayed water onto the wound, and cut it with a knife, then pus and blood flowed out, but the patient felt no pain. When the pus was drained, topical application of drugs would cure the patient." There is a close relationship between Zhuang medicine and sorcery. Isogeny and coexistence of medicine and sorcery are features of the journey of Zhuang medicine. It was very common to dispel pathogenic factors and treat diseases with sorcery in the history of Zhuang society. From the standpoint of medical advance, witchcraft medicine really hindered the development of Zhuang medicine. However, from the standpoint of historical materialism and dialectical materialism, witchcraft medicine is irreplaceable history in the emergence and development of Zhuang medicine.

2.2.4　Culture of symbol

A symbol is a sign with implication or symbolism. The German philosopher Cassirer said in *An Essay on Human*, "The human is a symbolic animal." A symbol is a conventional referent and a tool for thought expression for humans. The creation of symbols is related to cultural implication. People can understand or spread the information, emotion or attitude behind a symbol through interaction in their life. Namely, symbols are able to reflect the relatively stable ways of thinking, values and emotional appeals of an ethnic group in certain space and time. Every type of symbol system composed of instrumental symbols has special significance. Symbol creation, to some extent, means cultural creation. In the Zuojiang basin in Guangxi, numerous giant mural paintings with raw brushwork and austere beauty were found. Among them, the huge scale of the cliff paintings of the Huashan Mountains in Ningming County is second to none in China and rare throughout the world. According to research, those cliff paintings were made by Ouluo ancestors during the Pre-Qin Period. In terms of the cultural connotation of those cliff paintings, one idea is that they are charts of kung fu movements drawn by Zhuang doctors for disease prevention and health improvement. Ancient Zhuang medicine features methods for disease prevention and treatment, such as dancing, Tao Yin exercises, and Qigong. Some scholars have ranked those cliff paintings, jade pendants bearing Qigong inscription during the Spring and Autumn Period and the Warring States Period, and silk paintings of Tao Yin exercises in the Mawangdui Han Dynasty tomb in Changsha as the top three cultural relics of Qigong in China. Those cliff paintings on Huashan Mountains portray how ancient Zhuang people fought against diseases, and reveal the unique style and connotation of Zhuang medical culture.

2.2.5 Culture of oral inheritance

The interpretations of "koubei (oral inheritance or word of mouth)" can refer to in *Great Ancient Chinese Dictionary*, *Ciyuan* (*Chinese Etymology Dictionary*), *Great Chinese Dictionary*, and other reference books. The relatively explanation is that it is a metaphor for public oral praise. In addition, it also refers to public discussion, oral tradition and popular words in the society. Xie Aize, from Guangxi Hospital of Zhuang Medicine, considers "koubei" as "things taught orally (including things handed down in a family or succeeded from a master to his disciples) from generation to generation without cultural records". Zhuang medical material in the form of oral inheritance refers to Zhuang medical knowledge handed down orally through ethnic language. Zhuang's experience in folk medicine has survived thousands of years and remained with us till now, mainly because of the rich material inherited orally among Zhuang people. The material comes from doctor's records of their personal experiences, as well as oral narratives. For example, Luole (*Ocimum basilicum* L.), Foshou (*Citrus medica* L. var. *sarcodactylis* Swingle) and Jiulixiang (*Murraya exotica* L.) can treat abdominal pain and abdominal distension; Xiaohuixiang [*Schizonepeta tenuifolia* (Benth.) Briq.] and Shuitianqi (Lobedfruit Schizocapsa Rhizome) can treat stomachache; Huajiao (*Zanthoxylum bungeanum* Maxim.) and dried ginger can treat stomach cold; Root of Molihua (*Jasminum sambac* (L.) Ait.) and Xiangfuzi (*Cyperus rotundus* L.) can treat trauma and sprain and relieve pain. Some orally inherited Zhuang medical material usage spreads widely among Zhuang doctors, and it is inherited as a common sense among common people from generation to generation. For example, it is common knowledge in the Zhuang region to treat malaria with Banjiuzhan (*Premna ligustroides* Hemsl.), and they know Tianjihuang [*Grangea maderaspatana* (L.) Poir.)], Jigucao (*Abrus cantoniensis* Hance), Huanghuadaoshuilian (*Polygala fallax* Hemsl.), Wuniangteng (*Cuscuta chinensis* Lam.), and Buchulin [*Ardisia japonica* (Thunb.) Blume] are important treatment for hepatitis. After hundreds of years of development, oral inheritance of Zhuang medicine has unconsciously become a cultural atmosphere among Zhuang people without their awareness. The oral inheritance of medicine and treatment has a wide range and comes in a variety of forms, which is deeply rooted in the society. It has not only enriched and extended the knowledge base of Zhuang medicine to a large extent, but also created conditions for the formation of Zhuang medical theories.

2.2.6　Customary culture

A custom is an activity, a way of behaving, or an event which is usual or traditional in a particular society or in particular circumstances. Customary culture refers to cultural phenomena much related to people's life. It includes the popular and common preferences, customs, habits, practices, taboos and beliefs in people's material and cultural life, all of which are formed over long history, during absorption and transformation of a nation. Customary culture of medicine is an umbrella term for the knowledge and culture related to disease treatment and prevention and healthcare, emerging from the long-term production and life practice of a nation, and being accepted and passed on from generation to generation by the nation or society. In the long journey of development, Zhuang have developed rich customary culture of medicine, such as hygiene, sorcery and ancestor worship, disease prevention, healthcare, and plague and toxin prevention (for details, see Chapter 2.1). The customary culture of Zhuang medicine (diverse in cultural manifestations and also rich in connotation) has the typical characteristics of traditional Chinese medical culture as well as obvious cultural characteristics closely linked to the unique local environment, because it is the knowledge of disease treatment and prevention and healthcare accumulated by Zhuang people in different ways during ages of production and life practice in this unique regional natural, geographical and social environment, and in the context of ethnic culture.

2.2.7　Culture of ballad

Ballads refer to folk songs or music. Zhuang are good at singing and dancing. Zhuang ballads are rich in content, covering a wide range of topics about every aspect of Zhuang life. To be more precise, these ballads are about emotional exchange between men and women, Zhuang's ways of life, farming techniques, common customs, national conditions, social forms, and medicine. Zhuang ballads contain a great deal of content about medical affairs and healthcare (e.g., relationship between seasonal climate and diseases, marriage, birth, living conditions, house construction, and emotions), medical theories, disease symptoms, therapeutic methods, formula, effect of medicines, and so on. They have played an important role in the inheritance of Zhuang medicine. "Few people fall ill on the rainy Vernal Equinox, but epidemic diseases hit surrounding villages right after the wind and rain on the first day of the lunar month. East wind at the beginning of summer implies that few people get sick in the surrounding villages. People do not bother to prevent diseases if there is frost on the first day of the ninth lunar month. If there is no rain during the Double Ninth Festival or the three months of winter, severe drought will affect many patients, and natural disaster and disease will kill more people on the Renzi Day (based on the system of sexagenary cycle). Theft is rampant if west wind blows on the first day of the lunar month, and if it also snows heavily, disasters will come." The ballad tells of the relationship between climatic change and disease, and teaches people to pay attention to disease prevention when weather changes. It is written that "Acupoints on the hands are selected to treat fear of cold, those at the back are for fever, and lumps and skin damage are treated with a set of acupoints forming a plum flower shape around the affected part. Amyotrophy is treated with acupoints associated with the atrophic muscles. Pain or numbness is treated with acupoints along the affected part or at its center. Pruritus is treated with acupoints at the site of the first or biggest rash. But these alone are not enough, acupoints along the Longlu or Huolu should also be selected, according to practical requirements in treating diseases." This is a summary of rules for acupoint selection in Zhuang medicated thread moxibustion. In ballads, the records of actions of medicines fall into two categories. The first one is the summarization of general characteristics, for example, "Almost all herbs can be medicines — pungent flavor can treat sha diseases, bitter flavor can clear away heat, sour flavor can absorb sweat, and sweet flavor can tonify qi". The second one is the explanation of actions of specific Zhuang medicine, for example, "Nanshele (*Caesalpinia minax* Hance) can treat sha diseases, trauma, fracture, fishbone stuck in the throat, and scrofula". Zhuang ballads are just like an encyclopedia of the original ecology of ancient Zhuang.

2.2.8　Culture of medicinal food

Culture of medicinal food is a general experience and an important feature of medical culture of human beings. A Chinese legend has existed since ancient times, "Shennong tasted hundreds of herbs, and he got more than 70 types of poisonous ones in one day". In the early stages of human society, our ancestors, without adequate medical experience, realized that certain edible food could not only prevent hunger but also treat diseases. Then they gradually accumulated some preliminary experience in medicinal food. Therefore food comes before medicine, and the understanding of edibility promoted that of therapeutic value. The complementarity between medicine and food gave rise to the culture of medicinal food with national characteristics. The Zhuang nationality is one of the first Chinese ethnic groups to grow rice. Rice, the staple food of ancient Zhuang people, is also used as a sort of Zhuang medicine that can invigorate spleen, harmonize stomach, replenish kidney qi, and prolong life. It is processed into medicated porridge, wine, meal or cake. For example, the black glutinous rice wine of Hezhou City is famous, and the Guiping sweet wine made from black glutinous rice has the actions of invigorating spleen — stomach, replenishing qi and nourishing kidney. Zhuang ancestors not only found that cereal crops have an action of healthcare and can be used in dietary therapy, but also learned that most nourishing food plays specific therapeutic roles, such as fruits, vegetables, animals, and seasoning. "Orange can remove toxin in fish and crabs; taking powder of stir-baked fruit pits with wine can treat sudden sprain and contusion as well as lumbar pain; Zisu [*Perilla frutescens* (L.) Britt.] can allay hunger and fatigue; branches and leaves of Gouqi (*Lycium chinense* Mill.), sweet in flavor and neutral in nature, can clear heart and improve vision ..." The following experience has also been handed down in the Zhuang region: drinking fresh snake blood can treat wind-dampness; rat is so nourishing that "one rat is better than three chickens"; ant can also treat wind-dampness; and tokay gecko, sparrow, and cock testicle are nourishing and able to strengthen yang. Thanks to special climate and geographical environment, there are a great variety of edible and medicinal animals and plants in the Zhuang region. Abundant resources enabled the formation and development of culture of medicinal food.

2.2.9　Culture of reproduction

Reproduction is an old but ever-present topic in the journey of human beings. So to speak, the history of reproduction is as long as that of human survival on earth. As Engels wrote in the preface to the first edition of *The Origin of the Family*, *Private Property and the State*, production itself is of a two-fold character, "On the one hand, the production of the means of subsistence, food, clothing and shelter and the tools requisite therefore; on the other hand, the production of human beings themselves, the propagation of the species." In ancient times, human reproduction, a determinant of social development, was more important than the production of material goods. "Reproduction is an ethnic categorical obligation, just as death is the irresistible fate of an individual." So reproduction worship became a worldwide historical phenomenon. Zhuang, an ancient nationality with a long history, also have their own interpretations of human reproduction. Zhuang people believe in the Huaposhen (Flower Mother). She is the goddess of reproduction and also known as "Huawangshengmu (the Flower Goddess)". Zhuang people believe that children are flowers in the Flower Mother's courtyard, and their vicissitudes are entirely dominated by her. Families put paper flowers at the bedside when a new baby arrives, and mothers take their children to worship the Flower Mother during festivals. When children fall ill, the Flower Mother is also worshipped to obtain her blessing. Zhuang ancestors' worship of reproduction is also seen in their animal worship. There are many legends of frogs spreading in the Zhuang region. On the one hand, frogs are revered as the embodiment of men or women, because of their figure and strong reproductive capacity; on the other hand, frogs have been connected with the God of Birth in the Zhuang region — the Thunder God, and their image of strong reproductive capacity has been promoted. Frogs enjoy a unique position in the Zhuang culture of reproduction worship. In the archeological research of Luoyue culture, experts found that large phallic rocks around Damingshan Mountain have long been worshipped by local villagers. Also, we can clearly see two paintings of human sexual intercourse drawn by Zhuang ancestors, thousands of years ago, among the cliff paintings of the Huashan Mountains in Ningming County. They demonstrate Zhuang people's extraordinary worship of human reproduction.

2. 2. 10　Culture of sports

Zhuang ancestors realized quite early that physical exercise is able to improve constitution and prevent diseases. Among the cliff painting portraits of the Huashan Mountains in Ningming County, Guangxi, there are front-on and side-on action paintings portraying dance. In the front-on ones, people are doing half squat, raising their arms bending their elbows as well as their knees at 90 to 110 degrees. In the side-on ones, lines of people are bending their knees and stretching their arms up. According to expert research, both types of portraits demonstrate typical dance or kung fu movements. The position of dancing in early medical practice is confirmed by the paintings of Tao Yin exercises in the Mawangdui Han Dynasty tomb and the Five Animal Qigong attributed to Hua Tuo. Because of the special natural environment, it is often humid or rainy in the Zhuang region. Beriberi, wind-dampness and heavy body are commonly encountered diseases, which significantly affect their production and life. Therefore, Zhuang ancestors created dance movements that have actions of removing stagnation and soothing joints. They drew those dance movements and handed them down as methods for diseases prevention and treatment from generation to generation. Now, Zhuang people still love sports activities, singing and dancing. They often conduct traditional fitness activities during festivals, such as throwing embroidered balls, dragon boat racing, walking on stilts, dragon dance, lion dance, and catching sky lanterns. It is bound up with the important Zhuang medical idea of "prevention before disease onset".

References:

[1] Huang Hanru. Zhuang Medicine in China [M]. Nanning: Guangxi Nationalities Publishing House, 2000.

[2] Lan Richun, Liu Zhisheng, Qin Wenbo. A Discussion on the Relationship Between Luoyue Culture and Zhuang Medical Culture [J]. Journal of Medicine and Pharmacy of Chinese Minorities, 2008 (12): 1 - 6.

[3] Pang Yuzhou. Brief Account of Zhuang Healthcare Customs [J]. Chinese Journal of Ethnomedicine and Ethnopharmacy, 2008 (3): 3 - 5.

[4] He Xin. Semiology of Artistic Phenomenons: Culturological Explanation [M]. Beijing: People's Literature Publishing House, 1987.

[5] Lin Chen. Analysis of the Influence of Zhuang Sorcery Culture on the Development of Zhuang Medicine [C]. Proceedings Paper, the First China-Thailand Symposium on Traditional Medicines and Natural Medicines, 2006.

[6] Liu Keke, Zhang Mei. People, Symbols, and Culture [J]. Jiangsu Social Sciences, 2012 (5): 28 - 31.

[7] Xie Aize. Research on Orally Inherited Zhuang Medical Material [C]. Proceedings Paper, First National Academic Conference on Zhuang Medicine & National Forum on Experience in Ethnic Medicine, 2005.

[8] Mo Qinglian, Huang Ping, Huang Haibo. Discussion on the Role of Zhuang Folk Songs in the Inheritance of Zhuang Medicine [J]. Chinese Journal of Ethnomedicine and Ethnopharmacy, 2019 (21): 25 - 27.

[9] Karl Marx, Frederick Engels. Karl Marx and Frederick Engels: Selected Works, Volume 4 [M] Beijing: People's Publishing House, 1972.

[10] O. A. Wall. Sex and Sex Worship (translated by Shi Pin) [M]. Beijing: China Federation of Literary and Art Circles Publishing Corporation, 1988.

［11］Liao Mingjun. Zoolatry and Reproduction Worship ［J］. Journal of Guangxi University for Nationalities, Philosophy and Social Science Edition, 1995 (3): 23 – 28.

［12］Pang Yuzhou. Analysis of Connotation of Zhuang Medicine in the Cliff Paintings of the Huashan Mountains ［J］. Guangming Journal of Chinese Medicine, 2008, 23 (12): 1871 – 1873.

3 Zhuang Medicine，Philosophy and Religious Beliefs

3. 1　Zhuang medicine and philosophy

In ancient times，the Zhuang region had warm climate，plentiful rainfall，rolling rivers，thick forests，abundant wildlife，and numerous grottos. It was ideal for hominids to live and multiply. Since ancient times，Zhuang people have been living and multiplying in Lingnan，the vast and fertile land. They have been overcoming seemingly insurmountable obstacles and making unrelenting efforts to build a beautiful homeland. Different aspects of Zhuang ancestors' arduous journey of exploring and conquering nature are shown in research findings of recent archeological excavation，and in Zhuang folk tales about ancient times. In the struggle to conquer nature，Zhuang ancestors created material culture，and also developed elemental ideas，particularly simplistic views on the origins of the universe and all creatures including human beings. With the development of Zhuang society and deepening of practices，Zhuang ancestors were expanding their horizons and deepening their understanding. They had their own perceptions of nature and society，namely their own world view，which is a simple intuitive understanding. Zhuang's philosophic thinking is also a significant component of Chinese philosophic thinking.

Zhuang medicine has experienced a long history of formation and development. Its formation was based on hundreds of years of production，life and clinical practices of the Zhuang ancestors. For the conquest and control of nature，they had to explore the secrets of nature. Therefore，they formed an understanding of sensible external environment as well as ideologies closely related to living and multiplying，including their relationship with nature，human relations，and ideas about the human body.

3. 1. 1　Zhuang philosophical thoughts

Hegel said，"There comes a time to a nation when mind applies itself to universal objects，for example，in seeking to bring natural things under general modes of understanding，it tries to learn their causes. Then it is said that a people begins to philosophize."

When exploring the secrets of nature，Zhuang ancestors had their initial questions about the formation of nature and the origin of human beings. It was their reflections on heaven and humanity that gave birth to the simple and primitive philosophical thoughts with their own characteristics，which have remained with us till now in the form of Zhuang folk tales.

3. 1. 1. 1   Theories on the origin of the universe

There are many folk tales in the Zhuang nationality，most of which are spread in the form of long narrative poems represented by *The Creation of the Earth and the Sky*，*The Separation of Man and God*，*Menogga* （ "meroegga" in Zhuang language），*Buluotuo* （ "baeuqlozdoz" in Zhuang language），*The Legend of the Sun：a Journey toward the Horizon*，*Tekang Shooting down the Suns*，*The Story of Uncle Bu*，and *The Legend of Bronze Drum*.

Following is the outline of the ancient folk tale *Buluotuo*：a long，long time ago，when heaven and earth were one and the same，a cloud of gas，revolving faster and faster in the universe，formed a huge round egg with three yolks. After a subsequent explosion，the three yolks were separated into three pieces flying in three directions — the upper one as the sky，the lower one as the sea，and the middle one as the earth. There were three realms in nature — the sky as the upper realm supervised by the Thunder King，the ground as the middle realm supervised by Buluotuo，and the underground as the lower realm supervised by the Dragon King. The sky was low and the land was thin then. When people cut firewood，their axes often hit the sky. When they drove piles into the ground or spun，the ground was often broken through. So，Buluotuo asked beings in the upper realm to raise the sky to "as high as numerous pieces of Nanzhu (Phyllostachys Pubescens) so that no plait of hair could touch it"，and he asked beings in the lower realm to thicken the land to be "as thick as numerous rocky mountains so that no length of Huangteng (herba fibraureae recisae) could break it through". That is Zhuang ancestors' theory on the origin of nature. It is mythical，but it also contains the dawn of materialism and budding philosophical thoughts. The dawn of materialism is shown in Zhuang ancestors' understanding of the existence of inchoate gas before the formation of nature：the revolving gas formed a round egg，which exploded into three pieces — the sky，the earth and the sea，and then they gave birth to everything. There is a simple materialist view of nature in their materialistic explanation of the origin of nature. Also，there are budding thoughts of naive materialism and naive dialecticism in Zhuang's "theory of gas". In Zhuang ancestors' image, "gas", as the origin of the universe, is not static but spinning (movements) faster and faster (intensifying internal contradictions within an object), and it formed a huge round egg of small volume and large density. The explosion (qualitative change) of the round egg gave birth to the sky, the earth and the sea. With intuitional and concrete thought, Zhuang ancestors described motion, development and change of matter by revolution and explosion, and attributed the formation of the world to the movement and internal contradictions within an object. The view that the universe was formed through revolution and explosion is somewhat similar to the "nebular hypothesis" and the big bang theory in the field of modern cosmogony. The similarities originate from the underlying materialistic dialectics in thoughts on the origin of the universe, and Zhuang ancestors' dialectical thinking is a revelation of naive dialecticism.

3.1.1.2　Theories on the origin of human beings

With extremely inefficient modes of production, Zhuang ancestors generated some exaggerated ideas about "the riddle of the universe" by obtaining images through observation and simple and intuitive thinking. There are philosophical thoughts shining in those myths. Zhuang ancestors' descriptions of the origin of human beings can be categorized as "primary humans" and "regenerated humans".

In the first description, primary humans were created by the "Flower Mother Muliujia from soil". The Zhuang myth *Buluotuo and Muliujia* says, there was a swirling egg in the universe in ancient times, and it exploded into three pieces which were the heaven, the earth and the sea, namely the three realm. A beautiful flower grew up in the land of the middle realm, and then from it grew a woman who became the first human in the world. She was hairy all over her body and also smart, with disheveled hair. She wet the land, created humans with the wet soil, and divided the humans into male and female with chili pepper and carambola.

In the second description, "humans were regenerated through marriage between a brother and sister". The Thunder King, who supervised the upper realm, was in great anger and sent a great flood to destroy humans. Only one brother and sister survived, by hiding in a calabash gourd. To regenerate humans, the brother and sister married each other as it was the will of Heaven. The sister then gave birth to a fleshy lump which was cut into slices and scattered to the winds. Those falling into water became fish and shrimp, and those falling to the ground became humans. People got married, multiplied and survived.

The two theories interlink and are the results of different stages of historical development. The theory that Muliujia created humans from soil was born of Zhuang ancestors' unawareness of human reproduction through sexual intercourse. Based on the experience of fruit collection, they observed that flowers became fruit and believed that humans came from flowers. Nowadays, Zhuang still maintain flower totem worship. The theory that humans were regenerated through marriage between a brother and a sister reflected the stage of primitive group marriage. In Zhuang mythology, we can conjure up human evolution order: gas — the three realms including the sky, the earth and the sea — the Flower Mother Muliujia — primitive men — regenerated humans.

3.1.1.3　Relationship between man and nature

Over ages of labor and life practice, Zhuang ancestors realized the dialectical unity of man and the objective world. Humans need to adapt to the natural environment and conform to the objective laws, which is manifested in a series of idealistic worship and ceremony, in reverence for deities, for blessings and averting misfortune. However, from another perspective, people started the journey of self-awakening, as they adapted to the natural environment for development, through continuous transformation of the objective world. In Zhuang mythology, there are many heroes taking the lead in fighting against nature. For example, the hero Buluotuo led people to go-vern nature, after its formation, for the improvement of harsh environments. Together they sought old sago palm to hold up the heaven, and to support the earth; they used cunning tactics to force the Thunder God to go up to the sky for shelter; sent the flood dragon into the sea; banished tigers into the forest; and taught others how to knit clothes, grow plants and make fire, so that they could enjoy a good and prosperous life. As *The Story of Uncle Bu* relates, when the Thunder King refused to send rain, Uncle Bu went up to the sky to get even with him by grabbing his shoulders and placing a sword on the bridge of his nose. *The Legend of Thunder Drum* depicts people's brave fight against floods — the Teyi Brothers made drums to fight against the Thunder King. "The Thunder King relies on his drum to manifest his power. Let's make several drums, too. If the beats of our drums can drown out those of the Thunder King's drum, then he will lose and dare not lord it over us." In *Tekang Shooting down the Suns*, Tekang is a hero similar to Houyi in the Han nationality. Heroes like Buluotuo, Uncle Bu, the Teyi Brothers and Tekang are a miniature of the broad working masses' fighting against nature. Their stories seem bizarre and infantile, but they indirectly reflect people's enterprising spirit and eulogize people's courage to fight against nature. People's infinite worship and reverence for nature changed into defiance and struggle against deities（symbolizing the forces of nature）, which represents distillation of their naive materialism.

3. 1. 2　Basic characteristics of Zhuang philosophical culture

3. 1. 2. 1　The plain view of nature and worship of nature

In ancient times, Zhuang ancestors could not understand natural phenomena (e.g., thunder, lightning, wind, flood, drought, landslide, ground crack, and movement of the sun and the moon) because of their low social productivity and extreme lack of scientific knowledge. They imagined that there could be a certain of mighty and mysterious things behind those natural phenomena. Therefore, they attributed thunder to the Thunder God, lightning to the Goddess of Lightning, wind to the Wind Goddess, and rain to the Thunder King. They believed there were Dragon Kings in the seas, Mountain Gods in the mountains, Earth Gods in the ground, Moon Goddesses, Sun Gods, and so on. They also believed there were gods of vegetation, animals and birds. They anthropomorphized and deified the natural world and natural phenomena, which gave rise to their worship of nature.

3. 1. 2. 2　Belief in humanity's ability to conquer nature

Through continuous accumulation of experience in the long-term struggle against nature, Zhuang ancestors had developed a belief in humanity's ability to conquer nature. Their preliminary ideas about that ability formed after they gradually realized their own power in their struggle against nature, with the improvement of social productivity and deepening of their understanding towards nature. Those simple ideas are not directly reflected in their production and life, but are indirectly manifested in tales and legends. In those stories, they idealized real people and things, shaped heroic and deified figures, and won their fights against nature.

In their struggle against nature, they also realized that humans could change environments and overcome great scourges, such as fierce floods and savage beasts, as is recorded in the narrative poem *King Cenxun*. It is an ancient story about Cenxun in Jiangyan (now Tianzhou Town, Tianyang County, Guangxi). He saw that people were forced to move to the mountains as the frequent floods killed many people, but they were still attacked by venomous serpents and wild beasts there. Therefore, he vowed to prevent floods by water control and wipe out these threats. Across hills and rivers, he walked through Zhuang villages, where he observed springs and mountains, to find ways of preventing flood disaster. He also taught people about the scourge of floods and wild beasts. Finally he made a triumphant return after overcoming numerous challenges during his 720 days journey, and 1044 fights against serpents and beasts. After his return, he started to excavate the mountains, dredge watercourses, control mountain torrents and wipe out wild beasts. As a result, people could live and work in peace and contentment. The story tells us a truth: to control floods and wipe out wild beasts, people must first understand water streams, mountain terrain and lurking wild beasts, which requires an arduous journey for the observation of terrain, springs and the path of floodwaters. So in that sense, people had already vaguely realized it was necessary to seek out what must be done based on factual observation. In other words, they had already acquired a basic understanding that they first needed to know the properties and characteristics of water streams to control floods. That empirical knowledge is undoubtedly valuable given that it was developed by generation after generation of Zhuang ancestors thousands of years ago as the result of long-term accumulation of experience in their struggle and production. In brief, although the story is mythical, it reflects Zhuang ancestors' awareness of their own power and their emerging belief in humanity's ability to conquer nature.

3.1.2.3 Important role of sorcery culture in Zhuang philosophy

Mother Nature's secrets are boundless, and she is ever-changing. With very low productivity, Zhuang ancestors failed to explain natural phenomena (e.g., earthquake, flood and volcanic eruption) and even the common ones (e.g., sunrise, sunset, wind, rain, thunder and lightning). In particular, they felt mystified by night dreams, birth, death, old age and disease. Therefore, based on boundless imagination, they assumed that there must be supernatural powers and mysterious realms dominating nature and society. From their point of view, when these powers showed mercy to humans and nature, good things would come and help with their harvest and life and good weather made things grow better. However, when those powers became vicious and angry, they vented their fury on humans through disasters such as earthquakes and floods. So, based on imagination, they tried to look for supernatural powers and to leverage them to remove misfortunes, dispel plague, prevent diseases, end hunger, and make climate, animals, crops, health, and lifespan conform with their will for their peace of mind and spiritual sustenance. This was how sorcery culture came into being.

The emergence of sorcery culture had something to do with low productivity and existing animism in Zhuang ancestors' nature worship at that time. They personified and deified all natural phenomena. They believed that all things have a spirit, particularly forces affecting production, such as mountains, rivers, the sun, the moon, thunder, lightning, wind, rain, water, fire, and earth. They tried to placate natural forces and seek blessings from nature through sacrifice. They believed there were mountain, water and earth deities, to which they needed to offer sacrifice. Sorcery and religion were intertwined in those primitive beliefs as well as activities such as divination, sacrifice and soul deliverance rite.

Sorcery or witchcraft culture, with belief in ghosts and gods at its heart, plays a powerful role in Zhuang philosophy. It affects not only Zhuang folk religion and literary art, but also custom, medicine, diet, utensils, economic life, calendar, education, music, dance, art, crafts, exercises, etc.

3.1.3 The influence of Zhuang philosophy on Zhuang medicine

The Zhuang are an integral part of the Chinese nation. Because of the special geographical, political, economic and cultural circumstances where Zhuang people live, the Zhuang social and historical development has unique features, which had a great impact on the formation and development of Zhuang medicine. Zhuang medicine has distinct national and regional character. Its formation and development are inseparably bound up with the special social history, geographical environment, climate, economy, culture and folklore.

Different philosophical cultures may develop their unique modes of thought. The understanding of nature and the human body in Zhuang philosophy has deeply influenced and penetrated Zhuang medicine. Their beliefs about the relationship between man and nature include the synchrony of triple initial qi (heaven, earth and human). It is human beings, growing with the blessing of heaven and earth qi, that are the wisest of all creatures, and humanity has the ability to conquer nature, namely humans can change the natural world, based on the understanding of the rules of nature. The content, reflected in many orally inherited narrative poems, is studied in philosophy and also explored in Zhuang medicine.

3. 2　Zhuang medicine and religious beliefs

3. 2. 1　Taoism, Buddhism and Zhuang religious culture

After the period of Qin and Han dynasties, the central government strengthened the rule over the Zhuang region, and the political, economic and cultural exchanges between Zhuang and Han nationalities were enhanced. Taoism from Han nationality and other religions were introduced into the Zhuang region and integrated with the original culture of Zhuang. Therefore, Zhuang folk religions became complex and diverse with the interaction of Zhuang culture and artificially founded religions as well as with the mix of sorcery, Shi religion, Taoism and Buddhism.

3. 2. 1. 1　Taoism and Zhuang religious culture

Taoism, the earliest foreign religion introduced into the Zhuang region, began to arrive at Guangxi in the Eastern Han Dynasty from the Central Plains. According to the research of scholars in the field of Guangxi religions, famous Taoist priests in the Eastern Han Dynasty, such as Liu Gen, Hua Ziqi, Liao Ping, Liao Chong, Liao Fu, Dian Ao and Tuo Yu, all lived contemplative spiritual life in the Dujiaoshan Mountains of Rongxian County (current name). According to the record of *Local Records of Bobai County* (*Volume 240*, *Guangxi Local Records*) in the Emperor Jiaqing period of Qing Dynasty, "Ziyang Taoist Temple is 30 kilometers southwest of the city. Built by Liu Zongyuan in the Han Dynasty, it is in the south of Ziyang Rock." This shows that Taoism has been spread to Guangxi in the Han Dynasty. In the Eastern Jin Dynasty, Ge Hong heard that Jiaozhi (generally referring to South which involved in Guangdong, Guangxi, Vietnam and other places) was rich in cinnabar, so he applied as the leader of Goulou County (current Beiliu, Guangxi). After going to Lingnan, he wrote books and preached Taoism, promoting the spread of Taoism in Lingnan. In the Sui and Tang dynasties, Taoism expanded mainly into southeast Guangxi, and from there Taoism was gradually spread from southeast Guangxi to the Zuojiang basin, the Youjiang basin, and northwest Guangxi during the Song Dynasty, and it was slowly integrated with the primitive religions of Zhuang. Based on primitive beliefs, Zhuang people worshipped ghosts and gods, had an excessive liking for constructing excessive temples, and almost always turned to sorcerers instead of doctors when they got ill. Taoism came to the Zhuang region and suited Zhuang people's primitive beliefs and customs, meeting the needs of the Zhuang society. So interaction between Taoism and Zhuang primitive beliefs and culture was encouraged, which was good for the spread of Taoism in the Zhuang region and for the development of Zhuang philosophy.

Taoism was changed greatly after coming to the Zhuang region. By absorbing part of Zhuang primitive beliefs and Buddhism, Taoism freely developed its content and form to meet Zhuang people's psychological needs and beliefs in ghosts and gods. At that time, Taoists venerated Taishang Laojun （the Grand Supreme Elderly Lord）, and absorbed Zhuang primitive beliefs and Buddhism, by combining Taoism, Shi religion and Buddhism. In this way Taoism could be better accepted by the feudal ruling class and Zhuang society. A priest in Taoism （ "goengdauh" in Zhuang language） does not necessarily follow a monastic lifestyle. Taoist priests can marry, live in their own homes and hold other jobs. They cannot kill animals but they can eat meat excluding beef and dog. One major Taoist ritual is jiao, a rite of cosmic renewal, in which a Taoist priest dedicates the offerings. Taoist priests also perform Taoist funeral rites, hold ritual of soul deliverance, do Taoist chanting, give advice on Fengshui and selection of auspicious days, and help people avoid misfortunes. What they often do is chant of the Taoist scripture that is written in Chinese characters, usually without interpretation, so seeming very sincere. Their droning is monotonous and has incorrect pronunciation, so the folk call them "Namo".

3. 2. 1. 2　Buddhism and Zhuang religious culture

Buddhism is a foreign religion. It is believed in academia that Buddhism is spread from India to China by four routes: ①It is from northwest India to Persia, over the Pamirs and into Xinjiang, Gansu, Shaanxi, Henan, Hebei, etc. ②It is from northeast India to Myanmar then into Yunnan and Sichuan, the Yangtze River basin along the Han River and other parts of the Yangtze River. ③It is from India's Ganges river through Indian waters to Guangzhou, China or to Vietnam and then into the provinces of Guangdong and Guangxi. ④It is from the coastal area of India to Malay Peninsula, the South China Sea Islands, and finally into the southeastern coastal area of China. According to research on many cultural relics conducted by Guangxi scholars in the field of religious studies, by the end of the Han Dynasty Buddhism had been spread, across the seas, to Funan （now Cambodia） and then Hepu Port in Jiaozhi, whence it came to Guangxi via the Jiaozhi-Guangxi Corridor. Influenced by Zhuang primitive beliefs and culture, Buddhism became secularized and absorbed sorcery culture soon after coming to the Zhuang region. After the Song Dynasty, Zen Buddhism and Pure Land Buddhism were most popular in the Zhuang region. The essence of Zen Buddhism is that all human beings are Buddha, and that all they have to do is to discover that truth for themselves. The essential practice in Pure Land Buddhism is the chanting of the name of Amitabha Buddha with total concentration. Both Zen Buddhism and Pure Land Buddhism place less emphasis on obscure scriptures and more on people. With the combination of Zen Buddhism and Pure Land Buddhism and the integration of Confucianism, Taoism and Buddhism after the Ming Dynasty, Buddhist texts were summarized as easy-to-understand instructions on morality, and Guanyin (Goddess of Mercy) and Maitreya were the most common Buddha statues as they were better known by people, and the cultivation of moral nature was summarized as doing good deeds, making merit, and liberating all sentient beings from suffering. Therefore, Buddhist monks in the Zhuang region were permitted to marry, live in their own homes and hold other jobs. Also, they were allowed to eat meat except occasional vegetarian diet each month. *Record of Local Conditions of Baiyue* says, "Most Buddhist monks in Guangxi do not shave their hair, and they are allowed to marry and have children. So they are called 'monks at home'." According to *Touhuang Zalu (Miscellaneous Records when in Wilderness)*, "Southerners do not believe in Buddhism and there are few Buddhist temples in the south. Government officials assess monks in the temples for handling the temple lands and donations. There are few monks, but they all like hugging their wives and eating meat. They live at home and know nothing about chanting, praying and offering. Local people marry their daughters to monks and call them 'shilang' (a name for monks who marry and eat meat). People who get sick make round coins of paper and place them near Buddha statues, or ask monks to make offerings of food to the Buddha statues. The next day, people kill sheep or pigs to entertain monks, which is called 'breaking the fast'." The main activities of Zhuang monks included conducting Buddhist initiation rituals, funeral rituals and soul deliverance rites, holding ritual ceremonies for exorcism, divination, and fortune-telling. During ritual ceremonies in some Zhuang areas, there were Buddhist monks, Taoist priests and shamans. Replicas of Wenchang, Guanyin, Zhenwu, Guangong and Tudi temples are placed side by side or at the same altar. Buddhism in the Zhuang region was different from the orthodox Buddhism of the Han in Chinese areas as it became a region of orthodox Buddhism, Taoism and Shi.

In the Zhuang region, Buddhism was less influential than Taoism judging from the facts that how each of them was spread. Taoism is a local religion of China and its basic theories are intimately tied up with the mystical aspects and sorcery culture of primitive Chinese beliefs. Basically Taoism has embraced all the objects of nature worship in primitive religions. After coming to the Zhuang region, Taoism got involved in the production and life of Zhuang people in a comprehensive way. It integrated its beliefs with the gods and beliefs in the primitive religions of Zhuang as well as the new ones. Therefore, the integration of Taoism and primitive religions of Zhuang was rapid as Taoism took the gods in primitive religions of Zhuang as its objects of worship, and as primitive religions of Zhuang in turn leveraged rites and rituals of Taoism to carry out the practices that demonstrated their beliefs. Buddhism has a small influence in the Zhuang region because of multiple factors. According to *Records of Religions*, *Guangxi Local Records*, "Buddhism came to Guangxi early through seaways, but the vast areas along the spreading corridor were controlled by indigenous minorities with underdeveloped regional economy and isolated culture. Buddhism made very little difference there due to the overwhelming primitive shamanism." As a foreign religion, Buddhism is different from the Zhuang's worship of many gods. As much as possible, after coming to the Zhuang region Buddhism absorbed Zhuang gods and other content from the system of Zhuang folk beliefs, however, there was still inadequate communication and integration between Buddhism and traditional Zhuang culture. Buddhism came to Guangxi as early as the Han Dynasty. But there were few Buddhist temples in those areas inhabited by the Zhuang, with most of them in southeast Guangxi, northern Guangxi and other areas inhabited by Han people. Therefore, Buddhism was not spread widely in the Zhuang region, with a small number of Buddhists there. It did not mean the secularization of Buddhism failed there, but it reflected inadequate integration between Buddhism and traditional Zhuang culture, as well as incomplete involvement of social production and life of Zhuang. The spiritual needs of Zhuang people could not be satisfied by Buddhist views of the real world and future world and the problem-solving methodologies. Zhuang ancestors had a positive attitude on life and loved their lives. They begged gods for help when having insurmountable difficulties in their struggle for production. For example, they hoped that they could catch wild beasts without being hurt while hunting, and the Thunder King could send rain when water was exceedingly scarce at the time of spring planting. People worshipped gods for solving real difficulties in their real life. If it didn't work, people would punish gods and force them to meet their practical needs. For example, people asked the

Thunder King to send rain during a long drought. If their demand was not met, they would tie the god statue upside down, parade it through the village, let villagers whip it and splash water on it, and require it to go up to the sky and inform the Thunder King that people asked him to send rain before the deadline. Their beliefs were driven by pragmatism and were totally contrary to karma in Buddhism. Conversely, Zhuang primitive beliefs absorbed much of Taoism and Buddhism, and became new folk religious beliefs. When attending sacrifice offering ceremonies, Zhuang people did not care about which religion held the ceremonies, but whether the ceremonies were related to local and traditional Zhuang culture. What they really worshipped was the content of folk religion that contained different sources of beliefs and rituals.

Therefore, Buddhism did not make great progress on its own religious theories, and it could not adapt to the demands for production and life in Zhuang society after coming to the Zhuang region. It was not surprising that Buddhism had such a small influence.

3.2.2　Influence of Taoism and Buddhism on Zhuang medicine

3.2.2.1　**Influence of Taoism on Zhuang medicine**

As Taoism came to the Zhuang region, the thoughts of Laozi, Zhuangzi and other representatives were well-known among Zhuang people. From some Zhuang medical theories, it's clearly to be found that Taoism has an impact on Zhuang medicine, which has been deeply rooted in traditional Zhuang culture.

3.2.2.1.1　Influence of Taoist world-view and holism on Zhuang medicine

Taoist doctrine emphasizes life, and questions of life link Taoist thought. According to Taoism, humans need to follow the laws of nature in order to fulfill the ultimate purpose of living happily during old age. It is similar to the theory of "synchrony of triple initial qi (heaven, earth and human qi)" in Zhuang medicine, which is a paraphrase of "humans cannot act in defiance of heaven and earth" or "humans must act in obedience to heaven and earth" in the Zhuang language. The main concepts of the theory include: ①Human beings, growing with the blessing of heaven and earth qi, are the wisest of all creatures. ②The human life cycle — including growth, adulthood, aging and death — is nourished and constrained by the ever-changing heaven and earth qi. Human qi with heaven and earth qi are closely linked. ③Heaven and earth qi has created "rules" for human survival and health, but heaven and earth qi is ever-changing. The changing of night and day as well as seasons is normal, while abnormal changes are considered as disasters, such as the happening of earthquake, volcano, typhoon, flood and meteor shower. Humans, as the wisest of all creatures, can proactively adapt to the ever-changing heaven and earth qi. For example, people will make fire for illumination after dark, sweat during hot weather, dress appropriately and rug up during cold weather, and move to higher ground to survive a flood. The menstrual cycle has something to do with the waxing and waning of the moon. If people are able to proactively adapt to the changing heaven and earth qi, their body can maintain its normal state, which is necessary for survival and health. If not, they will suffer injury or fall sick. ④ Humans are a finite microcosm. According to Zhuang medicine, the human body can be divided into three parts: the upper part as heaven （"gyaeuj" in Zhuang language） including its extension, the lower part as earth （"dungx" in Zhuang language) including its interior and the middle part as human （"ndang" in Zhuang language). It makes people flourish when their body's heaven qi, earth qi and human qi interact with each other, move synchronously, and emerge naturally. There is a unity of the body's structure and functions. In general, heaven qi governs descending, earth qi governs ascending, and human qi governs harmony. Appropriate ascending, descending and harmony can balance qi and blood, yin and yang, maintain the normal state of zang and fu organs, and help the body adapt to the changing macrocosm. ⑤The unity of the body's structure and function, and the harmony of congenital qi and acquired qi, accumately enable the body to adapt, defend and consequently maintain health with the synchrony of triple initial qi.

Clearly, philosophic Taoist thought, such as "Tao is nature's way" and "the unity of heaven and man", is similar to the theory of "synchrony of triple initial qi （heaven, earth and human qi） " in Zhuang medicine.

3.2.2.1.2　Influence of Taoist "zhuyou exorcism" on Zhuang medicine

In addition to Taoist theories, Taoist "zhuyou exorcism" also has effects on Zhuang medicine. In ancient times, Taoists used "zhuyou exorcism" in prayer and sacrifice to ask ancestors for their blessings, as well as asking ghosts and gods for forgiveness. Also, it was used by witch doctors and Taoist doctors as a ritual therapy as they believed it could expel parasitic toxin. Taoist "zhuyou exorcism" was mainly used to treat diseases in addition to praying and resolving misfortunes. Such ritual therapy can move and transform qi by eliminating patients' negative emotions, including anxiety, tension and sadness.

According to traditional Zhuang beliefs, the soul, as a supernatural power protecting the life of an organism, can govern the spirit. If a man loses his soul, he will stop breathing and die as his body will stop functioning and growing. The soul, as the life essence of the body, can maintain health. A man experiencing "soul loss" will become sick, and he can be cured by a soul retrieval ceremony. Even now, there are still various popular activities carried out by witch doctors among Zhuang people, with "exorcism of ghosts and evocation of deities" as the main theme, and "praying for blessings of deities and health issues to go away" as the purpose.

3.2.2.1.3 Influence of Taoist "Fuqi and Daoyin exercises" on Zhuang medicine

"Fuqi" is a series of exercises for health cultivation, mainly relying on breathing techniques, and supplemented by "Daoyin" exercises and massage. Typically, "Daoyin" exercises involve movement of the arms and body, acting as a means of regulating qi and blood. Also, the important role of "prevention before disease onset" in health care and preservation is emphasized in Zhuang medicine. Zhuang people mitigate and treat some diseases through traditional dance movements. There is a lot of evidence to suggest that Zhuang people advocate Qigong, of which the practice of Daoyin is a precursor. For example, the cliff paintings of the Huashan Mountains in Ningming, dancing images and Qigong drawings on the Zhuang bronze drums and some traditional fitness activities still followed today during festivals and idle farming seasons both prove the popularity of Qigong.

3.2.2.2 Influence of Buddhism on Zhuang medicine

Buddhism came to Guangxi as early as the Han Dynasty, however, there were few Buddhist temples in those areas inhabited by the Zhuang. Historically, Buddhism was not spread widely in the Zhuang region, with a small number of Buddhists there. It had a smaller impact on Zhuang culture than Taoism. The spiritual needs of Zhuang people could not be satisfied by Buddhist views of the real and future worlds and the problem-solving methodologies of Buddhism, which does not mean Buddhism had no effect on Zhuang medicine. Buddhist teachings and thought have shared similarities with the thinking underlying Zhuang medicine.

For example, "the four great elements" in Buddhism are earth, water, fire and air. As the basic constituents of all matter, they give rise to everything including the human body. The body can stay healthy only when "the four great elements" within it maintain balance, otherwise it will get sick. The theory of "the four great elements" is similar to the theory of "synchrony of triple initial qi" in Zhuang medicine. The triple initial qi are synchronized through the inhibition, generation, coordination and other functions of Gudao, Shuidao, Qidao and relevant internal organs within the body. "Gudao" ("diuzgwnngaiz" in Zhuang language) mainly refers to the esophagus, the stomach and the intestines. The liver, pancreas and gallbladder form a part of the body's digestive system that is responsible for the absorption of nutrient in "Gudao". The body's "Shuidao" is the tract where water, the source of life, comes into and out of the body, and it allows the most direct and closest connection between the body and nature. The kidneys and bladder help regulate body water in "Shuidao". Gudao and Shuidao are congenetic but differentiated. After the essence of water and food is absorbed, Gudao allows defecation and Shuidao allows perspiration and urination. "Qidao" is the tract that enables the exchange between the body and natural qi, and the mouth and nose are inlets and outlets. The lungs are responsible for the exchange of gas in "Qidao". When the three tracts are unblocked and well-regulated, human qi with heaven and earth qi can remain synchronous, coordinated and balanced, namely we can stay healthy. However, if they are blocked or not well-regulated, the asynchrony of triple initial qi will cause diseases.

In addition to the similarities between the "the four great elements" in Buddhism and the synchrony of triple initial qi in Zhuang medicine, other Buddhists thought also had a positive impact on Zhuang medical ethics, for example, delivering all living creatures from torment, and healing the wounded and rescuing the dying.

3.2.3　Zhuang sorcery culture and Zhuang medicine

3.2.3.1　Zhuang sorcery culture

Zhuang ancestors' belief in ghosts and gods gave rise to sorcery culture. In the Zhuang region, there is still the custom of sorcery right up to the modern age, as sorcery took root there on the basis of totem worship in the primitive society. On the other hand, we can catch a glimpse of how Zhuang ancestors treated nature, society and the human body, and how these are related in Zhuang ballads, legends, folk tales and other forms of oral literature that have remained till now.

According to research on many ancient books, the cliff paintings along the Zuojiang River represent Zhuang ancestors' worship of the sun, the moon and stars, which still can be seen in the remaining fashion of sorcery in the Zhuang region. In terms of the influence of sorcery culture on Zhuang medicine, they were one and the same in the beginning, then they coexisted, and finally Zhuang medicine prevailed. In ancient times, Zhuang sorcerers were divided into female sorcerers and male sorcerers according to the gender. When there was sickness or disaster in the host family, the host would invite female sorcerers to ask immortals about the causes of the sickness or disaster. Then the host would pick an auspicious day to invite male sorcerers to carry out religious rites, where animals were killed for worship, immortals were urged to depart, people prayed for the ending of the disaster, and male sorcerers brandished swords, heated up a pot with oil, and drove away evil spirits. According to Zhuang folk tales, Zhuang people considered Sanjiegong as the God of Medicine as he was able to dispel pathogenic and noxious factors, protect their homes and defend their territories. They built temples for his regular annual worship, and there were Yaowang (the King of Medicine) Temples in large villages in the Zhuang region. That reflects the sorcery culture. According to archeological excavations, sorcerers had appeared in the Zhuang region ever since the Spring and Autumn and the Warring States periods. According to the research of Chinese archeologists, cliff paintings in the Zuojiang basin in Guangxi show sacrificial ceremonies with scenes of dancing crowds. In the center of those paintings, there are tall, imposing and front-on portraits of people with special dress, which are probably sorcerers and leading dancers responsible for sacrificial rites. The research establishes that the cliff paintings were created by Zhuang ancestors in the period from the Warring States Period to the Han Dynasty, with a history of over 2000 years. Zhuang ancestors took sorcery seriously. Many documentary records show there was a fashion of Yue sorcery in the Central Plains in the Han Dynasty. In *Records of the Grand Historian*, *Volume 12*, *Annals of the Xiaowu Emperor*, it is written that "Nanyue had been destroyed. Yongzhi, from Nanyue, said, 'Yue people believe in ghosts, which can be seen through sacrifice. Ghosts are influential and effective …' Therefore, Yue sorcerers were requested to build Yue-style temples, which have a table for sacrifice but no altar. In the temples, people offer sacrifices to both gods and ghosts, and practice divination with chicken bones." It is thus clear that the sorcery culture of Zhuang had a far-reaching influence. In the Qing Dynasty, there was still a fashion of sorcery in the Zhuang region, where the custom continues right up to the modern age.

3.2.3.2 Relationship between Zhuang medicine and Zhuang sorcery culture

Isogeny and coexistence of medicine and sorcery are features of the development of Zhuang culture, and they had a significant impact on Zhuang medicine. The long-term coexistence of medicine and sorcery is a feature of Zhuang medicine. Zhuang medicine was effective in treating some diseases, but in the form of witchcraft medicine, particularly for Zhuang people in the outlying mountain area before the founding of the People's Republic of China. In addition to dance movements, there appear to be depictions of diagnosis and treatment in the cliff painting portraits of the Huashan Mountains in Ningming, where we can see people performing witchcraft, holding instruments or being subjected to witchcraft. Considering the scenes of sacrifice in those cliff paintings and the features of Zhuang ancestors' sorcery culture, we can say there is evidence of treating diseases by witchcraft medicine in those cliff paintings. We can see relevant details in *Miscellaneous Review*, *Lingbiao Jiman* (*Records of the Barbarians of Lingnan*) by Liu Xifan, "The barbarians use herbs to treat trauma, carbuncle and all other diseases requiring surgery. It is often effective, but they also treat those diseases through superstitious activities." He witnessed the treatment and wrote, "I have seen a patient with carbuncle invite a Zhuang fellow to treat him. When the Zhuang fellow came, he asked the patient's family to place in the hall a rooster, a ten-cent silver coin, water and rice. The performer put the ten-cent silver coin into a bag, took off his straw sandals, placed them on the ground, got some water and cast a spell. Then he sprayed water onto the wound, and cut it with a knife, then pus and blood flowed out, but the patient felt no pain. When the pus was drained, topical application of drugs would cure the patient." That is an objective record of Zhuang medicine practices. To some extent, there is still such special form of treatment right up to the modern age. But now it is the relatives of patients who cast a spell. If we regard that form of therapy as a sheer superstitious activity, we will lose the proper medical part. Things like using some magic water and casting a spell cannot diminish the effectiveness of surgery and drug use in Zhuang medicine. According to some historical records on Zhuang people, "When people get sick, they don't take medicine but turn to worship only." It is a one-sided record that overstates the role of sorcery.

References:

[1] Huang Qingyin. Discussion on the Features and Research Significance of Zhuang Philosophical Thinking [J]. Journal of Guangxi University for Nationalities, Philosophy and Social Science Edition, 1995 (1): 36 – 39.

[2] Karl Marx, Frederick Engels. Excerpt of the German Ideology, Karl Marx and Frederick Engels: Selected Works, Volume 1 [M]. Beijing: People's Publishing House, 1995.

［3］Hegel. Lectures on the History of Philosophy, Volume 1 ［M］. Beijing: The Commercial Press, 1983.

［4］Editing Group for Philosophical Textbooks for General Courses in Institutes of Nationalities. Selected Works of Chinese Ethnic Philosophy and Social Thought ［M］. Tianjin: Tianjin Education Press, 1988.

［5］Li Fuqiang. Traditional Zhuang Culture from the Perspective of Anthropology ［M］. Nanning: Guangxi People's Publishing House, 1999.

［6］Zhu Mingsui, Xie Chunming. Records of Religions, Guangxi Local Records ［M］. Nanning: Guangxi People's Publishing House, 1995.

4 Zhuang Medicine and Rice-farming Culture

As Professor Liang Tingwang at Minzu University of China said in the article titled *Artificially Cultivating Rice and Rice-planting Culture*, "China is the first nation to grow rice artificially, while Yue people in the Jiangnan area (lands immediately to the south of the lower reaches of the Yangtze River) are the first to cultivate rice in China. They are the ancestors of Han people in the Jiangnan area and Kra-Dai-speaking peoples in South China and Southwest China (Zhuang, Dong, Bouyei, Dai, Li, Gelao, Shui, Mulao and Maonan people). The ancestors of Kra-Dai-speaking peoples have made tremendous contributions in making China the first nation to grow rice artificially." As China is the first nation to grow rice, rice-farming culture is an important cultural heritage for both Chinese civilization and world civilization. Rice-farming culture is also an important symbol of Luoyue culture. According to excavated relics and related research, wild rice was widespread in the area where the ancient Luoyue people lived. Luoyue people knew about wild rice from early times. They invented the method of artifical culturation of rice together with Cangwu and Xi'ou people, making tremendous contributions to the Chinese nation and people around the world.

4. 1 Rice-farming culture and its features

As Zhuang ancestors domesticated wild rice, Zhuang is one of the first ethnic groups to create the rice planting civilization in China. Modes of production determined types of civilization. Zhuang is a nationality with long rice-farming history. As Zhuang people call paddy field "naz" in their language, places with "naz" in their names can be found all over the Pearl River basin in China and throughout the whole Southeast Asia region. From the perspective of cultural ecology, Zhuang culture is a rice planting civilization that demonstrates the traits of regional culture when considered as a whole. Those places named with "naz" reflect rice-farming and ethnic culture, becoming a common symbol and historical imprint for all the people living there. Therefore, their culture is called "naz culture".

Zhuang ancestors lived in the Pearl River basin, a subtropical zone with a good climate and environment for growing rice. The basin has been a typical area of rice-farming culture since ancient times, and there rice agriculture originated with widespread wild rice. Zhuang ancestors have gradually understood the growth rhythm of rice after long-term collection of wild rice. In order to grow rice, they reclaimed land named "雒田 (Luotian)" along the valley water areas. The remains of rice from about 10,000 years ago were found in Yuchanyan Site in Daoxian County, southern Hunan Province and Niulandong Site in Yingde City, Guangdong Province. Historical documents, archeological discoveries and physical anthropology researches show that hominids in the area were the ancestors of Kra-Dai-speaking peoples. As Han, Yao and Miao people entered the area after the Qin and Han dynasties, Zhuang ancestors are proven to be the creators of rice planting civilization there. "雒田 (Luotian)", recorded in history books, is actually the word "麓那 (Luna)" in the Yue language, meaning the paddy field in the valley. Now, there are still many places with "麓" (雒, 六, 禄, 渌, 绿, 鹿, 罗) in their names in the vast Guangxi and Guangdong Pearl River basin where ancient Yue people lived. Also, there are numerous places with "那" ("naz" in Zhuang language, meaning paddy field) in their names. In some ancient Chinese books such as *Classic of Mountains and Sea*, *Classic of Poetry* and *Shuo Wen Jie Zi*, words like "耗", "膏" and "粳" are the transcriptions of Zhuang words for wild rice and rice grains. In those Zhuang "naz" places, there are counties, towns, villages, country fairs, arable valleys and parcels of farmland. They form a special cultural landscape of regional place names as a unique cultural pattern in the Pearl River basin. Naz-name places are distributed through the vast land from South China to Southeast Asia, forming "naz culture" with profound cultural connotations. In the long journey of development, the Zhuang nationality and its ancestors have formed a "naz-based" production pattern, lifestyle and cultural system featuring rice production, living near arable valley, having rice as a major staple food, and costume culture driven by rice-farming, with festivals based on, religions supporting, and art cultivated by rice-farming.

4.1.1 Naz-based production culture

The production culture mainly features stone axe with shoulders and big stone shovel culture. With the presence of those Neolithic tools, primitive agriculture emerged and wild rice was domesticated as cultivated rice. In adapting to the development of rice agriculture, Zhuang ancestors continued to create more complex and sophisticated instruments of production. Big stone shovel culture, emerging in the late Neolithic Age, reflects the rice production method of Zhuang ancestors and their utilitarian purpose. Since the 1950s, more than 60 significant sites of big stone shovel dating back some 5000 years were discovered in Yongjiang basin. The big stone shovels are polished, angular and exquisite with soft curves. Some of them have become amazing treasures as they have large size, appealing design and great polish. Developed from stone axes with shoulders, the big stone shovels were used for working in wetland and paddy field. Afterwards, they were used for sacrifice, reflecting Zhuang ancestral respect and worship of them, sincere prayer for bumper harvests, and enthusiasm in labor. The big stone shovels have marked the enormous progress in the productivity of Zhuang ancestors in the Neolithic Age, together with greater scale and level of development of rice agriculture. It indicates the further development of their awareness of worship, aesthetic standards and artistic creativity, which all originated from rice production.

4. 1. 2   Naz-based living culture

Zhuang ancestors lived near arable valley and formed the ganlan culture. In Zhuang language the house is called "lan" and when built on an underframe is called "ganlan". "Ganlan" means a house high off the ground. Zhuang settlements are mainly located around water-rich arable valley. Ganlan houses are built according to the mountain terrain around arable valley. A ganlan house is based on an underframe that is supported by wooden columns and high off the ground. It consists of two stories, with the upper layer for human habitation and the lower layer for rearing livestock or storing articles. Ganlan houses are built for humid, rainy and rugged environment among the mountains in South China. They can prevent damp, beast and thief intrusion. Also, they can provide good lighting and ventilation with optimal land utilization. *Liaoren Chapter*, *Book of Wei* says, "They pile up wood against trees and live aloft in the so-called ganlan houses. The size of ganlan houses varies according to the number of family members." In the long course of development, profound cultural connotations are reflected in the architectural process, structure, and functional characteristics of ganlan houses. As an important part of ancient architectural heritage, ganlan houses reflected how Zhuang ancestors adapted to the natural environment. This architectural form is still found in mountain villages in South China.

4.1.3　Naz-based food culture

Since the 1960s, archeological workers have discovered stone pestles, stone grinding rods, millstones, stone hammers, and other tools for processing grains in the early Neolithic Age Shell Mound sites located on both sides of Yongjiang, Zuojiang and Youjiang Rivers in Yongning, Wuming, Hengxian, Fusui and other counties (districts). Pottery shards were unearthed in Zengpiyan site in Guilin, dating back to the early Neolithic Age around 9000 years ago. According to genetic information, rice was the main grain for processing at that time as wheat and millet came later. Ethnoarchaeology shows that pottery was created for adaption to grain consumption. These indicate that people began to eat rice in the Zhuang region in the early Neolithic Age around 9000 years ago. Also they invented pestles, mills, hammers, pottery cups and other tools for processing and cooking rice. In *Greater Odes of the Kingdom: Gongliu* in *Classic of Poetry* (in which the first poems were written about 1100B. C.), it is recorded that "There are lots of grain in the barn, and rations are prepared for expedition (乃积乃仓，乃裹餱粮)." "餱粮" (or "糇粮") is a word from the Ancient Yue language, as a synonym of "粮" in North China. Now Zhuang people still call rice "糇" or "膏". It is revealed that Zhuang ancestors knew how to cook rice in ancient times. As rice was spreading across the Central Plains, it was recorded in *Classic of Poetry*. There is a saying from both the Zhuang and Dai, "There are fish in the water and rice in the paddy field." It reflects the fact that rice and fish were the staples of Zhuang ancestors. As their major staple food, rice is central to their food culture. They repeatedly screened and bred that glutinous rice which best adapted to the natural environment. Planted widely, it became an important food in their life and a main source of their processed grain products. Also, Zhuang ancestors use glutinous rice to make five-colored sticky rice, ciba cakes, zongzi, and other special food, leading to a preference for glutinous food.

4.1.4　Naz-based costume culture

The development of Zhuang ancestors' rice agriculture drove the development of their cotton and linen textile and garment processing industries. In the Zhuang region, there are rich resources of wild and cultivated bast fiber plants. Therefore, their linen textile industry has a long history. The stone and pottery spinning wheels were unearthed in the Neolithic cultural remains in the Zhuang region. They are tools for spinning thread from bast fibers. In *Treatise on Geography*, *Book of Han*, it is recorded that "Canton ... a place near the sea with abundant resources including rhinoceroses, elephants, hawksbill turtles, gems, sliver, copper, fruit, and cloth." According to Yan Shigu's note, "cloth refers to all kinds of fine cloth". In ancient China, cloth mostly refers to the fabrics of bast fiber plants including hemp, ramie, and kudzu. It is recorded in *Xiao Erya* that "hemp, ramie, and kudzu are materials for cloth", indicating that Zhuang people could weave cloth from bast fiber a long time ago. In the Warring States Period tomb excavated in Yinshanling site, Pingle County, Guangxi, there are weapons but no pottery spinning wheels in the male tomb, and there are pottery spinning wheels but no weapons in the female tomb, reflecting that Zhuang females mainly did the weaving, showing how the natural division of labor and linen textile industry had developed greatly at that time. *Yugong*, *Book of Documents* says, "In Yangzhou people are dressing in Huifu clothes, and they have textiles with wavy form in the baskets as tributes (岛夷卉服，厥篚织贝)". Yangzhou refers to the vast area from the south of the Huaihe River to the South China Sea. "贝（bei）" is short for "吉贝（jibei）", "劫贝（jiebei）" and "古贝（gubei）". "古贝（gubei）" is a transliteration. "织贝（zhibei）" refers to textiles made from cotton. The domestic Zhuang-Dong (Kra-Dai) languages including the Zhuang, Bouyei, Lingao, Dai and Li languages, Nung and Tay in Vietnam, Lao, and Thai all have cognate words for cotton. They are also related to "贝（bei）" in "吉贝（jibei）", "劫贝（jiebei）" and "古贝（gubei）". It reveals that planting and using cotton had been part of their life before those people of different ethnic groups moved to different places. Therefore, Zhuang ancestors are one of the first ethnic groups to grow and use cotton.

4. 1. 5　Naz-based festivals culture

Festival culture reflects the shared ethnic cultural identity. Zhuang festival culture is closely related to rice-farming, manifesting the mixture of material, behavior and concepts. It is the symbol of a rice planting civilization and Zhuang cultural community. Zhuang ancestors formed notions of worship objects for rice-farming, and then had festival activities centered around those objects. Taking Hongshui River area for example, people there celebrate the Frog Festival from the 1st to 15th days of the first lunar month, during which they offer sacrifices to the Frog God; they offer sacrifices before the cattle pen during the New Year; they hold a ceremony for starting farming after the Spring Festival; they offer sacrifices in the paddy field when they transplant rice seedlings in the 3rd and 4th lunar month; they hold a ceremony for worshipping rice seedlings and cattle soul during the Rice Seedling Soul Festival and the Cattle Soul Festival when rice seedlings turn green in the 5th and 6th lunar months; they celebrate the New Rice Tasting Festival when rice bears fruit and turns yellow in the 7th lunar month; and they celebrate the Ciba Cake Festival after the harvest around Frost's Descent in the 10th lunar month. Zhuang people have rites and Zhuang songs for each festival. In many regions, local Zhuang people hold solemn song fairs in arable valleys during rice transplanting and harvest in order to satisfy their pursuit of spiritual and material life.

4. 1. 6 Naz-based religious culture

Zhuang religions fall into three categories: primitive religions, indigenous folk religions (i.e., Mo religion and Shi religion), and artificially founded religions (i.e., Taoism and Buddhism). In primitive religions, the worship of nature, ghosts, gods, totem and reproduction might be handed-down forms cultivated by fishing and hunting culture as well as rice-farming culture. Only ancestor worship was "stubborn" and incorporated into the system of rice-farming culture. Ancestors were worshiped to ask for a prosperous and happy family, bumper rice harvests, and livestock proliferation. Also, the rice products were used when praying for prosperity. In indigenous folk religions and artificially founded religions, the core of their doctrines and rites also involves prayer for prosperous and happy family, bumper rice harvests, and livestock proliferation. Also, the rice products were used to pray for prosperity. In general, they were all integrated into the system of rice-farming culture. According to 29 scriptures in *The Mo Scriptures Buluotuo of the Zhuang Ethnic Group* (*Photocopy, Translation and Annotation*), material production is rice-centered. After heaven and earth were made, paddy fields, vegetable farms, ganlan houses, cattle, springs, waterwheels and granaries were created. Rice soul was invoked, next cattle, horse, pig, chicken, duck and goose souls, and last fish soul. This indicates the central position of rice.

4. 1. 7 Naz-based art culture

There is a strong atmosphere of rice-farming culture in Zhuang literary art, for example, in myths. Ancient Yue people worshiped frog, the most respected totem for the Zhuang nationality. In Zhuang myths, there are three great gods who are brothers and sisters. The eldest brother is the Thunder God in the heaven, the second brother is Buluotuo, the Earth God, and the third, the sister, is called Tu'e, meaning Water God (she is a combination of crocodile, rhinoceros and hippopotamus). The eldest brother committed incest with the third sister and they had an offspring (the Frog God). The Frog God lived with his father in the heaven before being sent to the mortal world. In the paddy field, he snatched insects and asked his father for water when there was a lack. Afterwards, he was respected as "ancestor". It is called "gungqsou" in Zhuang language, meaning "your grandfather". The three brothers and sisters represent fishing and hunting culture and the frog represents rice-farming culture. The evolution from fishing and hunting economy to rice-farming is interpreted in myths. The Zhuang myth about the source of rice seeds is named *A Dog Stole Rice Seeds*, according to which rice seeds were stolen from the heaven by a dog. Therefore, Zhuang people in northwest Guangxi formerly expressed thanks to dogs for bringing rice seeds by feeding them with the first meal of rice after harvesting new rice. Rice seeds were found as Zhuang ancestors noticed the wild rice seeds on their dogs when they went hunting. In a Zhuang flood myth named *The Story of Uncle Bu*, the Thunder King created a drought which caused cracks in the paddy field. Uncle Bu went up to the sky to force the Thunder King to send rain. Because of that, the Thunder King created flood for revenge. A great number of works concerning rice can be found in myths, folk songs and other forms of art. Rice-farming culture is reflected in the depictions of the Frog God with human body and frog head in the cliff paintings of the Huashan Mountains, as well as frog-relief bronze drums.

4.2　Zhuang medicine and rice-farming culture

A large number of archeological materials establish that Zhuang is a typical rice-farming nationality. According to research, basins of Zuojiang, Youjiang and Yongjiang Rivers in Guangxi are the original home of Zhuang ancestors including Xi'ou and Luoyue people, as well as one of the places where rice agriculture originated. Rice-farming culture is a fundamental cultural feature of Xi'ou and Luoyue nationality.

4.2.1　Rice-farming culture and the origin of Zhuang medicine

According to researches, primitive rice agriculture occurred in Guangxi Zhuang region in the early Neolithic Age of around 9000 years ago. Zhuang rice-farming culture continued to develop ever since, and now it still has a deep-rooted impact on every aspect of Zhuang social life. There is a close relationship between the origin of medicine and the development of primitive agriculture and stock farming. There are many legends on the origin of medicine. *Genealogical Annals of the Emperors and Kings* says, "The Fuxi clan ... numerous herbs were tried and nine needles were developed to save lives." *Shiji Gangjian* says, "Shennong tasted hundreds of herbs, then herbal medicines were first discovered." *Supplement to Records of the Grand Historian: the Stories of Three Kings* says, "Shennong tested hundreds of varieties of herbs with his holy red whip, and first tasted them. Then herbal medicines were first found." Many legends on the origin of medicine are about the Fuxi and the Shennong clans. Most people believe that the Shennong clan can be considered as the representative of primitive agriculture and the Fuxi clan can be considered as the representative of primitive stock farming, indicating that the origin of medicine is closely related to primitive agriculture and stock farming. These legends on the origin of medicine are portrayals of the origin of TCM and Zhuang medicine.

In the late period of clan society, tool making technologies had been improved in the Zhuang region, and impressive progress had been made in primitive agriculture and fishing and hunting economy there. With the development of primitive agriculture, Zhuang ancestors were able to start a long-term and detailed observation and more careful trials on more plants during crop cultivation. They turned some wild medicinal plants into cultivated ones, and knew about more species. With the emergence of fishing and hunting economy, Zhuang ancestors could acquire more fish and meat, and understand animal medicine. Zhuang medicines originated after repeated practice and observation and accumulation of experience.

4.2.2　Rice-farming culture, health preservation and disease prevention

Throughout ages of production and life practice, Zhuang people used their great wisdom to create time-honored Zhuang culture, and their popular traditional sports are closely related to rice-farming culture. Their distinctive sports events include bronze drum dance, carrying pole dance, windmill walking, frog dance, and throwing embroidered balls. Those traditional Zhuang sports events are closely related to nature, labor or skilled actions. Most of them reflect the farm work, sacrifice, customs and other aspects of rice agriculture. As an important part of Zhuang people's life, those events have been passed on from generation to generation.

Bronze drum dance was derived from the activities sacrifice and call to battle in Xi'ou and Luoyue tribes over 2000 years ago. There are lots of depictions of bronze drum dance in the cliff paintings of the Huashan Mountains in the Zuojiang basin in Guangxi. Those paintings were produced in the Warring States Period. After the Qin and Han dynasties, central governor strengthened the rule over Lingnan. With improved political stability and continuous social and economic development, people from different ethnic groups carried on extensive economic and cultural exchanges, including bronze drum dance. Many researches have revealed that bronze drum culture is derived from rice-farming agriculture. The decoration on bronze drums, simulating the sun, thunder, ripple, and frog, is closely related to rice-farming culture. For preserving bronze drums, Zhuang people tie the drum handles with straw, or place drums upside down and fill them with unhusked rice. Zhuang people call the practice "bronze maintenance". The functions of bronze drums include the enhancement of drum soul through filling with unhusked rice at home, communication with deities, or delivery of information. Zhuang ancestors created bronze drums primarily for cooking. Gradually, they became tools for pleasing deities, praying for rain, mustering people, ordering troops, and providing accompaniment to singing and dancing, etc. Also, they became a symbol of power and wealth. Rice-farming culture and bronze drum culture influenced and promoted each other in their formation and development. As Zhuang people said "The louder the drum is, the taller the crops will grow.", which is really relevant to rice agriculture, bronze drum dance now has become a popular traditional sports activity among Zhuang people. It can be seen in the Frog Festival every year in Donglan, Tian'e, Bama, Fengshan, and other Red River basins inhabited by the Zhuang. It involves one person beating the bronze drum while another uses a wooden box to improve resonance. They beat the drum to make euphonious sound and dance. They fully display their skills as they sometimes turn right and sometimes left with powerful and agile movements, or move fast or slow to the solemn, forceful, inspiring and rhythmic drumming. The simple, ancient and passionate movements of drum players reveal that Zhuang people are simple, resolute, brave and tenacious. Bronze drum dance can enhance people's strength, sensibility and endurance, and also cultivate their perseverance, courage, enterprise, desire for excellence, and other fine qualities.

The carrying pole is one of the earliest and most enduring tools used by people to carry a load. As a popular activity among Zhuang people, the carrying pole dance was derived from rice production and grain processing, with carrying poles as the instruments. Carrying pole dance was derived from rice pounding dance. Rice pounding dance is called "dwklongj" and "guhlongj" in Zhuang language, and Zhuang people also use the pole clunking sound to name the dance. The field for carrying pole dance can be either large or small. The number of performers should be even, for example, 4, 6, 8, or 10. When performing carrying pole dance, people around the bench hold the middle of the carrying poles with both hands, flexibly hit the bench with both ends of the carrying pole, in traditional rhythms. The traditional routines of carrying pole dance were designed based on Zhuang people's labor process, named pounding rice, happy family, happy reunion, transplanting rice seedlings, waterwheel irrigation, threshing, celebrating the harvest, etc. The dance movements include juggling the carrying pole, standing, squatting, marching, turning around, and jumping. In addition, it is accompanied by the sound of "keke" and the sound of drum-hitting and the rhythm is strong. Carrying pole dance is the imitation of actions in agricultural activities, including harrowing, transplanting rice seedlings, irrigating, harvesting, threshing, and pounding rice. The dance represents the process of rice-farming, and also summarizes the production activities of the entire year. Zhuang people pray for a harvest of the incoming year through that kind of dynamic and joyful performance.

It takes patience, care and perseverance to grow rice. Long-term rice-farming has cultivated the national character of Zhuang people, who are mild, introverted, hardworking, patient, cooperative, courteous, soft on the outside and hard on the inside. Rice is a crop that requires good care during its growing phases, including 10 periods or processing steps, such as returning green, tillering, panicle differentiation, booting, heading, milky ripeness, yellow ripeness, and full ripeness. Examples of good care include preparing rice seedling bed, seed presoaking, raising rice seedlings, ploughing, and transplanting rice seedlings. In the several months after transplanting rice seedlings, people must care for them like babies, for example, temperature observation, drainage, irrigation, fertilization, weeding, insect prevention, disease prevention, and lodging prevention. When harvest time comes, beast intrusion and rain should be considered. It takes patience for harvest. The paddy field is different from dry fields. Paddy fields should be located in sunny, flat and water-rich land near water sources. Therefore, people should settle down and stay put. This has cultivated the character of Zhuang people, who are mild, introverted, restrained, patient, and fond of a settled way of life. Now the landscapes of Guilin and Babao are marvelous, but they were surrounded by forests in ancient times. They were sunless, hot, rainy, and filled with miasma, insects, snakes and beasts. Life was hard there. In the Song Dynasty, Guangxi was still described as a "place of execution" (in *Lingwai Daida* by Zhou Qufei in the Song Dynasty). Guangxi was a place for banishing prisoners in the Tang, Song, Yuan and Ming dynasties. Shen Jianqi, a Tang Dynasty poet, in exile passed to Beiliu, Guangxi and wrote, "I heard about miasmic rivers and roads and now have come to Guimen Pass. Most people die before getting old there and few exiled people can return from there." Under such conditions, Zhuang people worked hard in the paddy fields in the heat and miasma. After a considerable period of time, Zhuang people became hard-working, soft outside and hard inside. They are not aggressive, but they are very brave in protecting the fruits of their labor. As *Chiya* wrote, "Ferocious and intrepid tusi soldiers have the greatest combat effectiveness." This directly indicates that Zhuang people are soft on the outside and hard on the inside. Both Han and Zhuang people rely on agriculture, therefore they can culturally communicate with each other easily. Zhuang people absorbed the Confucian idea of mild manner. They even adapted *the Twenty-four Filial Exemplars* into twenty-four long poems, in contrast with people of the Central Plains.

As discovered from the excavation of Hemudu culture, the ancestors of the Baiyue minority began to grow rice around seven or eight thousand years ago. During the period of Luoyue Kingdom, Zhuang ancestors were able to grow rice, and also planted cotton in large amounts, spun and wove cloth. This promoted the great development of rice-farming civilization. Zhuang people rely on rice for nourishment, and on cloth for protection against cold. Because rice grows from the earth, they are called "earth people". Ancient people called paddy fields as "naz", meaning the paddy field in the valley. The word "naz" contains the rich connotation of Zhuang ancestors' rice-farming culture. "Naz culture" gave rise to pottery culture and big stone shovel culture, which promoted cooking and hygiene. After Zhuang ancestors invented pottery, they cooked food provided by fishing and hunting. It was more beneficial to the development of tissues and organs including the brain. And it could prevent or relieve diseases of the stomach and intestines. It reflected that Zhuang ancestors began to have the concept of health preservation and disease prevention. Specifically, Zhuang ancestors had an amazing hygiene practice called "nasal drinking" as "the preventive treatment of disease". *Biography of Jia Juanzhi*, *Book of Han* says, "Fathers and sons of the Luoyue minority shower together in the same river and drink water through the nose." *Liaoren Chapter*, *Book of Wei* says, "Liao possibly belongs to an ethnic group of Nanman (Southern Barbarians)... They chew food in the mouth while drinking water through the nose." In the Song Dynasty, Fan Chengda said in *Guihai Yuheng Zhi*, "Southerners like nasal drinking through pottery cups and bowls. They drink alcohol by nose through a small tube. In summer, it is very pleasant to drink water through the nose, particularly for Yongzhou people." Zhou Qufei in the Song Dynasty wrote in *Lingwai Daida*, "Pour a small quantity of water in a ladle with an aperture, and add salt and several drops of Shanjiang (*Alpinia japonica* (Thunb.) Miq.) juice into it. Use a small tube, and insert it into the nose. Suck water into the head, and then it will flow into the throat. Rich people can use silver containers, tin containers come second, pottery third, and ladle last. Before nasal drinking ... then you will not feel choked by water. Exhale after drinking water, and the head and diaphragm will be cooled down, which is wonderful." Zhuang ancestors cooled down their heads and diaphragm through nasal drinking. Therefore, they were able to cool the body temperature down, prevent heatstroke, and defend against the miasmic toxin coming from the mix of the dampness, heat, and the rancidity of animals and plants. Now, nasal douche and nebulization are still applied in Zhuang medicine. They have certain therapeutic effects on nasal, laryngeal, and respiratory diseases.

4.3　Zhuang medical theories and rice-farming culture

4.3.1　Rice-farming culture and "Sandao" theory

Rice-farming culture is an important symbol of Luoyue culture, as well as an important cultural heritage for both Chinese civilization and world civilization. According to excavated relics and related researches, wild rice was widespread in the area where the ancient Luoyue people lived. Luoyue people knew about wild rice from early times. They invented rice cultivation together with Cangwu and Xi'ou people, making tremendous contributions to the Chinese nation and people around the world. Primitive rice shelling tools have been unearthed in Tingzixu site in Nanning. According to 14 dating, those tools can date back from 11,000 years ago, ranking only second to the carbonized grains of rice left by Zhuang ancestors in Dao County, Hunan province (previously Cangwu) between 20,000 and 11,000 years ago. Those grains are at least 2000 years earlier than 10,000-year-old rice in Wannian County, Jiangxi province. Early in the Luotian period, Luoyue people had known how to reclaim farmland, and they selected parcels of farmland along the valley water areas. According to *Ordered Annals of Nanyue*, *Records of the Grand Historian*, it is recorded in *Records of Guangzhou* that "There is luotian along the valley water areas in Jiaozhi. People there rely on the farmland, therefore they are also called Luo people." Qin Naichang, Guangxi ethnologist, said, primitive rice agriculture emerged in the Zhuang region 9000 years ago, therefore the Zhuang region is one of the places of origin for rice agriculture."

Rice is essential in Zhuang people's life, and has a profound impact on them. Therefore they have special beliefs about rice. (1) Nobleness of rice: Zhuang people believe that rice comes from the heaven, and it is the highest type among all cereal crops. Therefore, rice products must be used in offering sacrifice and in entertaining distinguished guests. (2) Rice soul: Zhuang people believe that there is the God of Agriculture in the farmland, and the God of Young Crops in the rice seedlings. Therefore sacrifice offering ceremonies are required before starting farming, and rice seedling soul should be invoked during bad harvests. (3) Interactions between rice and humans: the concept of interactions between heaven and mankind was widespread in ancient China, and it is reflected in *Classic of Changes*. Zhuang people have the same concept about rice. In song fairs in ancient times, young men and women simulated sexual intercourse in the farmland, believing that grain filling would be smoother. If a person in white was the first to go to the field, there would be crop failure and retribution. Some people believed that the more songs that were sung in the song fairs, the happier the rice seedlings would be and the better the harvest would be. Some people believed that straw or rice seedlings were able to repel pathogenic qi, so they hung them outside the door to exorcise evil spirits. Some people hung a handful of straw around their waists to repel wandering ghosts, so that they felt safe while walking. (4) Connection between rice and human life: it is widely believed by Zhuang people that rice represents human's life and it can increase longevity. When Zhuang elders have birthdays, their children need to add new rice into the longevity rice jars while Taoist masters chant. Therefore, birthday celebration is also called "replenishment of rice" by Zhuang people. They believe that the rice can be taken out to make congee and replenish longevity. However, the rice should not be used up, or it will imply the end of life. In Zhuang, a long and happy life is called "rice life" and a miserable life is called "(wild) vegetable life". Those ideas have not been changed much even until now.

The emergence of rice-farming culture has promoted the formation of Zhuang medicine, and deeply impacted its further development. Zhuang is a typical rice-farming minority. As rice-farming culture is directly linked to diet, the increasingly improved rice-farming technologies and diverse food have enabled Zhuang people to understand the role of diet in preserving health, warding off diseases and dispelling pathogenic factors. According to Zhuang medicine, "Dietetic invigoration is better than the use of tonifying medicines." It indicates that Zhuang medicine is closely related to rice-farming culture and diet. Also, rice-farming culture has contributed significantly to the formation of Zhuang medical theories. According to the research, the Zhuang nationality is one of the first Chinese ethnic nations to grow rice. Through practice and observation, Zhuang ancestors knew that rice grows naturally with the blessing of heaven and earth qi, and that grain crops nourish the body with heaven and earth qi within them. Humans live on "cereals", which are a necessary part of meals. Therefore the tract taking cereals inside the body and enabling digestion and absorption is called "Gudao" (literally cereal tract). Also, they noticed the importance of water and qi for the growth of crops. The lack or unbalance of water and qi is unfavorable for the growth of crops. Water and qi are also essential for the body. In the theoretical system of Zhuang medicine, there are two important tracts for exchanging qi and water within the body which are called "Shuidao" and "Qidao". As a core part of Zhuang medical theories, the theory of Sandao (Gudao, Qidao, and Shuidao) came from Zhuang ancestors' basic understanding of human and nature and accumulation of practical experience. Obviously it is related to Zhuang rice-farming culture.

4.3.2　Rice-farming culture and "yin-yang" theory

As the sun rises from east in the morning and sets in the west in the late afternoon, it brings brightness and warmth as well as darkness and silence to nature. The sun can rise again, and vitalize everything. Zhuang ancestors relied on sunlight in agricultural production, particularly in rice-farming. They hoped the sun would bring more light and heat to assure people of ample food and clothing and health. Naturally, they revered and worshipped the sun as "the Sun God". Therefore, they carefully observed the sun and studied its movement. Yin and yang are the description of its movement, which means life and death. When the day breaks, the yang cycle begins as the sun rises to bring light, and everything comes awake, which means life; When darkness falls, the yin cycle begins as the sun sets and everything falls asleep and becomes silent without light, which means death. Everything changes as the sun changes between life and death, i.e., between yang and yin. Naturally the sun was regarded as the master of the universe. Crops need heat and light from the sun to grow. The routine movement of the sun enabled peasants to follow a basic life pattern "waking up and working as the sun rises and going to sleep at sunset", as well as to have the basic sense of space and time. Therefore, people could know about the order of the universe from the sun, and identify everything in nature by the sun. Humans used the sun to determine the directions east and west, as well as day and night. Therefore, the sun was the major foundation for the sense of space and time. With the belief in "the Sun God", the primitive and basic concept of yin and yang developed into the yin-yang theory, which has a profound impact on traditional Chinese culture. As a systematic methodology, the yin-yang theory formed in the late Zhou, Qin and Han periods. However, its basic concept existed in the ancient Chinese belief in "the Sun God".

Rice grew in South China, where it was hot and yin and yang were interdependent upon each other. With the development of rice-farming culture, Zhuang yin-yang theory formed. According to the record of *Volume 17*, *Guangxi Local Records* in the Ming Dynasty, Zhuang people sincerely believed in yin and yang. Rice-farming culture brought Zhuang ancestors an early recognition of yin and yang, and gave rise to the concept of yin and yang in Zhuang medicine. The changes of everything in nature are revealed in the opposition, mutual rooting, waxing and waning, balance, and mutual convertibility of yin-yang. In Zhuang medicine, the concept of yin and yang is used to understand the birth, death, old age and disease of humans, the functions of zang and fu organs, as well as the relationship between humans and natural change. Gradually, the concept developed into the theory of "yin-yang basis" as a basic theory in Zhuang medicine.

References:

[1] Liang Qicheng, Zhong Ming. Zhuange Pharmacy in China [M]. Nanning:

Guangxi Nationalities Publishing House, 2005.

[2] Luo Shimin. The Memories of Daming Mountain: Historical and Cultural Study of Luoyue Ancient Kingdom [M]. Nanning: Guangxi Nationalities Publishing House, 2006.

[3] Su Bingqi. New Discussion on the Origin of Chinese Civilization [M]. Beijing: SDX Joint Publishing Company, 2009.

[4] Huang Hanru. Zhuang Medicine in China [M]. Nanning: Guangxi Nationalities Publishing House, 2001.

[5] Liang Tingwang. Discussion on Zhuang Rice-farming Culture and Social Development [J]. Journal of Wenshan Teachers College, 2006, 19 (3): 1 - 5.

[6] Liang Tingwang. Protection, Development and Utilization of Chinese Rice-farming Culture [J]. Journal of Hechi University, 2006, 26 (4): 63 - 68.

5　Zhuang Medicine and Customs

5.1　Zhuang customs

5.1.1　Introduction to Zhuang customs

Custom means the habits and mores. According to distinguished Zhuang scholar Liang Tingwang, a custom is a habitual way of behaving and thinking created by people based on the pattern of their life, their lifestyles, their natural conditions, and a certain level of social material production. Customs are associated with production, life, etiquette, seasonal occasions, society, belief, entertainment, literature and art.

Each place has its own way of supporting its own inhabitants. China is a vast country with many minorities. Its 56 ethnic groups are 56 flowers adorning its beautiful rivers and mountains. With different natural conditions and social environment such as distinctive features of productivity, and people's material and cultural life, each group has formed and carried with its unique behavioral habits and ways of life over the long course of development. *Yanzi Chunqiu*（*Yanzi's Spring and Autumn Annals*）says, "Habits differ within 100-li area and customs differ within 1000-li area." It reflects the difference of customs in different regions and nationalities. As one of the minorities in China, the Zhuang nationality has well-established customs, which are important forms of Zhuang people's spiritual and material life and behavioral patterns. Zhuang customs reveal Zhuang people's psychological characteristics, behavioral patterns and language habits in clothing, diet, living, marriage, burial, belief, production, transportation, trading, social organizations, culture and art. As a basic component of Zhuang characteristics, Zhuang customs unite Zhuang people and give them the sense of identity.

5.1.2　Features of Zhuang customs

Zhuang customs display the Zhuang characteristics. Firstly, they are closely related to ancient Yue people in language, literature, lifestyle and other aspects.

Secondly, they are less limited by feudalism. For example, women have their rights to speak openly in social life. Thirdly, they have regional differences. A custom usually has different forms in different Zhuang branches and regions. Zhuang customs are diverse, which might also have something to do with geographical situations. Fourthly, they are introverted and elusive. For example, Zhuang people do not impress others through distinctive appearance or individuality. Fifthly, they are greatly influenced by the customs of the Han nationality. The festivals of the Han and the Zhuang are closely related.

Zhuang culture gave rise to Zhuang medicine and promoted its development. Zhuang medicine and customs are also closely related. For example, Zhuang people worshipped ghosts and gods, and had an excessive liking for constructing excessive temples. That custom explains why witchcraft medicine and Zhuang medicine coexisted. Other customs associated with medicine include having the hair clipped short, tattooing the body, dressing in blue-black, nasal drinking, living in ganlan houses, and bone-collecting reburial. By learning Zhuang customs, we can know about Zhuang people's colorful spiritual world, material culture and behavioral characteristics, and also understand the foundations for the formation and development of Zhuang medicine as well as its indispensable culture base.

5.2　Zhuang medicine and drug fairs customs

5.2.1　Legends about drug fairs

There is a plentiful supply of evergreen vegetation and drug resources in the Zhuang region. On the fifth day of the fifth lunar month in each year, villagers in Zhuang region go to the drug fairs in the market town, where they either sell a variety of medicinal materials they have picked, or browse, smell and buy medicine. In Zhuang folklore, lush herbs exhibit strong efficacy and the best therapeutic effect during this Dragon Boat Festival. When people go to the drug fairs on that day, they can absorb the qi of medicine, prevent diseases, and consequently fall ill as rarely as possible throughout the year.

The formation of Zhuang drug fairs is associated with the folk tale called "Yeqi's Fight against the God of Plague". In ancient times, there was an old Zhuang doctor with excellent medical skills named Yeqi. He led Zhuang people to pick lots of herbs in the mountains, and to fight against "Duyi" (meaning one-thousand-year-old snake spirit in Zhuang language), the God of Plague hurting people on the fifth day of the fifth lunar month. The God of Plague Duyi is ferocious. It brought poison gas, plague, and venomous insects to villages. The whole village people could not beat it, let alone a single household. Yeqi treated villagers for years. He carefully observed Duyi, and found that it was especially afraid of Aiye (*Folium Artemisiae argyi*), Changpu (*Acorus calamus* L.), Xionghuang (realgar), Banbianlian (*Lobelia chinensis* Lour.), Qiyeyizhihua (*Paris polyphylla*) and some other herbs. Therefore, he taught people to pick those herbs to hang them on the door or store them at home, so as to fight against Duyi. Before Duyi came, people boiled herbs for drinking or showering, so that they could prevent plague or recover from illness. However, not all villages can pick all the required herbs. Yeqi suggested that people place their herbs on the street on the fifth day of the fifth lunar month, so that they could threaten the God of Plague Duyi and exchange required herbs and experiences in preventing and treating diseases. Duyi was discouraged and ran away, finding that people in different villages had stored a great number of herbs and stood together to fight against it. Yeqi was regarded as "the King of Medicine" as he taught people to pick and grow herbs. Afterwards, it became a Zhuang custom to go to the drug fairs. Now, drug fairs can be found in Jingxi, Xincheng, Longlin, Guigang and other areas inhabited by the Zhuang nationality. The drug fairs of Jingxi City during the Dragon Boat Festival are particularly large and famous.

5.2.2   Drug fairs and Zhuang medicine

The research establishes that the drug fairs of Jingxi City during the Dragon Boat Festival began during the Song Dynasty and its popularity prevailed through the Ming and Qing dynasties, with more than 700 years of history. During the Dragon Boat Festival, herb collectors bring their fresh wild herbs to Jingxi for trading and they mainly come together from local communities, such as Napo, Debao, Daxin, Funing (in Yunnan), and other nearby counties or regions. Zhuang people in nearby villages go to the drug fairs to absorb the qi of medicine with all their family, consult Zhuang herb collectors about medical knowledge, or get their required herbs. Drug fairs not only provide a great opportunity to exchange the knowledge of medicinal materials and disease prevention and treatment, but also reflect Zhuang's emphasis on medicine.

With a good mass base and excellent geographical environment, Jingxi drug fairs during the Dragon Boat Festival formed and developed. Zhuang people account for 99. 4% of the population in Jingxi City, which is one of the major areas inhabited by the Zhuang nationality. Local Zhuang people continue the custom of going to the drug fairs during the Dragon Boat Festival, where there are tens of thousands of people attending the Drug Fair Festival every year. Jingxi is located in the border area of southwest Guangxi and southeast Yunnan-Guizhou Plateau. Most part of Jingxi lies south of the Tropic of Cancer. It has the subtropical monsoon climate, with an average elevation of 800 meters. Its annual average temperature is 19. 1 degrees centigrade and its annual precipitation is 1600 millimeters. Its conditions are good for biodiversity. With superior geographical and climate conditions, Jingxi is abundant in Chinese and Zhuang medicinal herbs. With more than 3000 species, Jingxi is honored as the land of herbs. With rich resources, local people can pick and use various herbs and cultivate drug fair culture. Researchers have conducted field investigations and found that 564 types of medicinal herbs are traded in drug fairs, including rare medicinal materials [e. g., Tianqi (*Panax pseudoginseng* Wall. var. *notoginseng* (Burkill) Hoo et Tseng), and Gejie (*Gecko*)], bulk medicinal materials such as Jinyinhua (*Flos Lonicerae*), Yiyiren (*Semen Coicis*), and common genuine Zhuang herbs such as Zuandifeng (*Schizophragma integrifolium*), Jiujiefeng (*Pilea symmeria Wedd.* var. *salwinensis* Hand. -Mazz.), Huanghuadaoshuilian (*Polygala fallax* Hemsl.), Tengduzhong (*Parabarium micranthum* (A. DC.) Pierre), Jixueteng (*Spatholobus suberectus* Dunn), and Yanhuanglian (*Corydalis saxicola* Bunting). The development of Jingxi drug fairs during the Dragon Boat Festival has played an important role in exploring and utilizing local Zhuang medicinal materials.

5. 3　Zhuang medicine and traditional lifestyle

5. 3. 1　Tattooing

Tattoos were made by painting patterns on the skin, and using needles to insert dye (natural indigo was frequently used in ancient times) into the skin. Permanent tattoos were obtained after skin healing. Zhuang ancestors' tattooing custom is recorded in many historical documents. *Treatise on Geography*, *Book of Han* says, " (Yue people) cut the hair and tattoo the body in order to avoid the harm of flood dragon." As it is written in *Taiping Huanyu Ji* in the Song Dynasty, "People preferred forehead, face and body tattoos and tooth extraction in zhous (Prefectures) along the Zuojiang River and Youjiang River in Yongzhou. " Zhuang ancestors relied on hunting and fishing. In the rivers, lakes and seas in South China, there were many flood dragons (i. e. crocodiles) and they were a danger to fishermen. Fishermen revered flood dragons and painted them on the body to disguise as dragons, hoping that flood dragons would regard them as fellow dragons instead of hurting them. The custom of tattooing can be traced back to the totem images or signs of clans and tribes, and had the purpose of asking a blessing from the Totem God. Those totems can "avoid the harm of flood dragon" , and enable identification and distinction in communication and intermarriage. Later on, it became a fashion like decorative patterns on clothes and silver jewellery. Tattooing provided a boost to the formation and development of shallow needling therapy in Zhuang medicine, as it used shallow needling instruments, and more importantly, it was a religious activity, which motivated Zhuang people to tattoo their bodies.

5.3.2　Close-cropped hair

It is the custom of Zhuang ancestors to have the hair clipped short. According to *Xiaoyaoyou*, *Inner Chapters*, *Zhuangzi*, "A man in the State of Song purchased hats and sold them in the State of Yue. But hats were useless for Yue people because they liked cutting the hair and tattooing the body. " That means Yue people had the hair clipped short and they were free from Shufa and Jiaguan (tying the hair and wearing a hat). In *Treatise on Geography*, *Book of Han*, it is recorded that it was a custom for Yue people, from Wuyue to Nine Counties of Lingnan, to "have the hair clipped short" . From the cliff painting portraits of the Huashan Mountains in Ningming, Guangxi, it can be seen that Zhuang ancestors — Luoyue people — had the hair clipped short. Huang Xianfan pointed out in *A General History of the Zhuang* , "Both having the hair clipped short and tattooing the body were prevailing in areas near the sea or rivers in South China. They reflect primitive people's totem worship." Zhuang ancestors' original purposes for having the hair clipped short and tattooing the body were the same for the imitation of dragon, which revealed ancient Yue people's totem worship. There are considerations about healthcare in those customs. Those areas inhabited by the Zhuang nationality have the subtropical humid monsoon climate, with the annual average temperature of about 20℃. Those areas have long sunshine duration in summer and plentiful rainfall. Zhuang ancestors had the hair clipped short possibly because of damp and hot weather. It was easier and healthier for them to keep the hair short, so as to reduce the body temperature, keep the hair dry, and prevent hair from sticking to anything.

5.3.3 Tooth extraction

Like close-cropped hair and tattooing, tooth extraction was another kind of body decoration for Zhuang ancestors. The first type of tooth extraction is the removal of incisor teeth and the replacement with false teeth. *The Classic of Regions Beyond the Seas*: *South*, *Classic of Mountains and Seas* says, "Yi fought with Zaochi in the wilderness in Shouhua. On the east side of the Kunlun Mountains Yi shot Zaochi. Zaochi is a man with a chisel-like tooth about 5 or 6 chi long. *Yazhou customs*, *Taiping Guangji* (*the Extensive Records of the Taiping Era*) says, "Liao in Qiongya ... they remove their upper teeth and replace them with the teeth of dog. Some of those people have four teeth longer than other teeth, and they eat humans. People without those long teeth don't eat humans." People with the first type of tooth extraction eat people. The second type of tooth extraction is the removal of incisor teeth after one becomes an adult as the sign of adulthood or getting married. Zhang Hua wrote in *Various Customs*, *Bowu zhi* (*Records of Diverse Matters*), "When Liao's children grow up, their upper teeth are removed." Li Jing in the Yuan Dynasty wrote in *Customs of Minorities*, *Yuannan zhilue*, "When males in southern Xuzhou and northern Wumeng are fourteen or fifteen years old, their two teeth will be removed before marriage." *Guizhou customs*, *Taiping Guangji* (*the Extensive Records of the Taiping Era*) says, "Those people called Li or Wuhu have the same surname. Those men and women shower together in the same river. They eat their first children ... One of women's incisor teeth will be removed for marriage." (Guizhou here is the current Guigang City, Guangxi). *The Fanshe Caifeng Tukao* says, "Fanshe people there call marriage as joining hands ... Both men and women remove their upper teeth for their marriage ..." The custom of tooth extraction reveals the pursuit of simple "imperfect beauty", and reflects Zhuang ancestors' special aesthetic standards. This is also their special coming-of-age ceremony. In addition, the custom can encourage drug treatment. This is recorded in *Pingnanliao*, *Volume II*, *Records of the Southern Barbarians*, *New Book of Tang*, "Wuwuliao live in areas with miasmic toxin, but people who are poisoned cannot take drugs. Therefore they remove their teeth." This shows that Zhuang ancestors had a basic understanding of preventing and treating miasmic toxin before the Tang Dynasty. Severe miasmatic disease might lead to convulsions, coma, lock-jaw, etc. Therefore patients cannot take drugs or food, and that can be avoided by tooth extraction beforehand.

5.3.4　Nasal drinking

In ancient South China, some minorities including Zhuang had a peculiar custom — nasal drinking. Some scholars believe that nasal drinking is the simulation of elephants using their trunks to help them drink. Records about nasal drinking began in the Han Dynasty, when *Yiwu Zhi* says, "Wuhu is an alias of Nanman (Southern Barbarians). They live in a nest and drink through their noses." *Biography of Jia Juanzhi*, *Book of Han* says, "Fathers and sons of the Luoyue minority shower together in the same river and drink water through the nose just like animals." In *Lingwai Daida (Answer on Outer of the Five Ridges)*, Zhou Qufei in Song Dynasty elaborated on nasal drinking, "there is a custom of nasal drinking in the mountainous region where minorities dwelled in Yongzhou and villages in Qinzhou. Pour a small quantity of water in a ladle with an aperture, and add salt and several drops of Shanjiang (*Alpinia japonica* (Thunb.) Miq.) juice into it. Use a small tube, and insert it into the nose. Suck water into the head, and then it will flow into the throat ... Have a piece of preserved fish before nasal drinking, then you will not feel choked by water. Exhale after drinking water, and the head and diaphragm will be cooled down, which is wonderful." It shows that nasal drinking was common in areas inhabited by the Zhuang nationality (the mountainous region in Yongzhou and villages in Qinzhou). Nasal drinking can be applied to both water and alcohol. Lu You in the Song Dynasty wrote in *Laoxuean Biji (Notes in Old Study Room)*, "In Chen, Yuan and Jingzhou, people drink alcohol through the nose. They drink several litres of the alcohol with unknown ingredients called Gouteng Wine. When they get drunk, they sing and dance together." In that quote, both male and female Zhuang ancestors drank alcohol through the nose and sang and danced together. Lu Ciyun in the Qing Dynasty wrote in *Dongxi Xianzhi*, "The wine named Gouteng Wine (or Diaoteng Wine) is made from rice and grass seed. People drink it through hollow vines. It is interesting that many people drink it through the nose." It reveals that nasal drinking continued until the Qing Dynasty.

The Zhuang region is hot and rainy in summer, with the miasmic toxin coming from the mix of dampness, heat, and rancidity of animals and plants. It is known as "a miasmatic region". Zhou Qufei recorded in *Lingwai Daida* that Shanjiang [*Alpinia japonica* (Thunb.) Miq.] was used in Zhuang medicine for nasal drinking, which aimed at preventing and treating miasmatic disease and summer heatstroke. One method of nasal irrigation and aerosol inhalation has been handed down in the Zhuang region. Patients flush their nasal cavities with a decoction or inhale aerial fog produced by boiled herbs, so that some epidemic diseases can be prevented. This treatment has something to do with nasal drinking in ancient times. This peculiar custom of healthcare contains scientific knowledge such as physical cooling and mucosal drug delivery, and it has certain therapeutic effects on nasal, laryngeal, and respiratory diseases.

5.3.5　Chewing betel nuts

Betel nuts have a long history in Lingnan. People there grow and chew them. In the Eastern Han Dynasty, Yang Fu wrote in *Yiwu Zhi* (*Record of Foreign Matters*) that Yue people in Lingnan chewed betel nuts. Wang Ji in the Ming Dynasty wrote in *Rixun Shoujing*, "People in Lingnan like betel nuts." For Zhuang people, betel nuts are a must for betrothal gift and marriage. According to *Baishan Si Zhi* in the Qing Dynasty, "Local people value betel nuts for betrothal gift and marriage. Rich families usually prepare thousands of them. Sumu (*Caesalpinia sappan* Linn.) is used to dye them. 8 betel nuts are packed in reed leaves, and about 20 or 30 bundles are tied together with red thread." If a woman accepts betel nuts as the engagement gift, it means that she acknowledges the engagement. For Zhuang people, betel nuts are also important in entertaining guests. It is a prevailing custom to "serve guests with betel nuts instead of tea" in some Zhuang villages of Guangxi, such as Longzhou, Fangchenggang, Shangsi, Shanglin and Ningming. Xu Songshi wrote in *History of the People of the Yue River Basin*, "Zhuang people prefer betel nuts and Weiye (*Piper betle* L.), and this custom still prevails in Guangdong and Guangxi." According to *Annals of Shanglin Xian* in the Republic of China, "Betel nuts are also important in social activities, including tea parties and banquets." The Chinese words for "betel nuts (槟榔)" sound the same as "宾" and "郎", both of which are used to address distinguished guests to show respect. Judging from the medicinal value of betel nuts, they can repel foulness, expel miasma, promote circulation of qi, excrete water, kill parasites and resolve accumulation. Liu Xun in the Tang Dynasty wrote in *Strange Stories in Lingnan*, "People collect and eat tender and ripe betel nuts. They eat betel nuts with Fuliuteng (*Piper yunnanense* Tseng) and dust from tile-roofed house to repel miasmic malaria." *Annals of Pingle Xian* says, "With miasma in the air, chewing betel nuts is just like enjoying a feast." Prevention and treatment of miasmic malaria is one of the reasons why Zhuang people chew betel nuts.

5.3.6 Living in ganlan houses

Many ethnic groups in South China live in traditional buildings called ganlan houses, which developed from primitive people's nest building with distinctive ethnic and local characteristics. In historical records, they are also called gaolan, gelan, malan, etc. Those are the transliterations of words in minority languages. In the Zhuang language, ganlan house (gwnzranz in Zhuang language) is a kind of storied wood house, meaning "above-ground dwelling". The word "ganlan" can be found as early as *Book of Wei*, "Liao possibly belongs to an ethnic group of Nanman (Southern Barbarians)... They pile up wood against trees and live aloft in the so-called ganlan." Kuang Lu in the Ming Dynasty wrote in *Chiya*, "People use thatch, rope and wood to make houses, which is called malan, with the upper layer for human habitation and the lower layer for rearing livestock including cattle, sheep, dogs, and pigs." Tian Rucheng in the Ming Dynasty wrote in *Yanjiao Jiwen* (*Hearsay from the Borderlands of the Southwest*), "Zhuang people live in malan houses covered with hatch. Those houses have stories separated by planks, with the upper layer for human habitation and the lower layer for rearing livestock including cattle, sheep, pigs, and dogs." A great number of tombs from the Qin and Han dynasties were discovered in areas inhabited by the Zhuang nationality, including Hepu, Pingle, Guigang, Wuzhou, Zhongshan, Hezhou, Xing'an, Guilin, Xilin, and Du'an. The unearthed pottery models of ganlan houses indicate that Zhuang ancestors lived in ganlan houses, which still exist. Currently, Zhuang people still get used to living in that kind of building.

Ganlan houses feature two stories, upper layer for human habitation and the lower layer for storing articles or rearing livestock including cattle and pigs. Zhuang ancestors' invention of ganlan houses is associated with the natural environment in South China. It is hot and humid, characterized by plentiful rivers, lakes and vegetation. In the damp, hot and thick forests, miasma, as pathogenic poison gas, emerges in rotten plants and carcasses. There are also many venomous serpents and wild beasts in the forests. For the safety of people and livestock, Zhuang ancestors needed to design buildings that were able to prevent the cold and the heat and adapt to the natural conditions. *Records of Nanpingliao*, *New Book of Tang* says, "People live in storied ganlan houses to prevent miasmatic disease caused by poison gas from the earth, as well as poisonous herbs, chiggers and Gloydius halys." The upper layer of ganlan houses is for human habitation as it is wellventilated, cool, and filled with abundant sunshine. This is an adaptation for geographical conditions and weather change in South China. The design of the upper storey is able to prevent rheumatic disease and avoid miasma, wild beasts, insects and snakes as it is damp-proof and high. The lower storey is for rearing livestock or storing articles so that the livestock cannot run around and defecate everywhere. Therefore, environmental sanitation can be ensured in villages. With distinctive regional ethnic characteristics, ganlan houses reflect Zhuang ancestors' wisdom of sanitation and disease prevention.

5.4 Zhuang medicine and costumes

Topics about costumes usually involve clothes and ornaments, including tops, pants, skirts, caps, scarves, gloves, belts, shoes, socks, leggings, hairstyles, jewelry, bags, etc. Costumes of a minority can demonstrate its distinctive external image and spiritual connotation.

As an open and inclusive minority, the Zhuang nationality absorbed advanced culture from other ethnic groups through exchanges. In particular, Zhuang costumes have been deeply influenced by the fashion among Han people. In some fairly developed areas, Zhuang people dress like Han people and therefore look like them. However, those characteristic of Zhuang costumes still can be seen in some Zhuang regions, particularly in the outlying mountain areas in northern, western and southern Guangxi. Restricted by natural conditions, those regions are isolated with few external exchanges and experience slow changes in social life. Zhuang costumes there remain traditional. Zhuang people are industrious, wise, and passionate about life and work. Certainly they love beauty as everybody does. Their aesthetic taste and attitude towards life are reflected in the materials, styles, colors and other aspects of their traditional costumes.

5. 4. 1　Huifu clothes

Zhuang costumes are mainly made from bast fibers，cotton and bamboo. They are also called Huifu clothes. Ramie and kudzu were the first materials used for textile by Zhuang people. Bast fiber fabric is most frequently used in the Zhuang region，with a longer history than other fabrics including cotton. According to the research，the Zhuang region produced ramie cloth from the Han Dynasty. Ramie was a traditional product in Guangxi from the Song Dynasty. Guangxi is an important ramie region in China. Bast fiber fabric can help beat the heat. With it，the summer clothes can keep light and cool，which is good in the damp and hot climate in South China. Cotton is also called jibei（吉贝）or gubei（古贝），and cotton fabrics are called jibei fabrics（吉贝布）. Zhuang cotton fabrics were well-known in the Tang Dynasty. Poet Bai Juyi once used them to sew clothes and praised，"Gui fabrics（cotton fabrics）are as white as snow..." Since the Jin Dynasty，Zhuang people made bamboo fabrics. In the Tang Dynasty，the bamboo fabrics from Hezhou and other places had become tributes. It is recorded in the *Taiping Huanyu Ji* in the Song Dynasty that "Liao use bamboo to make fabrics..." Liao in the quote refers to Zhuang people in Yongzhou. According to *Jiaqing Yitong Zhi*（*Unified Gazetteer of the Jiaqing Reign Period*）in the Qing Dynasty，women in Pingle and Gongcheng could use bamboo to make clothes. It is clear that bamboo fabrics are special Zhuang products. Now there are an increasing number of synthetic fibers，but bast fibers，cotton and bamboo are still important materials for Zhuang costumes. Those materials are renewable natural products from plantable crops，which indicates that Zhuang people care about the environment and respect nature.

5. 4. 2　Clothes with left lapels and Tongqun dresses

Zhuang costumes are both practical and beautiful. In ancient times，clothes with left lapels were for men and tongqun dresses were for women in the Zhuang region. According to *Strategies of Zhao*，*Strategies of the Warring States*，"Ouluo people wear clothes with left lapels. They tattoo the body with dishevelled hair." *Volume 185*，*Old Book of Tang* says，"Those people called Nanpingliao have clothes with left lapels for men and tongqun dresses for women ..." In the Qing Dynasty，Zhuang men and women wore navel length shirts and long pleated or short skirts，with hair in a bun and wrapped. In modern times，Zhuang costumes have the following features：

tops are collarless clothes with right lapels and wide sleeves. They usually reach the waist only, but they reach the knees in some regions. They have colorful laces around the neckline, sleeves, front, and lower hems. Bottoms include long wide-leg pants, with laces of different sizes at the knees. Typically, a skirt is worn outside pants. On the skirt, there are embroidery patterns made from colorful floss, or batik bronze drum patterns. Also an apron is worn outside pants. Aprons have exquisite embroidery made from colored floss or silk thread. Middle-aged Zhuang women have their hair in a bun and wrapped, which can be seen from the book *Introduction to Zhuang Costumes* by Shi Jingbin. Zhuang costumes feature wide sleeves and pant legs, which allow flexible movement of limbs. This is practical and good for walking in the mountains and working in the paddy fields. Those embroidered or dyed lace patterns are mainly the shape of familiar natural things including flowers, trees, birds, beasts, insects, fish, mountains, rivers, clouds, the sun, the moon and the stars. Those simple and beautiful patterns reflect the Zhuang ancestors' love of nature and their belief that man and the universe should be in harmony.

5.4.3 Dressing in blue-black

Blue and black are typical colors of traditional Zhuang costumes. As the color of earth, black is the dominant hue of Zhuang costumes, representing solemnity. People wear black attire during important joyous festivals or those of sacrifice. Even now that the dominant hue still can be seen in Zhuang groups in Napo County, Longzhou County and other places, for example Black-clothes Zhuang group inhabiting Napo County in Baise City, and Zhuang people calling themselves "Budai" in Jinlong, Longzhou County, Chongzuo City. Blue is nature's color. In daily life, many Zhuang people wear blue clothes, kerchieves, dudous or aprons. Blue and black pigments, also called indigo, are refined from leaves of plants such as Songlan or Caodaqing (*Isatis indigotica* Fortune), or Mulan (*Indigofera tinctoria* Linn.), or Malan [*Baphicacanthus cusia* (Nees) Bremek.], or Liaolan (*Polygonum tinctorium* Ait.), family Cruciferae, Leguminosae, Acanthaceae or Polygonaceae. Indigo cloth is distinctive in tone and hue. *Bencao Shiyi* records, "Indigo can remove toxin when applied to heat sores." It reveals indigo has the actions of clearing heat and removing toxin. Therefore, blue and black Zhuang costumes fit the climate and environment in the Zhuang region as they have the actions of removing toxin and repelling mosquitoes and other insects.

5.5　Zhuang medicine and custom of plague prevention

5.5.1　Hanging Ai on the door

Zhuang people believe that Ai can repel pathogenic qi. Therefore, they hang Ai on the door, and wear Ai sachets to repel pathogenic factors. For feeble and ailing children, their parents usually make Ai sachets and let their children wear those sachets, which has the action of repelling pathogenic factors to ensure children's safety. When Zhuang women need to carry their children on their back for a long walk, they bring a twig of Ai. Families hang Aiye (*Folium Artemisiae argyi*) on both sides of gates when they think there are pathogenic factors in their houses. After attending burial ceremonies, people repel pathogenic factors by washing their hands with water and Aiye, or water boiled with pomelo leaves. Hanging Ai and drinking Changpu (*Acorus calamus* L.) wine are key activities for Zhuang during the Dragon Boat Festival. *Annals of Jingxi Xian* records, "On the fifth day of the fifth lunar month, all families hang Ai and changpu leaves on the door, and drink Xionghuang (realgar) wine to dispel plague." Early on the morning of the fifth day of the fifth lunar month, Zhuang people pick Ai before the rooster crow. They shape Ai leaves and roots to resemble a human or tiger (commonly known as Ai tiger), and center them on the lintel. They also shape changpu leaves like swords and hang them under the roof. Ancient people believe that tigers could devour evil spirits. Therefore they combine Ai and tiger to enhance their action of repelling pathogenic factors. On that day, they also heat up water with Ai leaves, changpu and garlic in it. Then they shower with the water, and scatter it around the house. In fact, it is a good sanitary practice in summer. The weather turns hot after the Dragon Boat Festival, and bacteria grow and multiply fast. Scattering water with Chinese medicinal herbs can effectively inhibit and kill bacteria and keep the environment clean. It is just like drinking changpu wine during the Dragon Boat Festival. *Clinical Manual of Common Zhuang Medicine* records, "Changpu (*Acorus calamus* L.) is pungent in flavor and slightly warm in nature. It can regulate the brain (ukgyaeuj), move and transform qi, and remove wind toxin, dampness toxin and miasmic toxin." It is able to resolve phlegm, dispel dampness, moisten lung and dispel wind-cold. It has an action of preventing external-contraction diseases in summer.

5. 5. 2 Wearing medicine

In ancient times, people used plants (including herbs) to cover body and to make clothes, which was called Huifu clothes. They found that it could prevent from and treat diseases to wear some varieties of plants. Therefore, they continue the custom of wearing medicine as ethnic culture. Zhuang people have the custom of wearing Huifu clothes, embroidered balls and sachets. In *Lingwai Daida*, Zhou Qufei in the Song Dynasty wrote, "On the third day of the third lunar month, men and women get together. They sing and throw embroidered balls. They make eyes contact with each other and look for love." According to the quote, young Zhuang people throw embroidered balls outdoors during the Spring Festival or song fairs in the Sanyuesan Festival. Embroidered balls are their love token. Many young people tie to each other in bonds of matrimony through the activity. Initially, sachets were mainly filled with wood dust, rice bran and herbs. According to the earliest historical records, there were different crop seeds inside embroidered balls, including beans, millet, cotton seeds, and grains. Later, people found that wearing sachets with herbs could prevent colds, improve health and make the body strong. Gradually, this became a popular custom for disease prevention and treatment. Typically, they wear medicine around the neck, the wrist, the chest or the abdomen. Feeble and ailing children can wear herbal bags around the neck or wrist to improve health and make the body strong. For that purpose, the bags should be filled with finely powdered herbs including Cangzhu [*Atractylodes Lancea* (Thunb.) DC.], Baizhi [*Angelica dahurica* (Fisch. ex Hoffm.) Benth. et Hook. f.], Xixin (*Asarum sieboldii* Miq.), Huoxiang [*Agastache rugosa* (Fisch. et Mey.) O. Ktze.], Peilan (*Eupatorium fortunei* Turcz.), Gansong (*Nardostachys chinensis* Bat.), and Shichangpu (*Acorus tatarinowii*). During periods when plague was prevalent, plague could be dispelled and other diseases prevented by wearing sachets around the neck as one of preventive measures. The sachets are filled with the powder of Guanzhong (*Cyrtomium fortunei* J. Sm.), Zaojiao (*Gleditsia sinensis* Lam.), Bohe (*Mentha haplocalyx* Briq.), Fangfeng [*Saposhnikovia divaricata* (Trucz.) Schischk] cinnabar, Aiye (*Folium Artemisiae argyi*), and Shichangpu (*Acorus tatarinowii* Schott.).

5. 5. 3 Isolation and repelling foulness

In ancient times, those families with plague patients hung red paper on the outside of the door as a symbol of no admittance. In order to repel foulness and miasmic malaria, they burned herbs in the room, including Cangshu, Baizhi, Aiye, and pomelo peel. During the prevalence of infectious diseases, those affected families usually refused guests, and visitors from different villages were not welcomed. When people returned home from distant places, usually they waited outside the village or even several miles away. Their families would bring clothes for them to change into. Those clothes taken off would be steamed or boiled to eliminate toxic factors and prevent pathogenic factors. If villagers died outside the village, their bodies would be placed outside the village for funeral arrangement instead of funeral at home. This was because ancient people didn't know whether people died of infectious diseases or not. They took action proactively to prevent toxin and diseases entering the village. The custom of isolation and repelling foulness indicates Zhuang ancestors' understanding of preventing infectious diseases including plague. They took effective measures including disinfection and isolation.

5.6　Zhuang medicine and customs of burial practices

5.6.1　Zhuang burial practices

Zhuang burial practices reflect their ethics. Zhuang people believe that funeral rites are important in their life, the forms of such rites vary in different regions. Funeral rites mainly include announcement of death, dressing and laying a corpse in a coffin, waiting, carrying a coffin to the cemetery, and burial. In some regions, people invite Taoist priests to chant. Their burial forms include cave burial, suspended coffin, in-ground burial, flexed burial, and water burial. In-ground burial is the most common form among Zhuang people.

5.6.2　Better understanding of human skeleton through bone-collecting reburial

In-ground burial is one of the major forms among Zhuang people. It includes single burial ("large" burial) and secondary burial ("small" burial or bone-collecting reburial). According to *Annals of Shanglin Xian*, "A coffin is buried shallowly in the ground. After three years, the coffin will be opened again and bones will be collected and placed in an earthen jar. This is called small burial. Rich families select the coffin made of superior materials. They bury the coffin after selecting an auspicious location. This is called large burial." It reveals that rich people choose large burial while the majority of ordinary people choose secondary burial (bone-collecting reburial). Typically bones are collected around the third Tomb-sweeping Day after the burial. Sometimes people pick an auspicious day to do that. Firstly, children and other relatives collect the skull from the coffin. Then other people are able to collect other bones. They clean the bones with straw, cloth, abrasive paper, or blade, and place them in a bamboo basket. Secondly, bones are placed in the jar from bottom to top of the body, with the skull on the top. Thirdly, people cover the jar with a lid and carry it to the family burial ground or other good place for burial and for a cemetery mound. Bone-collecting reburial demonstrates Zhuang's ancestor worship and recognition of Fengshui of cemetery hills. It also promoted the understanding of human skeleton in Zhuang medicine.

References:

[1] Pan Qixu, Qin Naichang. Encyclopedia of Zhuang Nationality [M]. Nanning: Guangxi People's Publishing House, 1993.

[2] Liang Tingwang. Records of Zhuang Customs [M]. Beijing: China Minzu University Press, 1987.

[3] Pang Yuzhou. Brief Account of Zhuang Healthcare Customs [J]. Chinese Journal of Ethnomedicine and Ethnopharmacy, 2008 (5): 3 – 5.

[4] Wang Baican. Traditional Zhuang Culture and Zhuang Medicine [C]. Proceedings Paper, First National Academic Conference on Zhuang Medicine & National Forum on Experience in Ethnic Medicine, 2005: 17 – 27.

[5] Shi Jingbin. Introduction to Zhuang Costumes [J]. Journal of South-Central University for Nationalities, 1990 (1): 26 – 29.

[6] Wu Huimin. Discussion on the Origin of Zhuang Ganlan Houses [J]. Study of Ethnics in Guangxi, 1989 (1): 89 – 94.

6　Zhuang Medicine and Ballads

6. 1　Zhuang ballad culture

Ballad is one of the oldest art forms coming with the emergence of human langua- ges, as well as one of the important genres of folk music. The Chinese word for ballad is "歌谣", the combination of "歌（ge）" and "谣（yao）". In ancient China, "歌 （ge）" was a song with musical accompaniment, and "谣（yao）" was a song with- out musical accompaniment. In modern times, songs with or without musical accom- paniment can be ballads（"歌谣"）. Ballads are short and contain succinct sentences. They have rhymes and special metrical patterns. Zhuang ballads, also called folk songs, are metrical works created orally by Zhuang people. According to the *Dictiona- ry of Chinese Folk Literature*, "The word '山歌（folk songs）' is used in South China to describe folk songs." As a part of literature, Zhuang ballads express people's thoughts, feelings, production and life through metrical languages. They are harmoni- ous in tone, natural in rhythm, and filled with Zhuang characteristics, providing a strong atmosphere of life. They deeply reflect Zhuang society, history, life, customs and practices.

Guangxi, inhabited by the Zhuang nationality, is regarded as "a sea of songs" "the land of folk songs". Guangxi people are known for being good at singing. They prefer to sing rather than to speak in their daily life, and they sing as part of the mat- ing ritual. Regarded as a minority with poetic thinking, the Zhuang nationality has created a wonderful Zhuang ballad culture over the ages of production and life practice. As one of the Zhuang cultures with the longest history, Zhuang ballad culture involves a series of cultural activities associated with Zhuang ballad.

6. 1. 1　The Zhuang language and cutting

Zhuang is a native ethnic group in the Pearl River basin in South China. The in- habited region extends east to west from Lianshan Zhuang and Yao Autonomous County in Guangdong province to Wenshan Zhuang and Miao Autonomous Prefecture in Yunnan province, south to north from Beibu Gulf of Guangxi to Congjiang County in Qiandongnan Miao and Dong Autonomous Prefecture in Guizhou. Zhuang people mainly live in Guangxi. As a nationality, an essential feature of the Zhuang is their common language — the Zhuang language.

6. 1. 1. 1   The language of Zhuang

The Zhuang language is a beautiful language with a long history. It was created by Zhuang ancestors in their life and production. The Zhuang language is of the Zhuang-Dai branch of the Zhuang-Dong (Kra-Tai) group of the Sino-Tibetan family of languages. It is divided by the Youjiang River and the Yongjiang River into southern and northern dialects. The areas of southern dialects are located in the south of the Youjiang and Yongjiang rivers, and Wenshan Zhuang and Miao Autonomous Prefecture in Yunnan province, while those of northern dialects are situated in the north of the Youjiang and Yongjiang rivers, Qiubei, Shizong, Funing, northern Guangnan, Lianshan, Huaiji and other Yunnan and Guangdong regions. There are seven sub-dialects in the north and five in the south. The sub-dialects have very similar pronunciation and vocabulary, while the different dialect groups are so different that people from different groups cannot understand each other.

6. 1. 1. 2   Writing of Zhuang

Zhuang people once had their own writing system, which faded after the First Emperor of Qin (Qin Shi Huang) unified China and promoted a unified writing system. An alternative script now called "The Old Zhuang Script" was adopted in the Tang Dynasty for social interaction amongst the Zhuang. They created it to record Zhuang speech by borrowing the writing, pronunciation and meaning of Chinese as well as six traditional classification principles. In the Song Dynasty, Fan Chengda wrote about the usage of the Old Zhuang Script in *Guihai Yuheng Zhi* "The distant and remote area has its own script to record even though its seclude location. " The Old Zhuang Script was named by Han people, and it was called "sawndip" by Zhuang people. "Sawndip" is a Zhuang word that means immature characters. Sawndip is not easy to use and it has never been standardized. Therefore, it didn't become a generally recognized Zhuang writing system. It was mainly used by Zhuang artists and shamans to record scriptures, folktales, myths, songs, notes, and places. Examples of works written in sawndip include *Liao Songs* in the Ming Dynasty and the famous *Buluotuo Poetic Scripture*.

6. 1. 2　Zhuang ballads

6. 1. 2. 1　Origin of Zhuang ballads

Yue people loved singing. Since ancient times, Zhuang people have been good at singing to express their emotions in production and life. This could date back to the primitive Zhuang society, when people worked and called out loud. In other words, people knew how to use different sounds to express their thoughts and emotions when language did not exist. Calling is not singing, but it gave rise to Zhuang ballads. One of the two main views on Zhuang folk songs is that it is about pairing marriage. It is believed that pairing marriage gave rise to folk song culture. The second view is about entertaining gods. It is believed that folk song culture was derived from religious beliefs. In order to seek blessings from deities to meet production and life demands, ancestors sang to praise and entertain them. The earliest written record of Zhuang ballads probably came from the Han Dynasty. According to the *Shanshuo Chapter of Shuo Yuan* (*Garden of Stories*) by Liu Xiang (a writer of the Western Han Dynasty), the *Song of the Yue Boatman* was a short song recorded in the state of Chu around 528 BC, when the prince Zixi, the Lord of E, on an excursion on his state barge, was intrigued by the singing of the Yue boatman. Wei Qingwen published the article *On the Relationship between the Song of the Yue Boatman and the Zhuang Language* in *A Collection of Essays Concerning the Languages of the Ethnic Minorities*, published by China Social Sciences Press, 1981. He pointed out in the article that it was a Zhuang folk song recorded through the prominciation of Chinese. Its pronunciation, grammar and parts of speech are the same as the Zhuang language, and it has the same rhymes and metrical patterns as existing Zhuang ballads. It seems that Zhuang ballads has a history of perhaps 3000 years.

6. 1. 2. 2　Content and forms of Zhuang ballads

Zhuang ballads are remarkably diverse, including ballads of lament (about long-term laborer, nagging wife, being single, grumbling about hardship, complaining about fate, etc.), love ballads (about wooing, compliment, courtship, expressing love, making friends, making a vow, farewell, etc.), folklore ballads (about congratulation, birthday celebration, ceremonies, toasts, greeting guests, lullabies, lamenting at funerals and the wedding day, etc.), labor ballads (about farm work, idle farming seasons, seasons, the solar terms, seasonal rain, drought, etc.), question-and-answer ballads (in antiphonal style), historical ballads, political ballads, children's ballads, and revolutionary ballads.

Differences between southern and northern dialects gave rise to different names of Zhuang ballads, including "Huan" "Xi" "Jia" "Bi" and "Lun". Zhuang ballads have various forms with distinct rhythms, beautiful tunes, and colorful lyrics.

(1) Huan

"Huan" ballads are popular on both sides of Hongshui River and its northern. They have various styles of lyric and construction. Their lyrics rhyme in the middle and at the end of lines, or at the beginning and end of lines. With simple structure, their lyrics are repeated. People can express their emotions easily and the theme can be highlighted through the special rhythms. People can recite, chant or sing these ballads harmoniously.

(2) Xi

"Xi" ballads are common across southern Guangxi. They are freer than "huan" ballads in styles of lyric and construction. The lines usually rhyme in pairs. However, it is not required that their lyrics should rhyme in the middle and at the end of lines, nor at the beginning and end of lines. Stanzas are not necessarily of the same length. The number of lines in a stanza is not fixed. They are typically sung in antiphonal style.

(3) Jia

"Jia" ballads are popular in Yongning, Fusui, Daxin and other areas co-inhabited by Han and Zhuang people. They are brief and usually describe love and life with strong rhythms, gentle tunes, and few embellishments.

(4) Bi

"Bi" ballads are found throughout northern Guangxi, including Hechi, Donglan, Bama and Rong'an. There are strict rules for tunes. Most lines of their lyrics consist of five characters. Their lyrics rhyme in the middle and at the end of lines, with gentle tunes and many embellishments.

(5) Lun

"Lun" ballads are popular among Napo, Chongzuo, Daxin, Ningming, Lingyun, and other Sino-Vietnamese border regions in southwest Guangxi. They are sonorous and lyrical with frequently and greatly changing rhythms and many embellishments. Their lyrics rhyme at the end of lines and most lines consist of five or seven words. They are typically sung in antiphonal style.

（6）Polyphonic folk songs

Polyphonic folk songs, containing two-part and three-part songs, are popular in 6 regions and about 30 counties in Guangxi. There are over 100 ways to sing them. They have special, simple and mature artistic styles with graceful tunes, simple textures, and clear lines.

6. 1. 2. 3 Zhuang song fairs

In the Zhuang language, song fair is called "haw fwen" "haw faengz" "roengz doengh" and "ok bo", etc. It is a social activity for singing and gathering at particular times and locations, as well as an event where people can meet, communicate, inherit culture, spread knowledge, and convey emotions. According to *Overview of Guangxi Counties* in 1934, there were 26 counties with song fairs across Guangxi. The origin of song fairs is related to ancient clans' modes of production, life patterns, festivals, sacrificial ceremonies, and exogamy. Song fairs, mainly held in spring and autumn, can be divided into festival song fairs and temporary ones. Festival song fairs are held during festivals, such as Sanyuesan Festival, Frog Festival, Cattle Soul Festival, and Lantern Festival. They are based on the farm work during seasonal occasions and are for praying for a good harvest or memorial. They are large and thousands of people attend them. People are passionate about singing and they usually sing for days on end. Closely related to life, temporary song fairs are mainly about labor, county fairs and weddings. They are small events where people can express their emotions, communicate, exchange experiences and spread knowledge. They enable people to sing even during the busy farming seasons. Therefore, singing is not only recreation during idle farming seasons, but also an integral part of life. Both Zhuang people's life and spiritual world are filled with songs.

There are inadequate written records of Zhuang ballads. However, they have been inherited orally since the Pre-Qin Period through song fairs across the Zhuang region. Song fairs play an important role in inheriting and promoting fine traditional Zhuang culture, communicating and expressing emotions, and encouraging the pursuit of liberty.

6. 2　Relationship between Zhuang medicine and ballads culture

6. 2. 1　Zhuang ballads and inheritance of Zhuang medicine

Languages and written letters contain most cultural elements. Two types of writing systems are used to record Zhuang medicine. The first type is Chinese characters. It was not until the First Emperor of Qin unified Lingnan in 214 B. C. that the Zhuang region started to be governed directly by a centralized feudal dynasty. For the development of Lingnan, the First Emperor of Qin continuously dispatched troops and ordinary people to Lingnan. With over 1.5 million people coming there, Lingnan started to be inhabited by both Zhuang and Han people. With extensive cultural exchanges between Lingnan and the Central Plains, Zhuang medical knowledge came to the Central Plains and became one part of TCM. *On Proper Therapies for Different Diseases Geographically*, *Suwen* says, "In the south everything between the heavens and the earth grows and develops, and yang qi is exuberant ... So, the therapy with nine kinds of needle also comes from the south." Zhuang region is included in "the south region" in the quote. A great number of records about Zhuang medicine can be found in TCM documents and Chinese historical materials, such as *Collected Commentaries to Classic of Herbal Medicine*, *Handbook of Prescriptions for Emergencies*, *Strange Stories in Lingnan*, *Lingwai daida*, *Yanbao zaji* (*Scattered Notes*), *Guihai Yuheng Zhi*, and other local chronicles and books of natural history in Guangxi. The second type is the Old Zhuang Script, which was not widely used. It was mainly used by Zhuang artists and shamans to record scriptures, folktales, myths, songs, adages, and play scripts. Therefore, no medical books and only a small number of fragmented Zhuang medical records were written in the Old Zhuang Script.

Without standard written characters through the history of Zhuang, the usage of the Old Zhuang Script was limited, while Chinese characters were introduced in the Qin Dynasty and they were not learned by ordinary Zhuang people. Therefore, the Zhuang nationality has relied on word of mouth to record history, customs, politics, economy, culture, production, life, and experience in preventing and treating diseases.

Language is a part of culture, and people rely on it to record ethnic culture. Zhuang people have their own language and in the Pre-Qin Period, Zhuang ancestors had already developed their own language culture. With good voice, Zhuang people are passionate about singing and even as babies they started to convey emotions through folk songs. They sing when they are happy, sad, accompanied or alone. They make impromptu songs based on their production and life. Singing is their way to express emotions, ask directions, visit friends, entertain guests, and choose mates. Having grown up in a sea of songs, Zhuang people learn singing in their childhood, sing in their youth, and teach singing at an old age.

Zhuang ballads are significant in the development of the Zhuang nationality. They are used to express emotions and ideas, and particularly record history. Liu Xifan said, "Zhuang men and women believe that singing is an important part of their life. He who cannot sing is not able to socialize well, is less likely to be loved and find a mate, and incapable of being knowledgeable. He will be as stupid as a pig." Zhuang ballads have diverse themes and rich content. They profoundly reflect every aspect of social life and the natural world in various forms. Love ballads can express emotions, historical ballads can describe history, and labor ballads describe technical skills. Also, there are ballads about astronomy, geography, medicine, healthcare and ethics. They convey Zhuang people's knowledge and reflect their wisdom. According to research, some Zhuang doctors have classified those Zhuang medical ballads they collected or made, and imparted them to their students. Those ballads are easy to remember. For example, Lu Jinshan, a senior Zhuang doctor in Liuzhou, has categorized collected and self-created Zhuang medical ballads into those about elementary Zhuang medicine, drugs, formulas, prescriptions for lung diseases, and secret recipes for diseases of liver and gallbladder.

Ballads are expressed in poetic languages, and they are essential for the passing down of Zhuang medical culture. They have played an important role in disseminating knowledge about hygiene and methods for diagnosis and treatment, as they are easy to understand and memorize, and are not limited by time or location. There is a song sung by an apprentice of Professor Lu Jinshan, "The Yufeng Mountain is located in Liuzhou, and Longtan Pond is under the mountain. People sing folk songs beside the pond, including medical folk songs. After Pangu created the world, the King of Medicine taught medical knowledge. Liu Sanjie, the Song Fairy in Guangxi, sang medical folk songs."

6.2.1.1　Hygiene in Zhuang ballads

Food, clothing, shelter and transportation are basic needs for healthy life and important aspects of hygiene. They are expressed in Zhuang ballads. For example, labor ballads [about seasons farm work, the solar terms, twelve months (in antiphonal style), and building house], life ballads (about ten-month pregnancy and twelve periods of each day), love ballads (about compliment, farewell and yearning), and folklore ballads (about lamenting at the wedding day and question-and-answer). Those songs tell about different aspects of daily life, including the change of diet and clothes according to season, relationship between health and house environment and orientation, changes and problems during pregnancy, etc. When people sing those songs, they can easily acquire the knowledge of hygiene in daily life.

(1) Narration of the history of marriage and promotion of pairing marriage

The development from incest to pairing marriage is described in the Zhuang epic *Buluotuo Poetic Scripture* and *Pantonggu* (a song in Yizhou and Jinchengjiang). During the incest period, "fathers-in-law slept with their daughters-in-law and sons-in-law slept with their mothers-in-law due to the lack of ethics." During the period of brother-sister marriage, "Fuxi and his sister Nuwa (a goddess in Chinese mythology) married each other as they are the only humans left on the Earth. When they lived together for three years and slept together for four years, Nuwa got pregnant. When she was nine months pregnant, at midnight she gave birth to her son, who looked like a grindstone. The couple were astonished: why their son did not look like a human child but a grindstone." *Pantonggu* tells that only exogamous marriage is good for survival and reproduction and consanguineous marriage is inappropriate. It is similar to a modern mountain song "Unrelated people can marry each other but intra-family marriages are unwise. According to scientific research, many mentally retarded children are from related parents. Consanguineous marriage is inappropriate, and its adverse consequences will last for a lifetime. Some people didn't believe it and married their relatives. As a result, they had mentally retarded children, and that was a disaster both for them and other people."

(2) Emphasis on pregnancy and creation of the related song

As fertility is essential for ethnic reproduction, there are "songs for ten-month pregnancy" in the life ballads in different Zhuang regions. The lyrics of *songs for ten-month pregnancy* summarize the development of the fetus, changes and reactions of pregnant women and relevant considerations. Those songs provide guidance for pregnancy and parturition. This is the main content of a song for ten-month pregnancy in Chongzuo: "The first month of pregnancy is a new start, like the spring for plants.

During the second month of pregnancy, women may start to be aware of being pregnant as they throw up ... During the ninth month of pregnancy, women should stay at home, since they might go into labor on the road if they go out. During the tenth month of pregnancy, women might suffer from unbearable abdominal pain ..."

（3）Construction of house and prevention of damp and beast

It is written in *Creation of Everything* in *Buluotuo Poetic Scripture* that Zhuang ancestors lived in the wild for a long time. It was hot, rainy and humid. There were many beasts in thick forests, threatening people's safety and health. Zhuang ancestors knew how to use wood to build nests and live in them.

This is described in a song, "In ancient times, people couldn't build houses, so they slept on the road or forest they passed by at night. Buluotuo saw everything and sent the King of Nest Clan to teach construction. Without iron and steel, trees in the mountains were used and tenon-jointed, and that was used to cover the house. People made houses and granaries, and then parents-in-law were separated from married couples."

Those above-ground ganlan houses could provide good lighting and ventilation, and prevent damp, beast intrusion and diseases. This is the adaptation to the damp climate in South China.

（4）House orientation and location

Zhuang people attach great importance to houses. In the process of house construction, they consider location, foundation, materials, structure and lighting. This is displayed in *Liao Songs* in Pingguo, Tiandong and other Youjiang River basins. *House Construction Song* in *Liao songs* is a long song about the whole process from negotiation to the construction of house, which is divided into twelve parts including discussion, cutting timber, excavation, making tiles, etc. Hosts and the invited singers sing it in antiphonal style. There are folk songs about the construction and functions of houses across the Zhuang region. For example, "Snakes live in deep holes, flood dragons live in deep pools, and people build and live in houses to keep out wind and rain. Dogs sleep in the doghouse, cats sleep by the fire, and people live in houses to settle down."

With the development of production, people found that the health was influenced by the environment and orientation of houses and the timing of house construction. Therefore, people gave careful consideration to those factors. It is written in a song, "Birds love high trees, and dragons love the sea. New houses near high trees and sea are splendid and able to bring good fortune. Father has built a south-facing house with adequate sunlight in the village, the house can prevent diseases, and cattle can find their way home. Father has built a house facing vast land in the south, situated on flat ground" "When the gate faces east, the house can get adequate sunlight, and lots of daylight on a cloudy day" "A new house near the mountain can bring good fortune" "If a new house faces the north, the domestic animals are all thriving and people can get peace. A new house with good orientation can bring luck in making money and for people."

(5) Climate care, disease prevention and healthcare attention

"Beginning of Spring is the first solar term in the year, and there is still spring chill even around Awakening from Hibernation, which is a threat to the old cattle. Feeble and ailing people should protect themselves against the cold, and strong people should be careful too ... Around White Dew, the autumn wind blows and rainfall is declining. After Beginning of Winter, there is less rainfall, and the cold wind makes people feel cold ...", "Few people fall ill on the rainy Vernal Equinox, but epidemic diseases hit surrounding villages right after the wind and rain on the first day of the lunar month. East wind at the Beginning of Summer implies that few people get sick in the surrounding villages. People do not bother to prevent diseases if there is frost on the first day of the ninth lunar month. If there is no rain during the Double Ninth Festival or the three months of winter, severe drought will affect many patients, and natural disaster and disease will kill more people on the Renzi Day (based on the system of sexagenary cycle). Theft is rampant if west wind blows on the first day of the lunar month, and if it also snows heavily, disasters will come.", "When the solar term changes in February and March, birds change their feathers and people change different types of clothes. They take off winter clothes and wear cool ones to go to the song fairs. It is muggy in February and March, clothes made from hand-made cloth are itchy, those made from machine-made cloth are coarse, but silk garments are cool ... In July around Beginning of Autumn, people need long sleeve tops as the sun changes its path southward, the nights get longer and the days get shorter. In October, the wind is cold and strong, and people warm themselves by firewood. They use bamboo spar to process cotton, wear cotton-padded clothes during the New Year and cover a quilt with cotton wadding in winter. " Those folk songs tell the relationship between climatic change, dressing and disease, and teach people to pay attention to disease prevention when climate changes. The mindset is closely related to basic Zhuang medical theories including the theory of "yin-yang basis" and the theory of "synchrony of triple initial qi".

6.2.1.2 Basic Zhuang medical theories in Zhuang ballads

Basic Zhuang medical theories are distributed in Zhuang ballads with dispersion. In daily Zhuang fairs, questions and answers include "Brother, you are so discerning that I want to challenge you, who created the world and who split yin and yang as well as day and night?" "Pangu created the world and split yin and yang as well as day with sunlight and night with moonlight." "The heaven god and earth goddess form a pairing, a male needs a female, and a scale needs a weight." This is not the theory of "yin-yang basis" in Zhuang medicine, but this has provided guidance for the clinical practices in Zhuang medicine.

Some ballads are summarized medical experience from Zhuang doctors. Most of them are known only by a small number of Zhuang doctors. With characteristic content, they have provided guidance for diagnosis and treatment. For example, "Acupoints on the hands are selected to treat fear of cold, those at the back are for fever, and lumps and skin damage are treated with a set of acupoints forming a plum flower shape around the affected part. Amyotrophy is treated with acupoints associated with the atrophic muscles. Pain or numbness is treated with acupoints along the affected part or at its center. Pruritus is treated with acupoints at the site of the first or biggest rash. But these alone are not enough, acupoints along the Longlu or Huolu should also be selected, according to practical requirements in treating diseases." This is a summary of rules for acupoint selection in Zhuang medicated thread moxibustion. Acupoints along the Longlu or Huolu should be considered, and there are different acupoints for fear of cold, fever, lumps and skin damage, amyotrophy and skin diseases. Chenlin, Pan Zhenxiang's son-in-law in Baise, showed us an excerpt from *Pattern Identification for Infant Diseases* by Pan Zhenxiang, a senior Zhuang doctor. In the ballad "抽兰密肚啼，睡红牙气畜；孩儿察色形，白头沙锁病", Pan Zhenxiang summarized common infant diseases. He believed that pattern identification for such diseases relies on the observation of infant's physique and color. The ballad is followed by writing about the manifestation, pattern identification, and treatment of discussed diseases. Those ballads are imparted by masters to their apprentices, and sometimes they are hard to understand without explanation from writers or experienced contributors.

6. 2. 1. 3 Prescription in Zhuang ballads

Belonging to a rice-farming minority, Zhuang people lay emphasis on the impact of climate and other factors on harvest. The pragmatic thinking is reflected in Zhuang medicine, in which therapeutic effects are emphasized. Therefore, they value the actions of medicines and the effects of prescription. Over several thousand years of medical practice, Zhuang people have accumulated and summarized the actions of common local medicines, and they have developed special principles for the composition of prescriptions. Ballad is an important way to record the actions of medicines and effects of formulas. Wei Bingzhi, a doctor in Donglan County, published *Folk Medical Formulas* in Guangxi Nationalities Publishing House in 1989. Based on his collected materials about Zhuang medicines, the book, written in ballads, contains 220 drugs in 17 categories. For example, "Nanshele (*Caesalpinia minax* Hance) can treat sha diseases; trauma, fracture; fishbone stuck in the throat, and scrofula" , and "Yeyutou (*Colocasia antiquorum* Schott) can treat exogenous cold diseases, common cold, and tuberculosis. Overdose might lead to poisoning, which can be treated with vinegar".

Folk songs about medicine actions can be divided roughly into two types. The first type is about the similar actions of medicines. For example, "Birds can tonify yang and replenish qi. Aquatic animals can tonify yin and blood. Animal placentas are very tonifying. Milk can replenish fluid. Corresponding parts or elements of the body can be replenished by eating bones, liver, kidneys, blood, tendons, brains, penises and testicles respectively. Those are unique skills for doctors" , "Lush and hairy leaves can stop bleeding, and hollow herbs can disperse wind. Thorny herbs can alleviate edema and draw out toxin. Leaves with sap can draw out toxin. Herbs with round stalks and white flowers are cold in nature. Herbs with square stalks and red flowers are hot in nature. Yellow root can clear heat and treat jaundice. Herbs with large nodes can treat trauma and bone fracture. Practice is required for morphological identification. Five flavors of herbs should be known well. Pungent flavor can promote circulation of qi and release exterior. Pungent medicines with aroma can relieve pain and treat snake or insect bite. Medicines with bitter flavor and cool nature can clear heat. Medicines with salt flavor and cold nature can soften hard mass. Most medicines with bland flavor can excrete water. Sweet and warm medicines can invigorate spleen." The second type is about the actions of a single Chinese medicine. For example, "Turenshen [*Talinum paniculatum* (Jacq.) Gaertn], sweet in flavor and mild in nature, can moisten lung, relieve cough, regulate menstruation, treat lack of breast milk, enuresis, carbuncle and boil. It has nourishing action for patients", "Yijianqiu (*Kyllinga monocephala* Rottb.) can treat malaria, trauma (for external use), and bacillary dysentery", "Gou Zaihua [*Vernonia patula* (Dryand.) Merr], mild in nature, can clear heat, alleviate edema, treat malaria, urticaria, and cassava poisoning", "Gougancai [*Dicliptera chinensis* (L.) Juss.], growing around vegetable patch, can clear heat, serve as a diuretic, treat dysentery, red eyes, sore and ulcer."

6.2.2 Emotional impact of Zhuang ballads

Conditions for life were harsh in the Zhuang region, which was known as "a miasmatic region". It was a place for banishing officials in many Dynasties. In Zhuang history, it is not until the First Emperor of Qin (Qin Shihuang) unified Lingnan in 214 B. C. that the Zhuang region started to be governed by a centralized feudal Dynasty, as well as by Zhuang rulers. Oppressed by them, Zhuang ancestors had a miserable life. Therefore, they continued to fight for their own rights. For example, Nong Zhigao left a revolt in the Song Dynasty, and Hong Xiuquan initiated an uprising in Jintian during the Qing Dynasty. Zhuang people's life was hard in the desolate land and they worked hard in the mountains on top of this dual oppression. However, they had a life full of laughter as they loved singing.

6.2.2.1 Singing folk songs as a social activity

Belonging to a rice-farming minority, Zhuang people lived in river valleys, basins and hills. Working in such an isolated geographical environment, they had few opportunities to socialize. Singing helped Zhuang ancestors cast off the fatigue of hard agricultural work in the vast, silent, mountainous region. Also, it helped boost morale and improve work efficiency. They needed to express their physical and spiritual needs and adapt to the real world, and this could be realized by singing. They communicated with others and expressed their emotions through songs during rare leisure time, traditional festivals and joyous get-togethers. They sympathized with and supported each other through emotional communication, and that was good for their mental health.

Zhuang people lived in a sea of songs. As a part of their daily life, singing folk songs was also a way to socialize and express emotions. That is recorded in a great number of Chinese historical materials. *Lingwai Daida* says, "Many Guangxi people can sing. They sing in sacrifice-offering ceremonies, marriage ceremonies, burials and farming." Zhuang people prefer to sing rather than speak in their daily life. They sing folk songs to express their emotions, demands of life and wishes, to make friends and find the right partners. Also, they use folk songs to record their history and culture.

As the excellent social platforms, regular large song fairs can be found across the Zhuang region. During song fair days, people in special costumes come together from different places. They sing and listen to songs, as a way to express thoughts and feelings, eulogize good things in nature and life, and criticize evils in life. In joyful song fairs, Zhuang people can get respect, friendship, sense of achievement, confidence and self-assessment.

Social identity and self-approval are good for physical and mental health as they can produce positive emotions, promote the circulation of qi and blood within the body. In the present day, singing is adopted by a great number of hospitals and institutions in treating depression.

6.2.2.2   Ballads can treat dysphoria, and regulate mood

Lingbiao Jiman says, "The barbarians have a hard life in the desolate land with hard work. They cannot treat dysphoria or regulate mood without singing." Zhuang people live in river valleys, basins and hills, and do farm work in isolated geographical environment. "Music can encourage people in adversity." They work and sing alone or together, for example, "A person who cannot sing will look old. The one who sings folk songs looks young, which is the same as Chinese chives in the backyard that turn green after being cut. Land needs ploughing to be softened, flowers need sunlight to be bright-colored, rice seedling needs fertilizer to be strong, and people need singing to impose. My heart is like a piece of sweet potato vine that can take root again in the soil. I am not happy when I cannot sing folk songs, but I am delighted again after I heard songs." "Cooked vegetables without oil are not soft, and boiled tea without sugar is not sweet. It can get rid of fatigue and make you happy for the whole day to work and sing." Singing can make people relaxed in hard work, and bring vitality to the vast, silent, and mountainous region. Also, it could help them relax, boost morale and improve farming efficiency.

In ancient times, conditions for life were harsh in the Zhuang region, which was known as "a miasmatic region". They suffered natural disasters and hardship. Zhuang people sang folk songs to smile at hardship and trouble. "I sing when walking, resting in bed. Songs are my betrothal gifts, and my food during the New Year", "I am not happy when I cannot sing folk songs, like unfrequented roads covered with moss", "Singing is heartwarming like hot tea. When singing I am carefree", "Firewood without sun drying will not burn easily, and people without singing will look old. You can sing to express all your emotions to get rid of sadness", "People cannot be poor for a lifetime, and air cannot be cold forever. If you sow the seed in the cold of winter, you will see flowers in spring", "Cold water is soothing, and mountain song is pleasing."

"Food can nourish the body, and songs can nourish heart", "There might be a lack of food and drink in a family, but the world will never be short of the sound of singing ..." Song is as important as dining for Zhuang people. They make impromptu songs based on production and life, usually in antiphonal style. *Lingwai Daida* says, "They love making and singing impromptu songs. Some of them can sing very well." The vivid metaphors and descriptions in the ballads can often touch singers and audience and make them optimistic and pleased in the seemingly monotonous life and work.

6.2.2.3 Singing folk songs can help move and transform qi and eliminate negative emotions

Emotional diseases are caused by disharmony of qi and blood in internal organs, particularly disorder of qi movement in the five zang-organs. *Listing and Analyzing Pain and Disease*, *Suwen*, says, "Hundreds of diseases are caused by qi disorder. Rage causes qi to ascend in reverse, excessive pleasure causes qi to flow slowly, sorrow causes qi dispersion, horror causes qi to descend, fright causes qi disturbance, and contemplation causes qi binding." Sorrow, melancholy, fright and other negative emotions can cause disorder of qi ascending and descending in the body. The subsequent imbalance of qi and blood in the zang and fu organs will finally cause diseases. Singing folk songs can help activate blood and unblock vessels, move and transform qi, energize people, eliminate negative emotions, and prevent and treat physical and mental diseases. *Second Volume*, *Book on Music* says, "Music can activate blood and unblock vessels, regulate essential qi, and prevent and treat physical and mental diseases."

Zhuang folk songs have rich content and diverse themes including love, folklore, labor, life, customs, lament and elegies. Lament songs are sad and indignant, they express people's desires for free life and life safety when they encounter problems in relationship, life, body, and ideal. Elegies, sung in funerals, are sad songs about the death of relatives.

Setbacks and misfortunes give rise to negative emotions including melancholy, resentment and deep sorrow. A lament song is the integration of emotional experience and music based on authors' experiences. It can express emotions better than spoken words. Some scholars believe that lament songs help authors and singers feel a sense of relief and comfort. Singing can cast off negative emotions. According to Wu Shangxian in the Qing Dynasty, "Treating emotional diseases with a floral excursion and music enjoyment is better than medication."

In addition, singing can change one's disposition and amuse ourselves. Confucius once said, "ethics and rites are most important for stabilizing a country and people to live in peace and contentment. Music is most important for changing old practices and customs." As the language of emotion, music can speak directly to your heart, and feed your heart and soul. Also, people can increase calm via beautiful melodies. The rapid pace of life and the fierce competition in the society contribute to the high incidence of emotional diseases. There are choruses of complaints in Finland, Germany and other countries, aiming at "writing and singing complaints". Singing those songs can make people feel a sense of relief, pleasure and calm.

Emotional pathogenic factors are important in TCM etiological theories. Some diseases might be caused by the change of any of seven emotions: joy, anger, anxiety, pensiveness, grief, fear and fright. The major etiological theory in Zhuang medicine is "pathogenicity of toxin and deficiency. " It reveals that toxic factors and deficiency are two major pathogenic factors that cause diseases. There is little emphasis on emotional pathogenic factors in the Zhuang etiological theory, as Zhuang people love singing folk songs, which can decrease diseases caused by a change in the seven emotions.

References:

[1] Lu Fei, Wang Dun. Poetic Thinking and National Psychology in Zhuang Song Culture [J]. Journal of Baise University, 2010, 23 (1): 31 – 35.

[2] Mo Qinglian, Huang Ping, Huang Haibo. Discussion on the Role of Zhuang Folk Songs in the Inheritance of Zhuang Medicine [J]. Chinese Journal of Ethnomedicine and Ethnopharmacy, 2009 (21): 25 – 27.

[3] Mo Qinglian, Dai Ming, Nong Minjian. Healthcare and Medical Records in Zhuang Folk Songs [J]. Chinese Journal of Ethnomedicine and Ethnopharmacy, 2009 (23): 5 – 6.

[4] Zhang Shengzhen. Commentaries on Buluotuo Poetic Scripture [M]. Nanning: Guangxi People's Publishing House, 1991.

［5］ Xiao Fengpei. Selected Guangxi Folk Literary Works: Rong'an Volume ［M］. Nanning: Guangxi Nationalities Publishing House, 1992.

［6］ Lei Qingduo. Selected Guangxi Folk Literary Works: Chongzuo Volume ［M］. Nanning: Guangxi Nationalities Publishing House, 1998.

［7］ Nong Minjian, Tan Zhibiao. Pingguo Liao Songs Annuals of Long Songs, Songs of March ［M］. Nanning: Guangxi Nationalities Publishing House, 2004.

［8］ Wei Bingzhi. Folk Medical Formulas ［M］. Nanning: Guangxi Nationalities Publishing House, 1989.

［9］ Mo Qinglian, Lin Yi, Dai Ming. Preliminary Discussion on Zhuang Etiological theories ［J］. Chinese Journal of Basic Medicine in Traditional Chinese Medicine, 2014, 20 （3）: 293 – 295.

［10］ The Editorial Board, Collections of Chinese Ballads, Guangxi Volume. The Editorial Board, Collections of Chinese Ballads, Guangxi Volume ［M］. Beijing: China Social Sciences Press, 1992.

［11］ Wei Suwen. Discussion on Zhuang Lament Songs ［J］. Ethnic Arts Quarterly, 1992 （2）: 114 – 124.

7 Zhuang Medicine and Local Festivals

7. 1　Zhuang festivals

Festivals were established by ancient people according to phenology and the periodic changes of weather and climate. Festival customs emerged with the formation and development of agricultural civilization, and involved a series of events about adapting to natural environment, interpersonal relationship, taboos, divination, worship, celebration, entertainment, etc. Held every year, festivals vary with the seasons. The festivals of a nationality are closely associated with local natural environment, production, life, and primitive belief. The same is true of Zhuang festivals, which have strong national characteristics in content and form. As major features and symbols of Zhuang culture, Zhuang festivals reflect Zhuang people's spirit of creativity, strong emotions, and unremitting pursuit and expectations of longevity, bumper harvests, peace, and prosperity.

7. 1. 1　Classfication of Zhuang festivals

Traditional Zhuang festivals can be divided into those concerning seasonal farming, religion and commemoration. All aim at praying for bumper harvests, abundant life, reproduction, prosperity, peace and happiness.

7. 1. 1. 1　Festivals about seasonal farming

As Zhuang is a rice-farming minority, its festivals are closely related to rice production. Festivals about seasonal farming include Frog Festival in the 1st lunar month, Kitchen God Festival in the 2nd, Farming-starting Festival in the 3rd, Cattle Soul Festival and Rice Seedling Festival in the 4th, Farm Implement Festival in the 5th, New Rice Tasting Festival in the 7th, Mountain Worship Festival in the 8th, and Harvest Festival in the 10th.

7. 1. 1. 2　Religious festivals

Religious festivals are mainly about ancestor worship, including Tomb-Sweeping Day and Buluotuo Birthday Festival in the 3rd lunar month, King Moyi Festival in the

6th, and Ghost Festival in the 7th lunar month. During those festivals, they worship ancestors in the halls of their home or in the ancestral halls in the villages. This reveals their belief and custom of ancestral worship.

7.1.1.3 Commemoration festivals

Commemoration festivals commemorate ancestors, particularly historical personages and events. The Sanyuesan Festival commemorates Zhuang Song Fairy Liu Sanjie, so it is also known as Song Fairy Festival; The Yabai Festival commemorates Zhuang heroine Yabai in the Song Dynasty; And the Liulang Festival commemorates Zhuang hero Nong Zhigao.

7.1.2 Features of Zhuang festivals

With a long history, festival culture is an important part of traditional Zhuang culture. Zhuang festival culture has developed its own unique characteristics.

7.1.2.1 Distinctive rice-farming agriculture

Situated in the subtropical zone with plentiful rainfall, the Zhuang region provides a good environment for rice growing. Zhuang people belong to one of the first groups to grow rice. Their daily life and production are closely aligned with rice-farming. Many of their festival activities are centered around seasons for production and rhythms of crop cultivation. For example, the Farming-starting Festival in the 3rd lunar month is a ceremony for starting spring ploughing. A village head places sacrificial offerings and burns incense beside a paddy field near the village, and kowtows to the heaven and earth, to pay respect to gods and ancestors. Then, he leads a water buffalo to plough once in the paddy field. This marks the official start of spring ploughing. After the ceremony, all families can plough. People established the Cattle Soul Festival on the 8th day of the 4th lunar month to thank and reward cattle for ploughing. On that day, cattle can have a rest, people bathe them in the river, give them fine feed, and clean cattle pens. On the New Rice Tasting Festival on the 7th day of the 7th lunar month, rice is almost mature. People pick those mature rice and hang three bunches of rice on the ancestral altar, and unhusk the remaining rice to cook with previous rice. After worshipping ancestors and then gods, family members taste and enjoy the earliest mature rice. Therefore it is called "the New Rice Tasting Festival". During the Harvest Festival in the 10th lunar month, all the late rice has been harvested and dried. People hold a grand ceremony for celebration of the harvest. They offer sacrifices to gods and thank them for their blessings. Both carrying pole dance and rice pounding dance are for celebration.

7.1.2.2　Strong sense of ancestor worship

Zhuang people believe that after ancestors die, their ghosts will remain in the world of the dead, and they bless their off springs to help them remove ill fortune and to keep them safe. During the festivals, Zhuang people worship ancestors in their home by providing offerings and burning incense and joss paper. On the Tomb-sweeping Day, they renovate and sacrifice ancestral tombs with wine, meat, and five-colored sticky rice, expressing people's yearning. On the Ghost Festival on the 14th day of the 7th lunar month, they burn paper clothes to keep ancestors warm, and burn ancestor money for use in the world of the dead. They also worship ancestors when they butcher chicken and duck or cook pork. Therefore, Zhuang people worship their own ancestors most of all, even though they follow animism and worship the Flower Mother and the Frog God.

7.1.2.3　Imprint of food culture

Festival celebration is called "gwnciet" in the Zhuang language and "gwn" means "eating", which is the core content of Zhuang festival celebration. During festivals, they prepare wine and meat in worship of ancestors and gods to seek their blessings. Also, they prepare nice food and drink to reward themselves and entertain relatives and friends. The core role of "eating" is closely associated with the saying "Food is the paramount necessity of the people" as well as with rice-farming. Rice agriculture was characterized by high farming techniques, long production cycle, and intensive labor in ploughing. People should work hard in every step in farming such as transplanting rice seedlings, fertilization, irrigation, and harvesting. In the heat of South China, people expended more physical effort to work in the paddy field under the blazing sun. In order to keep performing strenuous labor, people needed to rest, consume more nutrition, and improve life. Therefore, rest days for all people emerged, days during which people could rest. During festivals, all families prepared nice food to reward themselves, including wine, chicken, duck, fish, zongzi, ciba cake, and other desserts. Festivals have become happy days for resting, enjoying nice food and fruits of their labor. They serve as the symbols of family reunion, enjoyment of wonderful meals, relaxation of the body and mind, and felicity. The eating-centered traditional festivals have been inherited in Zhuang people's expectation, enjoyment and happiness.

7. 1. 2. 4 Group collaboration and unity

Zhuang ancestors fought against nature for ages. With low productivity, they formed the fine traditions of group collaboration, unity and mutual aid for the acquisition of means of livelihood, survival and development. The most important Zhuang custom in production is "vunzraeuh" or "doxraeuh", meaning "offer to help" in the collective labor of a clan society. Zhuang people helped each other in many aspects, including ploughing, farming, harvesting, building houses, marriage and burial. The spirit of group collaboration and mutual help is also reflected in festival activities. Most of the festival activities are celebrated by all people in the same village, including Frog Festival, Sanyuesan Festival, Buluotuo Birthday Festival, Drug Fair Festival, King Moyi Festival, and Harvest Festival. All villagers of all ages and sexes attend festival activities. They work together, organized by village heads. Taoist masters host worship ceremonies. At the end of festivals, people dine together at banquets. Collective festival activities can reveal the economic strength, organizing ability, popularity, and reputation of a village, so they can enhance the cohesiveness within and between ethnic communities.

7. 1. 3 Major Zhuang festivals

There are many traditional Zhuang festivals. Like those of other ethnic groups, they all have long histories. Some lovely legends are found behind many festivals.

1. Spring Festival

As one of the most solemn Zhuang festivals, the Spring Festival is at the beginning of the year. It lasts from the 1st to 15th days of the first lunar month. On the 15th day, the new year celebration ends after all families have eaten extra-large zongzi offered to ancestors and gods. In some regions, however, the new year celebration ends at the end of the 1st lunar month, and so the whole lunar month of celebration is called "the 1st lunar month celebration". "Cieng" in Zhuang language, which is the shortened form for the 1st lunar month, means the Spring Festival.

The first day of Lunar New Year is the most solemn Zhuang festival of the whole year. When the first rooster crow marks the beginning of a new day, people get up to welcome the new year. They wear new clothes and shoes, burn incense and candles before the ancestral tablets, lay out tributes and set off firecrackers. After the fireworks, children greet older people by saying "happiness and prosperity", and the older people will give children lucky money and fireworks. People of all ages and sexes dress up joyfully. Girls or recently married women go to rivers and springs to imbibe "smart water". It is said that the first person who gets the new water will become clever. Family members and neighbors visit each other. People pay a new year's visit to seniors, and adults give lucky money to visiting children. After the new year's visit, all families take their offerings to worship gods in the village temples. They pray for the safety of people and livestock, and for a bumper grain harvest.

On the first day of Lunar New Year there are many taboos across the Zhuang region. For example, sweeping is forbidden on that day, as rubbish removal from home implies the outflow of fortune. It is forbidden and ominous for most Zhuang people to see blood. Therefore slaughter is not allowed on that day, and on Lunar New Year's Eve people prepare chicken, duck and fish for the following day. It is forbidden to collect debt or borrow money during the New Year, as it is believed in some regions that debt or loan is inauspicious for production or business, and such business should be conducted before Lunar New Year's Eve or after the 15th day of the 1st lunar month.

During the Spring Festival, there are various cultural and recreational activities. Rice pounding dance is called "guhlongj" and "dwklongj" in Zhuang language. Zhuang people perform the dance during the Spring Festival to celebrate the New Year and anticipate a successful harvest. It is still popular in Mashan, Du'an, Wuming, Shanglin, Xincheng, Tiandeng, Pingguo, and other regions. Originally, Zhuang people performed the dance by using the wooden pestle to beat rhythmically in the wooden rice mortar. The Zhuang name "guhlongj" means "drum rice mortar". For convenience, they used carrying pole and bench to replace heavy wooden pestle and rice pounder. Therefore, people in certain regions call the dance "carrying pole dance" or use the pole clunking sound to name it. The gender and number of dancers are not fixed. People around the bench sing and beat the carrying poles. The audience cheer and shout for them in a celebratory atmosphere. Also they have lion dance, bronze drum dance, and martial arts.

2. Frog Festival

Frog Festival is celebrated in Donglan, Bama, Fengshan, Tian'e, Nandan and other counties. In Zhuang legends, the Frog Goddess controls wind and rain. On the first and second days of lunar new year, villagers along the Hongshui River worship the Frog Goddess for good weather, a bumper grain harvest, thriving livestock and prosperous families. According to legend, the Frog Goddess is the daughter of the Thunder King. She controls wind and rain and ensures good weather. One year, there was a young Zhuang man named Donglin. He was so heartbroken about his mother's death. The croak of the frogs outside the house agitated him, so he poured hot water onto frogs. Those frogs died, got hurt or escaped. Since then people did not hear the sound of frogs or see any rain, which was a big disaster. Donglin was frightened and asked Buluotuo for help. He was told that he should beg forgiveness of the Frog Goddess. Therefore, Donglin played the bronze drum on the first day of Lunar New Year, invited the Frog Goddess to celebrate the New Year in the village, and asked a thousand people to give a funeral for dead frogs. Subsequently, the mortal world was again blessed by the Frog Goddess with good weather, and from that time Zhuang people annually celebrated the Frog Festival and worshipped frogs.

The Frog Festival activity can be divided into three stages. The first stage is "looking for frogs". At the dawn of the first day of the first lunar month, people play the bronze drum and in large groups look for hibernating frogs. The first person who finds a frog is lucky and regarded as the "frog's bridegroom" (the Thunder King's son-in-law) and the frog leader for the year. The second stage is "worshipping frogs" and "carrying the frog in a sedan chair through the village". People take the first frog to the village, and put it into a small cage made from old golden Nan bamboo. They put the cage into the "flower house", which is carried by two singers through the village. Children crowd around the flower house, and frog songs are sung for good weather, longevity, and bumper harvests. People share New Year cake, zongzi, ciba cakes, rice cakes, colored eggs, cooked rice, and money. From the first day to the end of the first lunar month, during the day children carry the frog through the village and congratulate each family, then carry the frog to the frog pavilion at night where people perform frog dance and sing frog song to hold a wake for the frog. The third stage is "burying the frog", which is the climax of the Frog Festival activity. At the end of the first lunar month, people pick an auspicious time, follow the "frog's bridegroom", carry the "flower house" with the frog in it to the burial ground. Before burying it, the chief mourner will dig up last year's frog grave to examine the bones, and predict the year's harvest according to the color of the frog bones. Golden frog bones indicate good harvest, and people will cry out for joy and perform the bronze drum ritual. Grey or black bones indicate bad harvest, and people will burn incense and pray for removal of ill fortune. Then the new frog will be buried. After the burial, people of all ages and sexes will sing and dance to send the frog soul to heaven.

3. Flower Mother Festival

According to legend, the Zhuang ancestor Muliujia emerged from flowers. She managed the garden for human reproduction. As she brought flowers and children to women, she was regarded as the Flower Mother. People believed that women got pregnant because she brought flowers to them. The 29th day of the 2nd lunar month is the birthday of the Flower Mother (also it is said to be the 2nd day of the 2nd lunar month). On that day, Zhuang women bring chicken, duck, fish, joss sticks, candles, and joss paper for sacrificial ceremony in the Flower Mother Temple. Next come folk activities including sharing porridge, placing festive lanterns, and a parade. Then they walk as a group into the wild to pick and wear flowers, praying for fertility and the healthy growth of children. On that day, childless women in particular should walk into the wild to pick and wear flowers, and pray to the Flower Mother to bring flowers and children. After they get pregnant, they should ensure that their children have souls by inviting Taoist masters to chant and pray in the wild for flowers, and make a bridge ceremony above a ditch at the roadside, and receive flowers from the bridge. After the birth of children, the ancestral tablets for the Flower Mother should be placed beside puerperal beds for regular worship.

4. Tomb-sweeping Day

The Tomb-sweeping Day is a festival for renovating and sacrificing at ancestral graves. Zhuang people care a lot about Tomb-sweeping Day, which is a grand festival for remembering relatives, ranking only behind the Spring Festival and Ghost Festival. A special combination of food animals is used for tomb sweeping. Rich families hold sacrifice offering ceremonies with other branches of their clans, and they provide a banquet in cemetery hills and bypassers are invited. Typically tomb sweeping is carried out for 15 days before and after the Tomb-sweeping Day, during which time Zhuang people prepare essential food including five-colored sticky rice and ciba cakes (especially those made from Aiye). Typically, five-colored sticky rice is made for ancestor worship and entertaining relatives and friends. In the past, poor people could not afford rich food, including fish and meat, when visiting graves during the Tomb-sweeping Day. However, they must prepare a bowl of fragrant, sweet and five-colored sticky rice to worship their relatives.

5. Sanyuesan Festival

As a traditional Zhuang festival, the Sanyuesan Festival on the 3rd day of the 3rd lunar month is also called Song Festival or Gexu Festival. There are different explanations to the origin of the Sanyuesan Festival. It is said that Liu Sanjie was a smart Zhuang girl of the Tang Dynasty who was good at singing. She sang folk songs as a way to eulogize labor and love, and expose rich men's evils. Therefore, the rich men hated and feared her. On the 3rd day of the 3rd lunar month, Liu Sanjie cut firewood in the mountain. Rich men sent someone to cut off vines, which caused her to fall off a cliff and died. In memory of Liu Sanjie, people sing on the 3rd, 4th, and 5th days of the 3rd lunar month, and gradually song fairs formed. In another explanation, it is said that for hundreds of years, people have been getting together on the 3rd day of the 3rd lunar month in Qiaohualing, Anchui Township, Rongshui Miao Autonomous County. Liu Sanjie was leaving Sanjiang Dong Autonomous County for Liuzhou City. She passed by Qiaohualing in a boat and sang for three days. In memory of her, the 3rd day of the 3rd lunar month has been identified as the song fair day. On the Sanyuesan Festival, all families make five-colored sticky rice and colored eggs for celebration. The Sanyuesan Festival typically lasts two or three days in an open space near the village. A song booth is made from bamboo and cloth for entertaining singers from other villages. Singers are mainly unmarried youth, who leverage singing to express emotions and choose mates. If a young man and a young woman fall in love, they will exchange love tokens as expressions of love. The scale of song fairs varies from a thousand to tens of thousands of people. They go to song fairs for the singing competition or just for enjoyment. The song fairs are filled with boisterous crowds and the sound of song. Songs in these fairs have a broad range of topics including astronomy, geography, folk tales, farm work during seasonal occasions, social life, ethics, relationship and marriage. There are other interesting activities in the song fairs including throwing embroidered balls, smashing colored eggs, sparkler-grabbing, shoe plank race, bamboo pole dance, Zhuang opera, Taoist master opera, tea-picking opera and other singing and dancing activities. Throwing embroidered balls is a major recreational activity, and embroidered balls are also love tokens. When a young woman takes a fancy to a young man, she will throw her embroidered ball to him. Nowadays, throwing embroidered balls is a form of team sport. The purpose of smashing colored eggs is simply to have fun and express love. In 1985, the People's Government of Guangxi Zhuang Autonomous Region set the Sanyuesan Festival as the Guangxi cultural and arts festival.

6. Cattle Soul Festival

Zhuang people believe that cattle are holy creatures instead of ordinary beings.

According to legend, the cow was born in heaven on the 8th day of the 4th lunar month. Therefore, that was the birthday of the King of Cows. In ancient times, the land was filled with rock, loess, dust and sand with no vegetation. That had an enormous influence in human life. The King of Cows was sent by the Jade Emperor to the world to plant grass. The Jade Emperor instructed him to plant one handful of grass seed every three steps, but he planted three handfuls of grass seed every step. High seed density led to overgrowth of grass everywhere. The farmland was also affected, doing harm to rice seedlings. Therefore, the Jade Emperor sent him to the world to eat grass and plough the fields as punishment. In the world, he lived on grass, ploughed the fields throughout the year, and gained respect. People appreciated his hard work and so worshiped the cattle soul on the 8th day of the 4th lunar month, the birthday of the King of Cows. That is the origin of the Cattle Soul Festival. The Cattle Soul Festival is also called "Cattle King Festival" and "Unyoking Festival". On that day, cattle owners let their cattle have a rest, clean their cattle, and renovate cattle pens. The elder in the village make comments on all ploughing cattle and encourage people to love them. All families make five-colored sticky rice, and wrap it with loquat leaves to feed cattle. Cattle owners put a low table outside the cattle pen, place offerings, burn joss sticks and candles, and worship the cattle soul.

7. Medicine King's Day

Medicine King's Day is a traditional Zhuang festival, the 5th day of the 5th lunar month, and it is also called Drug Fair Festival. According to legend, the King of Medicine was a Zhuang doctor. He discovered medicinal herbs and treated people. Also he taught people the knowledge of growing and picking herbs and treating diseases. There were Yaowang (the King of Medicine) Temples in large villages throughout the Zhuang region. People worship the King of Medicine, and pick herbs for preventing diseases on the Dragon Boat Festival, the 5th day of the 5th lunar month. In Longsheng Pan-Ethnicities Autonomous County, Guangxi, Zhuang people pick Wujiu [*Sapium sebiferum* (L.) Roxb.], Tianjihuang [*Grangea maderaspatana* (L.) Poir.], Hulucha [*Tadehagi triquetrum* (L.) Ohashi], Yuanbaocao (*Hypericum sampsonii* Hance) and other herbs in the mountains on that day. They boil those herbs for showering, believing it can smoothen and clean skin and avoid scabies. Zhuang people in Jingxi City establish drug fairs to sell herbs on that day, when there are about 2000 booths in the drug fairs and over 30,000 admissions. Hundreds of medicinal materials are listed, including Huanghuadaoshuilian (*Polygala fallax*

243

Hemsl.）, Huzhang （*Reynoutria japonica* Houtt.）, Sumu （*Caesalpinia sappan* Linn.）, Gusuibu （*Davallia mariesii* Moore ex Bak.）, Shidagonglao ［*Mahonia fortunei* （Lindl.） Fedde］, Daluosan （*Ardisia crenata* Sims）, Xiaoluosan （*Ardisia punctata*）, Jinbuhuan （*Abrus mollis*）, Jiaogulan ［*Gynostemma pentaphyllum* （Thunb.） Makino］, Shichangpu （*Acorus tatarinowii*）, Daxueteng ［*Sargentodoxa cuneata* （Oliv.） Rehd. et Wils.］, Chuifengteng （*Clematis meyeniana*）, Tugancao （*Fordia cauliflora*）, Tuniuxi （*Achyranthes aspera* L.）, Tudangshen （*Campanumoea javanica*）, Tudanggui （*Angelica oncosepala* Hand. -Mazz.）, Jiubiying （*Ilex rotunda*）, Diulebang （*Claoxylon indicum*）, Jiujiecha （*Sarcandra glabra*）, Jinguolan ［*Tinospora sagittata* （Oliv.） Gagnep.］, Tianqi ［*Panax pseudoginseng* Wall. var. *notoginseng* （Burkill） Hoo et Tseng］, and Yanhuanglian （*Corydalis saxicola* Bunting）. In Zhuang folklore, lush herbs exhibit strong efficacy and the best therapeutic effect during the Dragon Boat Festival. When people go to the drug fairs on that day, they are able to absorb the qi of medicine and prevent diseases. At drug fairs, people like buying and learning medicines for preventing and treating diseases and increasing knowledge. On the Medicine King's Day, all families make zongzi in the shape of a goat horn, and ciba cakes containing Aiye. They dispel pathogenic factors and prevent plague by boiling vinegar and burning pomelo peel in the room, as well as by hanging Ai and calamus on the door.

8. Liulang Festival

Liulang （June Man） Festival or Qilang （July Man） Festival is a traditional Zhuang festival on the 6th day of the 6th lunar month. During the festival, people will not do farm work for three days, and that is the same as in the Spring Festival. All families in the villages happily set about butchering ducks and chickens, cooking five-colored sticky rice, and holding sacrificial ceremonies. According to a legend, Zhuang hero Nong Zhigao broke a siege, and then in June and July people celebrated it wherever he had passed by. Emperors of the Song Dynasty resented Nong Zhigao and prohibited people commemorating him. Therefore, Zhuang people started to commemorate their hero in the Liulang Festival in June and Qilang Festival in July. Sacrifice offering ceremonies start after wine, meat and other food are prepared. After the village head offers praise to Zhuang leader Nong Zhigao, all families can put bamboo couches out in front of the door for worshipping and praying. On the evening of the festival, villagers work together to expel the evil spirits. They butcher chickens, ducks, dogs and so on. They shape straw into different evil spirits, beat drums and strike gongs, then Taoist masters chant to expel evil spirits. Grand sports activities are held in some Zhuang villages, including sparkler-grabbing, playing basketball and horse racing. On that day, Zhuang women make and compare five-colored sticky rice, particularly for color. On the second day, they visit their parents' home taking five-colored sticky rice.

9. King Moyi Festival

King Moyi Festival is a traditional Zhuang festival on both sides of the Liujiang and Longjiang Rivers on the 2nd day of the 6th lunar month. It is also called Wugu Temple Festival. King Moyi, also named "Tongtian Dasheng", is a god with Zhuang characteristics in the god system of Shigongism. According to a legend, the 2nd day of the 6th lunar month was the birthday of King Moyi. He saved Zhuang people and gave blessings for bumper grain harvests. Zhuang people were so grateful that they built temples in front of the village and placed memorial tablets in the home. Every year, people offer chicken, duck and pork to worship him. Every six years, people in the same village raise money by butchering pigs and sheep. One member of each family should attend the spectacular sacrifice offering ceremony in the King Moyi Temple. The village heads host the ceremony, where Taoist priests are invited to chant. Twelve dishes are placed on the sacrificial altar, representing the 12 months of the year. They are made from different parts of pigs and sheep including the flesh, liver, intestines and bones. Joss paper can be burned and other rites can continue after all twelve dishes are laid out. When the ceremony is completed, those dishes will be shared.

10. Ghost Festival

The Ghost Festival, which is also called Zhongyuan Festival, is a sacrificial Zhuang festival on the 14th day of the 7th lunar month. It is also called Mid-July Festival or July Festival. It ranks only second to the Spring Festival for Zhuang people, and involves ancestor and ghost worship. According to legend, Zhuang ancestor Buluotuo died on the 14th day of the 7th lunar month, so people worshipped him from generation to generation on that day. From the 14th to 16th days of the 7th lunar month, people offer sacrifice at the altar, including pork, whole chicken, whole duck, rice noodles, steamed sponge cakes, ciba cakes, and sticky rice. They have their meals after worshipping ancestors and re-heating offerings. It is said that wandering and haunting ghosts are the homeless ghosts of those who suffered unnatural death. In order to avoid being harmed, people worship ancestors as well as wandering ghosts on that day. They butcher chickens and ducks, steam cakes, make pancakes, and cut colored paper as clothing tops, bottoms, shoes and socks for all seasons. After home sacrifice, at nightfall they go to the river for outdoor sacrifice. They burn joss sticks, candles and paper clothes, and scatter the ashes in the water. On that day, married women should visit their own parents, but return after celebrating the festival, instead of staying overnight.

11. Back-hitting Festival

Back-hitting Festival is a traditional Zhuang festival, called "Bunong" in western Guangxi. "Back-hitting Festival" in Zhuang language also means "tasting the new rice". On the night of the festival, people taste new rice, the youth attend back-hitting activity, so it is called "Back-hitting Festival". The festival is held on the 15th day of the 7th lunar month. All families butcher chickens and ducks, make tofu, steam new rice, worship ancestors, gather together and enjoy meals. Also they feed dogs and cats with rice to thank them for defending the home and catching mouse and rat. After dinner, young men and women dress up, gather together in the grain-sunning ground or grassland, and participate in the back-hitting activity under the moonlight or around the fire. Men and women interact with each other by stepping on each other's feet, hitting each other's heels, and hitting each other's backs, chanting and speaking Zhuang words, which means "taste new rice and find a partner". Old people and children come to watch them and cheer them on. There are happy laughter and cheerful voices. According to the custom, if a man hits a woman's back first, it means that the man has fallen in love with the woman. If a woman hits a man's back first, it means that the woman is in love with the man. If a man and a woman hit each other's backs, it means they have both fallen in love with each other. Since they like each other, they chase each other and run outside. They sing to each other, play the leaf instrument, and perhaps exchange love tokens.

12. Mid-autumn Festival

Mid-autumn Festival is held on the 15th day of the 8th lunar month, which is believed to be an auspicious day as the moon is the fullest and brightest of the year. On that day, men travelling or residing far away return home and enjoy the happiness of a family reunion. All families eat mooncakes, steam cakes, butcher chickens and ducks, prepare lavish dinners, gaze at and worship the moon. They wish for family reunion and harmony. There are different activities across the Zhuang region during the festival. In Debao and Jingxi, Zhuang people hold an event to invite the Goddess of the

Moon to come down to earth and share their happiness. In western and northern Guangxi, young people hold song fairs and sing together searching for love. Therefore, it is also called Mid-autumn Song Festival in many regions. Children use pomelo peel to make masks and lanterns, play spinning whip top, walk on stilts, dress up, and play other games happily.

13. Birthday Celebration Day

Birthday Celebration Day is held to offer congratulations to the elder on the 9th day of the 9th lunar month, which is associated with the Zhuang saying "9 divided by 9 equals one, and people living to 100 will become immortals". It was derived from birthday celebration for the elderly. All families celebrate the festival whether they have old family or not. Those with old relatives pay greater attention to the festival. Sons need to have old people's heads shaved and help them wear new clothes. Married daughters need to return home with a chicken and several kilograms of rice as "replenishment of rice" meaning long life. During the banquet, descendants should show their filial piety by feeding the elderly before dining. For people aged over 60, descendants should offer congratulations to them by butchering chickens and ducks and providing a longevity rice jar. Descendants need to replenish the jar with rice on the 9th day of the 9th lunar month every year until it is filled up. Only when the elderly get sick will the rice in the jar be cooked. However the rice jar should not be emptied.

14. Harvest Festival

In the tenth lunar month, all the late rice has been harvested and dried. People hold a grand ceremony in celebration of the harvest. They offer sacrifices to gods and thank them for their blessings. Both carrying pole dance and rice pounding dance are conducted for celebration. For this festival, all families prepare nice dishes and invite relatives and friends. More guests make the banquets livelier and the hosts happier, indicating good harvests in the next year.

15. Chinese New Year's Eve

Chinese New Year's Eve on the 30th day of the 12th lunar month is the busiest festival in a year. On that day, all families gather happily, and rice is cooked for the following 1st day of the 1st lunar month. The cooked rice is for celebrating bumper grain harvests in anticipation. On that night, all families butcher pigs and chickens, put up New Year couplets, make new clothes, zongzi, New Year cakes, swelled candy rice and pancakes. They offer pig's heads, capons and fruit to worship ancestors solemnly, and enjoy the New Year's Eve dinner together. Then, adults gather together around the fire and stay up late or all night on New Year's Eve. Children stay up all night to play games. All families hang firecrackers on the outside of the door and set off them when they hear the first rooster crow. It is auspicious and called "firecrackers against crow". People place offerings beside the cooking ranges to welcome the Kitchen God. People set off firecrackers until daybreak whenever they hear the rooster crow.

7. 2　Relationship between Zhuang medicine and festivals

7. 2. 1　Relationship between yin-yang theory and the Ghost Festival

The Ghost Festival or July Festival is a sacrificial Zhuang festival on the 14th day of the 7th lunar month. It ranks only the second in importance to the Spring Festival for Zhuang people, containing ancestor and ghost worship. As the name describes, the activities of the Ghost Festival are linked with "ghosts". According to legend, Zhuang ancestor Buluotuo died on the 14th day of the 7th lunar month. They believe that people become ghosts in the world of the dead after they die, and they are allowed to return to and stay in the world of the living to visit their kinsfolk from the 7th day to the 15th day in the 7th lunar month. Therefore, from generation to generation people worship their ancestors on that day. It is said that wandering and haunting ghosts are homeless ghosts who suffered unnatural death, and they want to repossess the human body. In order to avoid being harmed, people worship both ancestors and wandering ghosts on that day. There are a great number of water areas in South China. It is said that rivers run through both the world of the living and the world of the dead. The joss paper and clothes for ancestor worship are conveyed by ducks across the Naihe bridge. Therefore, people eat ducks on the Ghost Festival, which has become an indispensable part of the festival over time. Situated in the subtropical zone, the Zhuang region is actually in the rainy season in the 7th lunar month. Frequent mountain torrents kill many people as they fall off cliffs or drown. The older generation use "wandering ghosts" to warn people, particularly reckless teenagers, not to play near the mountain streams or rivers for fear of accident.

Zhongyuan originates from Chinese Taoism, according to which the 15th day of the 1st, 7th and 10th lunar months are Shangyuan, Zhongyuan and Xiayuan respectively. In the theory of yin and yang, the interaction of yin and yang happens on the 1st and 15th days of each lunar month. On the 1st day of a lunar month, yang qi, yang spirit, heaven gods, and life gods are predominant, whereas on the 15th day of a lunar month, yin qi, yin spirit and earth gods are predominant. Therefore, people worship goddesses, lunar deities, earth gods and ancestral spirits on the 15th day.

Zhuang inhabit in subtropics with high average temperature and four distinct seasons. The sun and the moon move back and forth with the changing of night and day as well as the changing of season. These natural phenomena gave rise to the yin and yang concept in the Zhuang nationality. Strengthened by the cultural influence of the Han nationality in the Central Plains, that concept is widely applied in their production and life. It is an argument for explaining the complex relationship between nature and the body's etiology and pathogenesis. According to the record of *Volume 16*, *Guangxi Local Records* in the Ming Dynasty, Zhuang people sincerely believed in yin and yang. In *Illustrations of Acupuncture for Sha Diseases*, attributed to famous Zhuang doctor Luo Jia'an, exuberant yin and declined yang, exuberant yang and declined yin and exuberant yin and yang are used as the general principles of pattern identification in classifying sha diseases. The Ghost Festival is extremely important for the Zhuang nationality, and yin-yang theory in Zhuang medicine is closely related to Zhuang festival customs in daily life. The dead and the living are in the worlds of the dead and the living respectively. As the saying goes, "yin and yang separate humans and spirits". Zhuang people worship ancestors in the Zhongyuan Festival around the 15th day of lunar month, when the yin qi and yin spirit are predominant. Ducks, as food on that day, have a unique function — messengers between the worlds of the dead and the living. This reveals that yin-yang theory in Zhuang medicine is not unfounded but originated from Zhuang people's understanding of nature. It is derived from Zhuang production, life and thinking, and is deeply based on Zhuang culture.

7.2.2   Theory of synchrony of triple initial qi and agricultural festivals

Zhuang is a typical rice-farming minority. Rice farming is deeply ingrained in daily life and production. Zhuang festivals celebrating seasonal farming follow the laws of nature, and they are centered around seasons for production and rhythms of crop cultivation. After the Spring Festival and resting in the 1st lunar month, the spring ploughing begins in the 2nd lunar month. After spring ploughing, the Sanyuesan Festival falls in the 3rd lunar month for entertainment, and people can sing, dance, and enjoy the idle farming season. People appreciate cattle for their hard work in spring ploughing, and worship the cattle soul on the 8th day of the 4th lunar month, the birthday of the King of Cows. That is the origin of the Cattle Soul Festival in the 4th lunar month. In the tenth lunar month, all the late rice has been harvested and dried. People hold a grand ceremony to celebrate the harvest. They offer sacrifices to gods and thank them for their blessings. That is the origin of the Harvest Festival in the 10th lunar month.

Zhuang people believe that humans, as part of the natural world, should live in harmony with nature. Humans, the wisest of all creatures, can resolve conflicts with nature by understanding and leveraging the laws of nature. Humans adapt to the change of season through spring ploughing, summer planting, autumn harvest, and storing of grain for winter. The arrangement of Zhuang agricultural festivals reveals that Zhuang ancestors have understood and conformed to laws of nature. Zhuang people's life is balanced and seasonal, reflecting their belief that "humans should live in harmony with nature".

Zhuang people respect nature and follow the laws of nature. We can see the budding concept of the Zhuang medicine theory of "synchrony of triple initial qi (heaven, earth and human qi)", which is a paraphrase of "humans cannot act in defiance of heaven and earth" or "humans must act in obedience to heaven and earth" in the Zhuang language. The heaven, earth and human parts of the body should remain coordinated and balanced, so the body can be healthy. That is the synchrony of triple initial qi, which is first proposed in *Review of Academic System of Zhuang Medicine* by Qin Baolin, a prestigious Zhuang doctor in Guangxi. Professor Huang Hanru, a famous expert in Zhuang medicine, systematically expounded the synchrony of triple initial qi as a theory about the relationships between humans and nature, and relations within the body.

The synchrony of triple initial qi was derived from the understanding of nature in Zhuang medicine, and it is closely related to Zhuang ancestors' views on the origin of nature, and a simple world-view. The heaven and the earth should remain synchronous and balanced, or there will be natural disasters. The heaven, the earth and humans should remain synchronous and balanced, or people will get sick. That is a rule consciously or unconsciously followed by Zhuang ancestors and applied to the arrangement of agricultural activities. As it is sung in *Chuanyang Songs* (songs to teach moral conduct, as the moral scripture of the Zhuang), "Ploughing work should be done in the 1st and 2nd lunar month. The 2nd and 3rd lunar month is a good time for ploughing and weeding. Early seeding brings strong rice seedlings, and late seeding leads to dead seedlings." In addition to adaption to the laws of nature about agricultural activities, people should proactively transform the natural world and do well in production for good harvests. "Identity of object and self" can bring increased production and harvest, health and relations peace for people.

7. 2. 3 Application of Zhuang medicine and the Medicine King's Day

Long long ago, Zhuang people started to fight against all health hazards including diseases. Disease prevention and removal of pathogenic factors are reflected in many Zhuang festivals.

Medicine King's Day has the richest connotations among all Zhuang festivals, expressing Zhuang people's understanding of disease prevention and treatment, herb cultivation and collection, and understanding of the functions and usage of medicines. Among the activities of Medicine King's Day, Jingxi drug fairs during the Dragon Boat Festival have the longest history and the greatest influence. The research establishes that the drug fairs of Jingxi City during the Dragon Boat Festival began during the Song Dynasty, and its popularity prevailed through the Ming and Qing Dynasties. *Annals of Zhinizhou (Jingxi Gounty)* records, "On the fifth day of the fifth lunar month, all families hang Ai and calamus leaves on the door, and drink Xionghuang wine to dispel plague." On the 5th day of the 5th lunar month in the sweltering midsummer, the hot and damp weather promotes the breeding of poisonous insects and the prevalence of plague. As the roots and stems of some plants mature, it is a good time for picking herbs, which can exert their best effects. On the fifth day of the fifth lunar month, Zhuang people pick Ai. They shape Ai leaves and roots to resemble a human or tiger (commonly known as Ai tiger), and place them centrally on the lintel. They shape calamus leaves like swords and hang them under the roof. On that day, they also heat up water with Ai leaves, calamus and garlic in it. Then they shower with the water, and scatter it around the house. There are scientific reasons for this festival custom. According to *Zhuang Pharmacy in China*, Ai can dispel cold and dampness, regulate qi and blood, relieve pain and blood, and repel mosquitoes, flies, ants and other insects as it is rich in volatile oil, and aromatic. According to *Clinical Manual of Common Zhuang Medicine*, it can regulate the brain (ukgyaeuj), move and transform qi, and remove wind toxin, dampness toxin and miasmic toxin. Garlic also has the actions of removing toxin and killing worms. These ideas explain why Zhuang people heat up water with Ai leaves, calamus and garlic in it, shower with the water, and scatter it around the house. In this way they can kill worms, disinfect the living condition to control the source of infection, and help prevent and treat diseases in summer. Even now there are about 2000 booths in the drug fairs and over 30,000 admissions. Hundreds of medicinal materials are listed, including Huanghuadaoshuil-ian (*Polygala fallax* Hemsl.) and Tianqi. Drug fairs have promoted the development and utilization of genuine Zhuang medicines.

7.2.4　Health preservation and festival activities

7.2.4.1　Healthy diet and disease prevention and treatment

Zhuang festival culture is closely integrated with food culture. "Eating" is always a core part of Zhuang festivals, which can be described as "festivals on the tip of the tongue". This highlights an ever-present topic in characteristic Zhuang festival culture: food is the paramount necessity of the people. Diverse Zhuang festival diets contain knowledge about dietotherapy and healthcare. During the Spring Festival, all families prepare zongzi. Zongzi made from Chinese chestnut and pork are traditional and typical. Zongzi are wrapped in the leaves of phrynium (*Phrynium capitatum* Willd.) which can clear away heat, act as diuretic, treat hoarseness, laryngalgia, oral ulcer and alcoholism. After being cooked for half a day, the medicinal components of the leaves are absorbed by the sticky rice. The Chinese chestnut is warm in nature and sweet in flavor. It can nourish stomach, invigorate spleen, tonify kidney, strengthen lower back and sinews, promote blood circulation, stop bleeding, and remove edema. Eating delicious zongzi in festivals can intake nutrition and also enjoy the healthcare and therapeutic functions of phrynium and Chinese chestnuts as food and medicine. The five-colored sticky rice is a kind of traditional Zhuang food for entertaining guests during festivals, particularly on the 3rd day of the 3rd lunar month, when almost all families prepare it. It has rice in five colors: black, red, yellow, purple, and white. For Zhuang people, it symbolizes good fortune and bumper grain harvests. The sticky rice is dyed using natural plants. Yellow dye is from Shanzhizi (*Gardenia jasminoides*) or Jianghuang (*Curcuma longa* L.), black dye is from maple leaf, red and purple dyes are from different types of Honglancao [*Peristrophe baphica* (Spreng) Bremek.], called "gogyaemq" in Zhuang. According to *Zhuange Pharmacy in China*, Shanzhizi (*Gardenia jasminoides*), cold in nature and bitter in flavor, can clear heat, remove toxin, purge fire, cool blood, stop bleeding, and act as diuretic. Jianghuang (*Curcuma longa* L.) is bitter, pungent and warm. It can break blood stasis, move qi, dredge channels and relieve pain. According to *Clinical Manual of Common Zhuang Medicine*, Honglancao [*Peristrophe baphica* (Spreng) Bremek.] is bitter, pungent and cold. It can regulate Longlu, remove heat toxin and wind toxin, and also generate blood. It is written in *Lvshantang Leibian* in the Qing Dynasty , "It can generate blood and promote circulation of blood. " According to the *Compendium of Materia Medica* , "Maple leaf can help diarrhoea and sleep, strengthen sinews, and tonify qi. Long term usage can improve health and extend lifespan." Therefore, five-colored sticky rice, as a common food, can clear heat, remove toxin, tonify blood, strengthen sinews and bones, and prolong life. It is evident that Zhuang people are wise in health preservation.

7.2.4.2　Mental health and spiritual consolation

One of the important parts of Zhuang festival activities is ancestor worship. Zhuang people believe that ancestral spirits can influence and bless their offspring, so they worship their ancestors including Buluotuo, the founding ancestor of the Zhuang nation. Lacking science and technology in ancient times, Zhuang ancestors believed that frog was a holy creature that can control the forces of nature. In real life, the sound of frogs in spring informs people of the coming of the season for seeding and transplanting rice seedlings, and therefore, the frog became a totem that Zhuang ancestors worshipped. The totem worship aimed at praying for good weather and harvests. The worship of the Flower Mother aimed at praying for reproduction. Ancestral worship aimed at expressing family affection and yearning, and at asking blessings for offspring. Sacrificial ceremonies are good for a healthy life as they give people psychological comfort, spiritual purity, hope for the future, and positive attitude towards life.

7.2.4.3　Relaxation, rest and recovery

Good rest can boost productivity. Modern people emphasize a proper balance between work and rest. Busy in rice-farming, the hard-working and wise Zhuang ancestors leverage festivals to rest for mental and physical benefits, to gather strength and prepare for further work. They enjoy fine food, and visit relatives and friends. During festivals, young people look for the right partners through recreational activities including singing in antiphonal style, back-hitting, and throwing embroidered balls. Such activities help young women and men obtain spiritual pleasure, coordinate yin and yang in the body, maintain psychological health and achieve family happiness. Such activities can please people of all ages and sexes, permitting venting of emotions, improving the mood, and forgetting worries and troubles, all of which are good for health and longevity.

7. 2. 4. 4 Health and intelligence improvement and mood regulation

Zhuang festivals include diverse sports activities, including lion dance on the first day of Lunar New Year, throwing embroidered balls on the Sanyuesan Festival, sparkler-grabbing, bamboo pole dance, and shoe plank race. Currently, most Zhuang villages have basketball courts, where games are held during festivals. With simple equipment, these activities are easy, interesting and popular among Zhuang people. With Zhuang characteristics, they can also improve health, make the body strong, increase intelligence and regulate mood. They show how optimistic and united Zhuang people, emphasize health preservation and love their life through exercise.

References:

[1] Qin Cailuan. Reconstruction and Innovation of Zhuang Festival Culture [J]. Study of Ethnics in Guangxi, 2012 (4): 66－72.

[2] Pan Qixu, Qin Naichang. Encyclopedia of Zhuang Nationality [M]. Nanning: Guangxi People's Publishing House, 1993.

8　Zhuang Medicine and Food

The Zhuang nationality is the most populous among China's ethnic minorities. Zhuang food culture is influenced by geographical environment, climate conditions, customs, social environment, etc. With diverse food materials in the Zhuang region, Zhuang people prefer local green food, and have created a colorful food culture. Their food can not only allay hunger, support life, but also satisfy people, make the body strong, and prevent and treat diseases. In its long history, Zhuang food culture has been closely related to Zhuang medicine. They harmonize with each other, and influence and promote each other.

8.1　Features of Zhuang food culture

Zhuang is a typical rice-farming minority. Situated in a humid and rainy subtropical zone, Zhuang people grow a variety of crops and fruits that are available in all seasons. Wise Zhuang people work hard in unique natural conditions. Gradually, they have formed an age-old food culture with various food. Zhuang staple food include rice, corn, taro, sweet potato, cassava, buckwheat, black rice bean, white rice bean and mung bean, etc. There are a great variety of corns in the Zhuang region, and waxy corn is one of the excellent varieties. Like sticky rice, tasty waxy corn can be used to make zongzi and ciba cakes. Traditional animal food for Zhuang people includes pork, chicken, duck, fish, goose, lamb, beef, horse meat and wild birds and beasts. Vegetables in the Zhuang region include radishes, beans, melons, bamboo shoots, mushrooms, agric, Chinese cabbages, mustard, water spinach, rutabaga and Chinese kale. Zhuang people particularly love mountain products, including famous and precious bamboo shoots, tremella, agric, and mushrooms. The Zhuang region is known as "the land of fruit", as there are many kinds of fruits. There are over 120 kinds of fruits recorded in *Guihai Yuheng Zhi* in the Song Dynasty. Zhuang people like sugar cane, kumquat, pomelo, orange, almond, pineapple, jackfruit, banana, lychee, longan, wampee, olive and mango, etc. In the past, Zhuang people mainly drank low-alcohol wines made by themselves, including rice wine, sweet potato wine, and cassava wine. Rice wine is used for celebrating festivals and entertaining guests as the main drink.

The Zhuang region is rich in flora and fauna. In ancient times, Zhuang ancestors had food made from edible animals and plants from the sky, water and the earth. In their long history, Zhuang food customs have formed distinct characteristics.

8. 1. 1　Preference for glutinous food

Rice is the staple food of the Zhuang nationality. Guangxi is home to wild rice, and Zhuang ancestors are one of the first ethnic groups to grow rice. Since the Han Dynasty and perhaps earlier, rice has been Zhuang ancestors' staple food. According to grain quality, rice can be categorized as hsien rice, keng rice, and glutinous rice. Of these glutinous rice is sticky. Compared with most ethnic groups whose staple food is rice, Zhuang prefer food made from glutinous rice, which accounts for a large proportion of the Zhuang staple food. Glutinous rice is mainly used in making Zhuang festival food, including zongzi, ciba cakes, rice cakes, five-colored sticky rice, tang-yuan, and fried dough. Zongzi and five-colored sticky rice are particularly characteristic of Zhuang food.

Zongzi, called "zongba" in Zhuang, is made in a variety of ways. In Ningming, Guangxi, Zhuang people make surprisingly large zongzi, the same size as a traditional square table for eight people. The zongzi is filled with a boneless cured pig's leg and wrapped in Chinese banana leaves. It is used for ancestor worship on the Lunar New Year's Eve. After ancestor worship, kins share the extra large zongzi to show that they are united and harmonious. In Wenshan Zhuang and Miao Autonomous Prefecture in Yunnan province, Zhuang people make "horse-hoof-shaped zongzi" for festivals. The zongzi is wrapped in large leaves that are 30 centimeters long and 10 to 15 centimeters wide. It looks like a horse hoof, thick and big at one end and thin and long at the other. Therefore people call it "horse-hoof-shaped zongzi". The following steps should be followed to make "horse-hoof-shaped zongzi": soak washed sticky rice for more than 30 minutes; burn last year's dry leaves for zongzi to make ash; mix the ash evenly with drained sticky rice; mix the sticky rice with shredded ham, jujube, pork, salt (or sugar), and other fillings; wrap it with leaves; then boil the zongzi. "Horse-hoof-shaped zongzi" looks grey and yellow, with tender, soft, delicious and fragrant taste. It can be stored for a long time and eaten directly or after being heated. It is used for festivals and served as gifts for market day, song fair, and other activities.

Five-colored sticky rice, with different Chinese names, is essential Zhuang food for Sanyuesan Festival. On the 3rd day of the 3rd lunar month, all families make five-colored sticky rice in memory of the Song Fairy Liu Sanjie. Before being steamed, five-colored sticky rice is divided and soaked separately in dyes of Honglancao (*Peristrophe baphica* (Spreng) Bremek.), maple leaves and other natural plants to make five colors of rice being red, yellow, black, purple, and white (undyed). People shape and present the different colors of sticky rice in attractive ways. The natural dyes can flavor and help preserve sticky rice. Each different color of sticky rice has special functions, for example, yellow sticky rice is used when visiting graves or entertaining ghosts.

In addition to making festival food, people also use sticky rice to make special staple food, such as pumpkin rice. People cut the lid off an old pumpkin and scoop out the insides. They fill it with sticky rice, preserved meat and other foodstuffs. They add some water and stir, then replace the pumpkin lid. The pumpkin is roasted over a slow fire until its rind looks brown. Then it is covered with embers to ensure thorough cooking. People cut up the pumpkin and eat the contents.

Like other ethnic groups, Zhuang people use sticky rice to make wine. In *Strange Stories in Lingnan*, Liu Xun has recorded how Zhuang people in the Tang Dynasty made wine, "They wash and dry a kind of rice, and mix it with medicines and make it green powder. They cook it and then shape it like dough. They use fingers to thrust into its center, place it on the bamboo mat, and add leaves of Gouqi. It is like making distiller's yeast. Vines are used to hang it and the amount of sticky rice used for making wine each year is stable and determined. In South China, it is ready after seven days in spring and winter and five days in autumn and summer. It is put into an earthen jar and burned with cow dung." Since the Ming and Qing dynasties, making wine is popular in the Zhuang region, where almost all the wealthy families make wines. In addition to high-degree alcohol, Zhuang people also drink low-degree sweet wine, which is easy to make by mixing cooked sticky rice with distiller's yeast and waiting for several days of fermentation. When they want to enjoy the sweet wine, they cook it with water, and the grain is edible too. Zhuang people believe that eggs boiled with sweet wine and brown sugar have nourishing action for puerperae.

8. 1. 2　Preference for uncooked food

The preference for uncooked food is a long-standing Zhuang tradition. Zhuang people eat uncooked plants and animals, even live ones. In the Tang Dynasty, Zhuang ancestors ate live baby mice. According to the second volume of *Chaoye Qianzai* (*Draft Notes from the Court and the Country*) in the Tang Dynasty, "In Lingnan, Liao enjoy baby mice with honey. They feed newborn red mice with honey. They put the squeaking baby mice on the bamboo mat and use chopsticks to eat them." In modern times, Zhuang people preserve the tradition of uncooked or undercooked food. In *History of the People of the Yue River Basin* from the Republic era, Xu Songshi wrote about Zhuang diet, "Zhuang people prefer undercooked food. Fan Chuo wrote in *Manshu* that food for people outside the Central Plains includes pigs, sheep, meat of cats, dogs, donkeys, mules, leopards, rabbits, gooses and ducks. However, the food is undercooked, which is different from the Central Plains. Nowadays, people in Guangxi and Guangdong have similar customs ... In addition to uncooked sliced raw fish and lettuce, they eat undercooked common vegetables, chicken, duck, and beef." The most famous uncooked Zhuang food includes uncooked blood and sliced raw fish.

Common uncooked blood is from pigs, sheep, chickens or ducks. Zhuang people believe that uncooked blood can replenish blood and tonify qi. Some scholars believe that the custom, as entertaining etiquette, originated from the primitive belief that blood was mysterious. Zhuang people believe that sheep blood is the best and the most nourishing uncooked blood. In *Yuexi Ouji*, Qing Dynasty Lu Zuofan mentioned that the blood from the hearts of goats in Zuojiang is superior to the blood from other parts, which is good too. This is how Zhuang people eat uncooked blood: they get blood from pigs, sheep, chicken or ducks, pour the blood that is still warm in clean plates, keep stirring it to avoid coagulation, and mix it with hot, spiced, cooked meat and internal organs until it thickens.

Sliced raw fish is a delicacy used for entertaining guests during festivals. *Hengzhou Zhi* in the Qing Dynasty recorded how people prepared and ate sliced raw fish: live fish was sliced and eaten by using chopsticks with spice, vegetables and vinegar. Nowadays, Zhuang people generally use fresh and tender carp for sliced raw fish. They scale and bone, clean and slice the fish, mix it with sesame oil, salt, monosodium glutamate, green onion, garlic and ginger. When they eat the sliced raw fish, they dip it in vinegar, wampee or soy sauce. Experienced people eat it with peanuts, sesame, coriander, Chinese toon sprouts and Chinese mahogany, so that it becomes crispy, smooth and refreshing.

8.1.3 Preference for pickled food

Zhuang people adore pickled food. In the Republic era, Liu Xifan wrote in the fourth chapter *Lingbiao Ji Man*, "Pickled food is common among barbaric ethnic groups. They pickle both planted and wild vegetables. In the 5th, 6th, and 7th lunar months, the barbarians farm and eat the pickle food for all meals. Almost everyone cooks only rice then." Common pickles for Zhuang people include Chinese cabbages, mustard, radishes, cowpeas, jack beans, papayas, peppers, ginger, bamboo shoots and Chinese onion bulbs. Of these the pickled bamboo shoots are the most famous. According to the ninth volume of *Baishan Si Zhi* of the Qing Dynasty, "People pick bitter bamboo shoots in April and May, remove their shells, put them into an earthen jar with pure water. After a long fermentation time, they become sour and smelly, but these people think they are fragrant and cook them together with small fish, making a delicacy. The bamboo shoots soaked for years can treat febrile diseases. They are so effective that these people cherish them."

In addition to planted and wild vegetables, Zhuang people pickle meat, fish and shrimps. According to *Annals of Tongzheng Xian* in the Republic era, "People in different mountain villages in western areas like to butcher a whole pig and share the flesh. They put meat and sticky rice flour into jar. It becomes edible after more than ten days without cooking, and it improves over time. It is called sour meat." In the Republic era, Liu Xifan wrote in the fourth chapter of *Lingbiao Ji Man*, "When people butcher cattle and hogs, they pickle bones with vegetables, and eat them after fermentation." Preserved fish is typical Zhuang pickled food with a long history. Song Dynasty Zhou Qufei wrote in the sixth volume of *Lingwai Daida*, "Southern people make preserved fish that can be stored for as much as ten years. They preserve fish with salt and flour, and put them in an earthen jar that can be sealed with water and an inverted bowl around the mouth. People keep adding water to maintain the seal. The fish is dotted with white spots after several years, as if it is rotten. Both wine and preserved fish, particularly the long-preserved fish, are served as gifts for relatives."

8.1.4 Preference for sour and spicy food

Most ethnic groups living in the mountains in Southwest China are exceedingly fond of sour and spicy food. As Zhuang proverbs go, "If you haven't eaten sour food for three days, you can't even walk normally"; "Sour food is an integrated part of diet"; "Cuisine can't be good without spicy flavor"; "Spicy food is necessary for entertaining guests".

Like other ethnic minorities in southwest, Zhuang people love sour and spicy food. In Wenshan Zhuang and Miao Autonomous Prefecture in Yunnan province, Zhuang people love sour "Laoba Soup". When making Laoba Soup, people cool down the water in which rice has been cooked, put it into a jar, and mix it with salt and clean pieces of green vegetables, Chinese and other cabbage, and other vegetable leaves. After the jar is sealed for one or two days, the rice water and vegetable leaves ferment and become sour. Laoba Soup is made after mixing and cooking fermented rice water, vegetable leaves, and fleshy smoked meat or fried preserved meat. Also, tofu and other mate-rials can be added to make different soup flavors. Sour and refreshing Laoba Soup can relieve summer heat. As it is hot from the period of transplanting rice seedlings to the 8th lunar month, Laoba Soup is common on the tables. The cooled soup from pickled vegetables can also be a refreshing drink, which provides relief from summer heat.

Zhuang people's preference for sour and spicy food is associated with their living environment and produce. Most Zhuang people live in humid mountain areas. Sour and spicy food can help dispel coldness and dampness. As Zhuang people often eat sticky rice that is hard to digest, sour and spicy food can help digestion and absorption.

8. 2   Customs and etiquette in Zhuang dining

People developed customs and etiquette in dining as one of the most obvious forms of rites and activities governed by strict norms. Dong Zhongshu in the Han Dynasty, a master of Confucian classics, wrote in *Tiandaoshi*, *Chunqiu Fanlu* (*Rich dew of the Spring and Autumn Classic*), "Lasciviousness and absence of rites will cause misconduct, diet without rites will cause combat, and misconduct and combat will in turn cause turmoil." Like other ethnic groups, the Zhuang nationality has developed a set of colorful dining etiquette and customs.

8. 2. 1   Everyday dining etiquette

Compared with other ethnic minorities, the Zhuang nationality is greatly influenced by the traditional culture of the Han nationality, and the influence can be witnessed in Zhuang's everyday dining etiquette, including views of respecting the old and cherishing the young, harmonious social hierarchies, and the superiority of men over women. For example, the elderly are particularly respected at table. People should use both hands to provide a bowl of rice from either side of the elderly. After the meal, a bowl of tea or water should be given to the elderly for rinsing the mouth. Zhuang people believe that the hearts and livers of chickens and ducks are nutritious, and their breasts and tails are fat and tender. Therefore, these parts are particularly provided for the elderly. At table, Zhuang men and women usually sit around separate tables, following the old maxim — it is improper for men and women to touch each other's hand in passing objects. Their seating arrangement is also strict: parents should have the main seat, children have the seats on both sides of the main seat, and daughters-in-law have the farthest seat from the main seat.

8.2.2   Entertaining etiquette

Zhuang is a hospitable minority with many related document records. Ming Dynasty Kuang Lu wrote in the upper volume of *Chiya*, "They hospitably serve guests, whether known or unknown, with meat and wine." Qing Dynasty Min Xu wrote in *Yueshu*, "People hospitably entertain guests with dishes." According to *Annals of Shanglin County* in the Republic of China era, "When relatives or friends visit families that are not well-off financially, those families still hospitably entertain them with wine, and even give more cordial reception for guests from afar." Zhuang people in Longzhou have the custom of asking guests to stay. When there are visitors at home, the hosts will prepare food and drink and lay out dining table and tableware, indicating that guests are invited to have dinner which they should not refuse. If the guests still want to go, the hosts will feel humiliated.

In many Zhuang villages, the guests of any family are regarded as the guests of all families for the whole village. Several families take turns at inviting the guests to have dinner and they should have dinners and taste the dishes in turn to avoid discourtesy. When Zhuang people entertain guests, they ask elder and distinguished guests to have the main seats. They must prepare wine to show solemnity. Particularly, they have the custom of "cross-cupped wine". When they drink cross-cupped wine, they don't use cups but bowls. They drink each other's wine in white porcelain spoons, looking into each other's eyes sincerely. In order to show respect to guests, hosts use chopsticks to select food from each plate served for guests, then other people can choose food from the plate. Zhuang hosts never allow the guests' bowls to be empty as they keep hospitably selecting the best food for them. Zhuang hosts believe that the higher the food is in their guests' bowls, the more respect is shown. In some Zhuang villages, people use one chopstick to spear several pieces of meat and put them into the guest's mouth, and this is called "meat infusion". Some guests, who come to Zhuang villages for the first time, try their best to eat up all the food in their bowl to avoid embarrassment. However, hosts keep adding food for them, because they feel happy if guests cannot finish all the food. They will feel themselves bad hosts with bad food if guests finish all the food in their bowls.

8.2.3　Dining etiquette for life rituals

In marriage, funeral, birthday and other rituals, diet plays an irreplaceable role with important meaning. Therefore, people emphasize diet in these life rituals. Of the various life rituals, marriage is the most solemn one, with food customs throughout the whole marriage celebration from relationship, engagement to wedding. In Jingxi, Debao, Napo, Daxin and other places, a young woman's family should prepare a feast to entertain the visiting son-in-law early in the first lunar month of the following year if the young woman has been in a relationship with the young man for a while. It is called "question and answer banquet for son-in-law". In the banquet, the young woman's family invites a respectable and informed village senior to question the son-in-law about general knowledge including agriculture, daily life, religion and history. The question and answer session is carried out in a natural and harmonious dining process. The performance of the son-in-law will directly influence the engagement outcome.

In Zhuang engagement etiquette, betel nuts can serve as engagement gifts. According to *Baishan Si Zhi* in the Qing Dynasty, "Instead of engagement cards, people use one box of betel nuts and one pair of rings for engagement." Zhuang people eat oval and orange betel nuts for digestion. In *Helin Yulu* (*Jade Dew from the Forest of Cranes*) by Luo Dajing in the Song Dynasty and *Baishan Si Zhi* in the Qing Dynasty, it is written that the reason why Zhuang people prefer betel nuts is for the prevention of miasmic malaria. Zhuang people use betel nuts as engagement gifts because they are delicious and represent the respect for the woman as the Chinese pronunciation for "betel nuts（槟榔）" sound the same as "宾"（bin）and "郎"（lang）, both of which are used to address distinguished guests to show respect.

For villages along the Hongshui River and the Liujiang River, a bride should turn her back to the burning incense and sit in the middle of the central room before entering the sedan chair. A bowl of rice from the husband's family is held by a person who has both parents and at least a son and a daughter. The wedding celebrant chants, "After the wife eats her husband's white rice with sugar and meat, her descendants will become Number One Scholars." Other people answer, "Yeah! Great!" The person holding the bowl puts a piece of Chinese onion, a chicken drumstick and a piece of brown sugar aside in the bowl, and provides the bride with three mouthfuls of rice. The bride spits out all the rice on to the skirt prepared by the sister-in-law. The person holding the bowl gives her a pair of chopsticks, and she passes them over her shoulders on to a younger person behind her without looking back, meaning "I will never look back".

In the marriage ceremony, Zhuang women and men sit around seperate tables, but they can sit in any seat of their table. One of the Zhuang customs for the marriage ceremony is that everyone can get a portion of food, whatever their age. An infant who still needs breast feeding can also get a portion, which will be brought back by their parents. Such etiquette reflects Zhuang people's ideas of equality. In some Zhuang villages, however, male guests can have good seats while female guests can only sit on bamboo mats. This reflects the discrimination against women in Zhuang society, which is rare now.

Zhuang dining etiquette for life rituals apart from marriage is also diverse. In Anping, Daxin, Guangxi, the Zhuang custom for birth is unique. One dan of sticky rice, and 20 duck eggs should be provided by the grandmother of mother's side. The son-in-law's family should invite all children in the village to walk around the house and cry out, "Baby, let's go farming ..." Then each child will be provided with one roll of sticky rice and one duck egg. In some places in western Guangxi, the eldest sons of seniors aged over 60 should feed their fathers when the seniors celebrate their birthdays.

8.2.4 Dining etiquette during festivals

There is also some special etiquette observed in Zhuang dining during festivals. For example, people eat zongzi but no vegetables during the Spring Festival, as they believe that grass will grow wildly and out of control in the fields and influence the harvest next year if they eat vegetables during the Spring Festival. On Sanyuesan Festival, Zhuang people eat five-colored sticky rice and five-colored eggs. Five-colored eggs are chicken, duck or goose eggs in five colors. Everyone eats just one colored egg, and each child hangs a string of five-colored eggs for playing game. On Mid-Autumn Festival, Zhuang people admire the moon and eat mooncakes. Children use pomelo peel to make strange ghost head props, and dress up before taking mooncakes from the tables of wealthy families. Young men and women symbolically steal some fruit and vegetables in the field, believing that eating them can improve eyesight.

8.3   Relationship between Zhuang medicine and food

8.3.1   "Sandao" theory and food culture

In Zhuang medicine, Gudao, Shuidao, Qidao and relevant internal organs within the body are the places for the generation, storage and circulation of nutriments maintaining vital activities within the body. They are interlinked and work in coordination. Also, they perform their own functions cooperatively and help nourish the whole body. They ensure normal physiological activities with the synchrony of triple initial qi— heaven, earth and human. Gudao is the tract for the digestion and absorption of food, and the distribution of nutriments; Qidao is the place for the generation, distribution and storage of human qi; and Shuidao is the place for the generation, storage, distribution and circulation of body water. Fresh air, high-quality water sources, and natural and green food in the Zhuang region have played an important role in the normal operation of Gudao, Qidao and Shuidao. This can improve the body's resistance to diseases and maintain the body's healthy state. In Zhuang medicine, the five zang-organs collect essence for nourishing the body, and the six fu-organs distribute the essence of water and food and the excretion of waste matters. The functions of the five zang-organs and the six fu-organs rely on Gudao, Qidao and Shuidao. Zhuang people particularly emphasize the regulation of Gudao.

They have a well-balanced diet, which explains why there are many long-lived Zhuang people. The emphasis of the regulation of Gudao in Zhuang medicine is similar to the concept in TCM that the spleen and stomach provide the material basis of the acquired constitution. Zhuang diet features low fat, animal protein, salt, sugar and calories, as well as high vitamin and cellulose. Zhuang people rely mainly on local green food including coarse food grain and vegetables. One kind of corns in Bama is full of nutriments including high fat and protein. Hemp seed oil in Bama is the only vegetable oil soluble in water in the world. In addition, they have a light diet and they are not particular about food. Their food intake is low in calories. Their well-balanced diet and good ways of life are important for unblocking Gudao and keeping it working well. People usually evaluate their health condition based on whether the functions of Gudao are normal or not.

8.3.2　Medicated diets and food culture

Zhuang medicated diet is made from medicines, food and spice according to Zhuang medical theories. It is delicious food with local and ethnic characteristics that can prevent and treat diseases, improve health and promote longevity.

In Zhuang medicine, medicated diet is reasonably applied as a dietotherapy based on the overall analysis of patients' symptoms, causes of disease, and constitution. The principles for dietetic invigoration vary according to the change of season. Zhuang medicated diet particularly maintains the original taste and flavor of food and medicinal materials, while combining food with the nature and flavor of medicinal materials for better therapeutic effects and healthcare. The cookery methods for medicated diet include steaming, boiling, stewing, frying, and simmering. Some spices are added to improve color, smell and flavor, and to increase the appetite.

Fruits provide the raw materials for making unique Zhuang medicated fruit diet, including haw jelly cake, pineapple cup and grenadine juice. There are also many methods for cooking rice, including famous rice cooked in bamboo tubes, rice rolled in lettuce and five-colored sticky rice.

Nowadays, Zhuang people keep developing modern medicated diet based on the traditional one. Canned medications, healthy drink, medicated candies, medicated dessert, and medicated wine are increasingly popular at home and abroad. Zhuang medicated diet will make greater contribution to disease prevention and treatment as well as extending life.

8.3.3　Health preservation and food culture

Zhuang health preservation is based on the unique experience developed from the long-term Zhuang medical practice implementing Zhuang medical theories. As the saying goes, dietetic invigoration is better than the use of tonifying medicines. Zhuang health preservation emphasizes the role of diet in making the body strong, preventing diseases, improving health, and slowing down aging.

In Zhuang medicine, to tonify deficiency with animals' flesh and blood is an effective way. Deficiency refers to the clinical manifestations resulting from the functional decline of zang and fu organs. This is caused by insufficient healthy qi due to congenital medical condition, acquired disorder or disease. According to Zhuang medicine, the clinical manifestations of deficiency are common in chronic and senile diseases, and during the recovery phase after removing pathogenic toxin. Human beings are miracles, and are the wisest of all creatures. It is believed in Zhuang medicine that the most effective way to tonify deficiency is using animal medicine, as animals have flesh and blood as well as emotions, and like attracts like. Therefore animal meat and blood have long been used to strengthen and nourish the body. Traditional animal food for Zhuang people includes pork, chicken, duck, goose, lamb, beef, horse meat and fish. According to *Dictionary of Chinese Materia Medica*, "Mutton can replenish qi, tonify deficiency, warm the middle or the body from lower. It can treat consumptive diseases, marked emaciation, soreness and weakness of waist and knees, postpartum deficient cold, abdominal pain, cold colic in abdomen and vulva, deficient middle qi and regurgitation." Sliced raw fish is nutritious and delicious, and all Zhuang families make sliced raw fish during the Mid-Autumn Festival. Blood from pigs, cattle, ducks, chickens, sheep, gooses and other animals can tonify and nourish qi and blood. Sheep blood is sweet and bitter in flavor and cold in nature. It can remove toxin, cool blood and stop bleeding, promote blood circulation, dissipate blood stasis, gelsemium and other herb poisoning, hematemesis, massive haemorrhage, retention of placenta, trauma, etc. Blood sausage is made from cleaned pig intestines infused with pork blood, minced meat, fine glutinous rice, Chinese onions and garlic. Blood sausage can be a staple food and it is able to tonify deficiency. Regularly eating the famous Guangxi dish "Sanqi chicken" can treat nutritional anemia and prevent stagnant dysmenorrhea. Some animals can be used to tonify deficiency, including black-bone chickens, sparrows, mice and snakes. Black-bone chicken is sweet in flavor and neutral in nature. It can tonify liver, kidney, blood, and yin, and clear deficiency-heat. Therefore it can treat deficiency of both liver and kidney, consumptive disease, and syndrome of yin blood insufficiency, syndrome of endogenous heat due to yin deficiency, metrorrhagia, leukorrhea, and other syndromes of deficiency. Medicated food made from sparrow and mutton can treat infertility due to cold in the uterus. Infertility due to deficient cold in the uterus can be treated with medicated food made from goat meat, sparrow meat, motherwort herb, and black soya bean. According to Zhuang medicine, people should often eat snake soup if they suffer from years of pain in neck and joints and their joint pain increases with weather change. People with dry cough related to lung yin deficieney should eat lotus root cooked with pork, old female duck or partridge meat. In addition to deficiency syndrome, other syndromes complicated by stasis are also treated with animal flesh and blood to reinforce healthy qi and remove stasis. Common yam rhizome and beef porridge is often used to help reinforce healthy qi.

Medicated wines are also employed in Zhuang medicine for disease prevention and health improvement. Zhuang people live in Lingnan, where the terrain is so tough that miasma emerges and converges among the misty hills. Yang is exuberant and yin is congealed there, dampness is accumulated and heat emerges. The region is haunted by filthy-attack diseases and miasma. Because of the hot, cloudy, damp and rainy weather, many diseases are associated with dampness pathogen. *Bencao Shiyi* records, "White spirit can promote blood circulation, regulate stomach and intestines, moisten skin, and expel dampness." Zhuang ancestors were good at making wine, including rice wine, sweet sticky rice wine, sweet potato wine, cassava wine, and other low-degree wines. Drinking an appropriate amount can dispel dampness, expel miasma, warm and dredge meridians, and allay fatigue. Rice wine is a must for entertaining guests during festivals. The rice wines containing chicken gallbladder, chicken giblets or pig liver are respectively called chicken gallbladder wine, chicken giblet wine and pig liver wine. Chicken giblet wine or pig liver wine should be drunk completely, while the chicken giblet or pig liver should be chewed slowly as a dish for dispelling the effects of alcohol. Sweet potato wine can help prevent hyperlipemia and hypercholesterolemia. Sweet sticky rice wine has the action of tonifying qi and nourishing blood, and Zhuang people get used to welcoming guests with it. Longan wine is made from longan, a special kind of fruit in Guangxi. It can tonify blood, improve intelligence, nourish heart and tranquilize mind. Emblic wine can help prevent and treat hypertension and hyperlipemia. Tokay gecko wine is particularly characteristic. Tokay gecko, salty in flavor and mild in nature, can tonify lung and kidney, treat coughing dyspnea, tonify kidney yang, benefit essence and blood, treat menostaxis, and dredge Shuidao. Tokay gecko wine is made from tokay gecko (finished product) and white spirit. It can tonify lung, treat dyspnea, warm kidney, assist yang, treat coughing dyspnea and chronic bronchitis due to lung and kidney yang deficiency. Zhuang people often drink it as medicated wine for health care and treatment. Sanshe wine is also a famous medicated wine. It is made from specially processed cobra, Chinese rat snake, krait (or many-banded krait), and herbs. The white spirit containing cobra gallbladder can dispel wind-dampness and remove dampness toxin.

In Zhuang medicine, beverages are applied in removing toxin and preventing diseases. Pathogenicity of toxin and deficiency is the etiological and pathogenetic theory of Zhuang medicine. Toxin is considered as the main cause of diseases. In the Zhuang region with its special climate and geographical environment, toxin refers to tangible poisonous substances (e.g., snake venom and poisonous insects, herbs and trees), intangible toxin (e.g., heat, fire, wind, and dampness toxin) and all pathogenic factors. As miasma emerges in the hot Zhuang region, people there easily suffer from shanghuo (or yeet hay), predominant yang, and dampness-heat. Therefore, special drinks in the Zhuang region are those able to clear heat, relieve summer heat, expel miasma, and dispel dampness. Zhuang people like to use betel nuts, Chinese hawthorn leaves, and fermented rice water to make drinks. In spring and summer when diseases are prevalent, Zhuang families have betel nuts in their home for boiling in water to make a drink that can expel miasma. Also, Zhuang people often soak dry Chinese hawthorn leaves in boiling water. After it cools down, people drink it to quench thirst and relieve summer heat. In Zhuang villages, all families make fermented rice water to soak peppers, cowpeas, tender bamboo shoots and garlic. In hot summer, drinking fermented rice water can help quench thirst, relieve summer heat, and treat gastrointestinal diseases. Appetite can be increased by adding fermented rice water into dishes. Dry emblic pulp makes emblic tea, which can prevent and treat hypertension, hyperlipemia, bronchitis and pharyngolaryngitis. Bean jelly and juice are traditional Zhuang refreshers in summer. They are sweet, refreshing, and thirst-quenching. Cinnamon tea, sugarcane drink and other drinks are simple and convenient, and they can clear heat and help get rid of yeet hay. In the damp and hot Zhuang region, people suffer from dampness. Papaya soup and papaya cup are popular as they have the action of removing dampness-heat. Jigucao (*Abrus cantoniensis* Hance) and Gougancai (*Dicliptera chinensis* (L.) Juss.) decoction can remove heat and dampness toxin and treat jaundice. Corn contains glutathione, which can help control cancer. In Bama, a village in Guangxi famed for longevity, Zhuang people eat corn as the staple food and make corn soup as a drink.

References:

[1] Feng Qiuyu. Features of Zhuang Food Culture [J]. Journal of Medicine and Pharmacy of Chinese Minorities, 2009 (11): 77 - 79.

[2] Liu Pubing. Preliminary Discussion on Zhuang Food Culture and Customs [J]. Journal of Nanning Polytechnic, 2007 (12): 1 - 4.

[3] Tang Zhenyu, Pang Yuzhou, Lan Lixia, et al. Preliminary Discussion on Principles of Zhuang Health Preservation [J]. Chinese Journal of Basic Medicine in Traditional Chinese Medicine, 2015 (1): 21 - 22.

[4] Zhu Hua. Annals of Zhuang Medicine in China [M]. Nanning: Guangxi Nationalities Publishing House, 2003.

[5] Ye Qinglian. Basic Zhuang Medical Theories [M]. Nanning: Guangxi Nationalities Publishing House, 2006.

[6] Lan Yuying. Preliminary Discussion on Etiological and Pathogenetic Theory of Zhuang Medicine [J]. China Journal of Traditional Chinese Medicine and Pharmacy, 2010, 25 (12): 2147.

9　Zhuang Medicine and Dwelling

9.1　Evolution of Zhuang dwelling

The housing conditions of Zhuang people and their ancestors are closely associated with the special natural environment and level of productivity. Zhuang people built their houses with local materials according to the terrain. They dwelled in mountain caves, lived in nests in the trees, and finally developed ganlan houses.

9.1.1　Dwelling in mountain caves

Mountain caves were the first places of residence for early humans. As there are many mountains and caves in Lingnan, suitable caves are readily available. *Nanman Chapter*, *Book of Sui* records, "Nanman (Southern Barbarians) have no leaders and live in mountain caves." Dwelling in mountain caves is also mentioned in *Taiping Huanyu Ji* of the Song Dynasty. Mountain caves, as shelters from wind and rain, are the simplest and most convenient places of refuge.

9.1.2　Living in nests in the trees

In primitive society, Zhuang ancestors lived by picking fruit and hunting. "Liao people live near the mountain forests. Without chiefs, they live by hunting and also eat insects." Lingnan was humid, rainy and rugged, where venomous serpents, wild beasts, and natural disasters constantly threatened people's safety. In order to survive in the natural world, Zhuang ancestors constantly looked for the optimum dwelling environment. Gradually, they began to live in above-ground dwellings to avoid venomous serpents and wild beasts. *Wudu*, *Han Feizi* says, "In ancient times, there was not a very big population. People suffered from the attack of numerous beasts, insects and snakes. A sage invented shacks in the tree to avoid attack. Therefore people loved and esteemed him, chose him to be the ruler, and called him Youchao." Jin Dynasty Zhang Hua wrote in *Bowu Zhi*, "Southern people live in nests, and northern people dwell in caves to escape the cold and the heat." *The Commentary on Wenshui*, *Water*

Classic also discussed living in nests in the trees. *Linyi Ji* records, "Wenliang people live in the wild without houses. They live in places with trees, and live on fish and raw meat..." *The Tianxia Junguo Libing Shu* (*Merits and Drawbacks of All the provinces and Counties in China*) says, "Liang people live in tree dwellings in the mountains." *Volume two*, *Geography*, *Book of Sui* says, "Li people live in nests in the mountains, and do farm work." *History of Song* says, "Li people live in nests and speak like birds." Wenliang, Lang, and Li people refer to Zhuang ancestors, who lived in trees.

9. 1. 3　Ganlan houses

With the improvement of production, Zhuang ancestors gradually changed from living in trees to living in raised dwellings, and finally developed ganlan houses. Ganlan houses are primitive and unsophisticated residential buildings that still exist in the Zhuang region, mainly in remote and inaccessible mountain villages. *Records of Pingnanliao*, *Old Book of Tang* says, "People live in multi-storied ganlan houses." *Pingnanliao*, *Records of the Southern Barbarians*, *New Book of Tang* says, "People live in multistorey ganlan houses to prevent poisonous herbs, chiggers and Gloydius halys." As people started to raise livestock, the above-ground upper layer of ganlan houses was used for human habitation, and the lower layer for rearing livestock. Song Dynasty Fan Chengda recorded in *Guihai Yuheng Zhi*, "People live in malan houses covered with hatch, with the upper layer for human habitation and the lower layer for rearing cattle, hogs, and other livestock." Primitive ganlan houses were built with bamboo and wood, covered with thatch or bamboo. With the progress of society and the development of economy, the materials of ganlan houses changed from bamboo and wood to soil, tiles, bricks and stones.

According to structure, ganlan houses can be categorized into five types: fully raised long-pole ganlan, half-raised ganlan, low-pole ganlan, on-ground ganlan, and transversal type ganlan. According to building materials, they can be broken down into four categories: wood, wood-bamboo, wood-stone, other.

9. 1. 3. 1　Fully raised long-pole ganlan

This type of ganlan houses is one of the most primitive architectural forms that still exists in the Zhuang region. Such ganlan houses are mainly distributed in the mountain villages in northern Guangxi (Longsheng Pan-Ethnicities Autonomous County, Sanjiang Dong Autonomous County, Rongshui Miao Autonomous County), central Guangxi (Xincheng), western Guangxi (Jingxi and Xilin) and eastern Guangxi (Hezhou). In particular, the most complete and typical ones are in Longji 13 villages in Longsheng Pan-Ethnicities Autonomous County. Most of them are built on steep mountain slopes independently or some of them joined together. They are arranged in close order but no fixed layout is shown for the entire village, each of which consists of 20 to 50 houses. They feature wood structure and are fully raised long-pole structures. Poles, walls and frames on the foundations on high slopes all use timber. The roofs are covered with Chinese-style tiles (or cedar bark or thatch), forming overhanging gable or half hip-and-gable roofs. The plank floor is built on stilts, with the first layer for rearing hogs, cattle and other livestock or storing articles, and the second layer for human habitation. The second layer can be reached by a wooden ladder, and is separated by planks into rooms. The third layer is half attic on plank floor, used for placing grain and articles. Each layer is about 2.0 to 2.4 meters in height.

9.1.3.2　Half-raised ganlan

This type of ganlan and fully raised long-pole wooden ganlan are usually in the same village. They have basically the same beam frames. Such ganlan houses are built on steep mountain slopes, with the three front rooms built on high stilts. People live on the second plank floor. The two rear poles are built on top of the platform level with the second plank floor, at a height of about 2 meters above the ground. With three quarters above-ground floor and one quarter ground floor, thus it is called half-raised ganlan. In addition, in some other places the back wall of a half-raised ganlan is made from stone or brick, forming a stone-timber or brick-timber structure.

9.1.3.3　Low-pole ganlan

The low-pole ganlan represents those ganlan houses whose ground floor of a low-pole ganlan is as low as one meter. This type of ganlan house is mainly distributed in western Guangxi (Pingguo, Longzhou, Jingxi, and Daxin) and northern Guangxi (Donglan, Tian'e, Rongshui Miao Autonomous County). Most of them are built on the root of the mountain.

9.1.3.4　On-ground ganlan

This type of ganlan is common in Zhuang villages in Rongshui Miao Autonomous County. It is built on flat ground with plank or cob brick walls and overhanging gable roof. Bays and other rooms are separated with planks. The lower storey at ground level is for human habitation, and the upper floor for storing grain and other articles. Because of terrain, wooden poles are used to support overhanging joists and eaves. Belvederes and corridors are built between poles or on the ground before the door. The corridors without foundations remain a feature of traditional ganlan houses.

9. 1. 4   On-ground buildings

On-ground buildings are widely distributed in towns and villages where transport is convenient and Han and Zhuang people live together. Their form and structure vary by region, with similar basic structures— earth or stone or brick walls, wood purlins, blue roofing tiles, overhanging gable roofs, three bays as main rooms, two storeys with the lower storey for human habitation (on the ground), the upper storey as mezzanine level or second floor, and the central hall as central bay. Some on-ground buildings remain the "chuandou" type timber constructions. In Ningjiang, Xincheng County, the partition of the wing reaches the pediment, and some ganlan houses have features similar to traditional ganlan cloister.

9. 2   Features of Zhuang residence

9. 2. 1   Layout of Zhuang residence

The internal layout of Zhuang residence strictly follows one rule: the shrine should be in the center and the fireplace comes second. Located on the central line, the shrine has the most prominent position in a house. It reveals the solemnity of ancestor worship and the influence of family traditions. People hope that their ancestors' miraculous brightness can illuminate the entire house. In order to place incense burners, a traditional square table for eight people is put before a shrine. Strangers must not move the incense burners without permission, since it would be considered as disrespect of ancestors. Such behavior would lead to the host's displeasure or even reproach. Two seats are placed on each side of the table. The left seat is for the master of the house, and any other person who sits there will offend the head of the family. The right seat at the other end is for guests. The fireplace, as another important part, can be set to one side or the rear of the hall. Its place comes second to the shrine as people cook and eat at the fireplace. Generally, Zhuang people set up a sacrificial altar near the fireplace or cooking range to worship the Kitchen God to pray for blessings and a bumper grain harvest. The living area is at the back of the house, accounting for a small part of the total area. The front section of the house is a hall for celebrations and social activities. On either side there are wings, and the wing that opens onto the hall is for guests. The households' bedrooms are in the second half of the house in the wing that does not open onto the hall. Generally people don't live in the area behind the shrine, where only the master of the house can live. See Figure 9-1 for the layout of Zhuang residence.

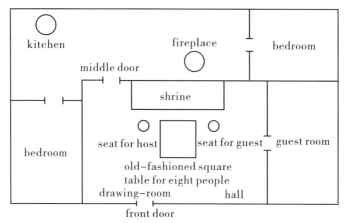

Figure 9-1　Layout of Zhuang residence

The area of ganlan houses, particularly fully raised and half-raised ganlan houses, is large, with a width of about 20 meters and depth of about 10 meters. The entrance is on one side of the first floor, and the second floor can be reached by a wooden ladder. A belvedere with length about 7 meters and width about 2.5 meters is built before the gateway. Wooden benches are placed on the belvedere so that people can put down rain gear and tools before entering the house or can rest. A ladder leads to a hallway opening into a large hall which is open on both sides. The hall is about 18 meters in length and 8 meters in width. A fireplace is set on both sides. Families usually use the fireplace on the right side, and the one on the left side is used for marriage, funeral arrangements, or other days of celebration. A capacious hall is ideal for gatherings, banquets and other group activities, so people don't need to go outside (large flat ground areas are rare). On the side with the frequently-used fireplace, there is a wall surface with cooking vessels and tableware. There are bedrooms or storerooms separated by planks at the rear and on the left side, with customary layout.

In Longsheng, for example, an antechamber leads into the central room, with spirit tablets facing the entrance. To the rear of the spirit tablets are bedrooms. The bedroom in the middle is for father/father-in-law, while the one on the left is for mother/mother-in-law to avoid women committing blasphemy against ancestors. If father-in-law lives in the middle bedroom and mother-in-law lives in the left one, there is a door joining their rooms. The rightmost room is for the daughter-in-law. Rooms on either side of the hall are for children, with the right side for sons and the left side for daughters who will remain in those rooms when visiting home after getting married. One of the obvious features of the layout is separate rooms for a couple. In "Longji 13 Villages", the layout of the house features girl's rooms beside the ladder at the right corner, and that helps girls contact the young men. See Figure 9-2 for the layout of Zhuang residence in Longsheng. In Baise, a hall runs along the middle of a ganlan house, with the rear end of the hall serving as a kitchen. The left and right wings are bedrooms. The front section of the left wing is for father and the rear of both wings is for descendants. When families divide, the oldest son retains his room, signifying inheritance. Other sons have to build their own houses.

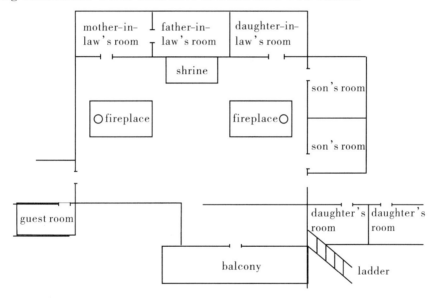

Figure 9-2 Layout of Zhuang residence in Longsheng

In Baiding Township, Tian'e County, the ancestral altar and two fireplaces in Zhuang residences are distributed in the shape of the Chinese character "品". Different from Longji, the bedrooms of parents are not behind the ancestral altar, but in the left rear corner. Common rooms are behind the ancestral altar and are available for daughters-in-law and unmarried daughters. This indicates that people in the outlying mountain area in western Guangxi are less influenced by the view that women are inferior.

In addition, belvederes and corridors are built on either side for enjoying the coolness. At the front of one side, there is a balcony made from bamboo and wood, for drying grain. Windows in the walls provide good lighting and ventilation. Halls and fireplaces are located in the central bay. On one side there is no attic, but rooms separated by planks as storerooms, or sometimes bedrooms for guests. Therefore, a residence can satisfy many aspects of the whole family's daily life, including drying grain, pounding rice, drinking, cooking, eating, entertaining guests, and gathering.

Low-pole and on-ground ganlan houses are narrower, smaller, lower and less practical than fully raised long-pole and half-raised ones. Usually there are three bays about 13 meters wide, and 10 meters deep. Simple in structure and low in cost, they give easy access and can basically meet the whole family's living requirements.

Zhuang people believe that the main door can bring in wealth and treasure, and reject ghosts. Therefore the main door is usually in the middle, facing the shrine, in the hope that ancestral spirits can bless and protect the entrance and bring good fortune. But customs vary with regions. In some regions, the door is not in the middle but on the left side as people believe that "ancestors cannot rest in peace and the family cannot be prosperous and happy if the door opens on a view of mountains". In other regions, there is no back door as it's believed that back door allows the outflow of money. If a back door is necessary, the front and back doors cannot be in line, or else money will come in via the front door and exit through the back door. Various customs indicate that the door is related to the good and bad fortune of a family. Therefore, Zhuang people paste written spells on the door frame to protect against evil influences, and hang mirrors, scissors or other magic weapons to reject evil spirits.

With the improvement of living standards and the mixing of Zhuang and Han nationalities, many Zhuang people now live in modern houses and consequently ganlan houses are decreasing over time. However, the layout of houses remains some special Zhuang customs.

9.2.2 Administrative offices in the Tusi system

There is a rigid hierarchy in the tusi system in the Zhuang region. The native chieftains (called tusi) imposed limitations on Zhuang people's house construction to distinguish the tusi from common people by quality of residence. According to Qing Dynasty tusi in Shangying, Xiangdu and other places, ordinary people were not allowed to build houses with decorative dragons, phoenixes, or with steps higher than tusi's. Therefore, tusi's houses had much greater scale, layout, quality and decoration than those of ordinary people.

Following the lifestyle of official families of Han nationality, tusi in the Ming and Qing Dynasties built Tusi yamen complexes with Zhuang characteristics, including well-preserved Tusi yamen in Xincheng, built in the Daoguang Era, and tusi halls built in the Qianlong Era. They have the features of both traditional Zhuang culture and culture of the Central Plains. The integration of Zhuang and Han building technologies is revealed in their Han-style layouts, masonry-timber structure, carved beams, painted rafters, and colorful paintings.

Described as "Zhuang Palace Museum", they are among the largest and best preserved tusi buildings in China and Asia. With an area of over 40,000 square meters, they consist of yamen, mansions, pools, parlours, temples, cemetery, etc. Founded in 1582, they all have masonry-timber structures with the wood components made from valuable timbers. They absorb the advantages of Ming Dynasty architecture, which can be seen in the design of eaves, ridges, paintings, screens, poles, and other details. Tusi yamen is composed of screen wall, front gate, main hall, second hall, third hall and backyard. On either side are east and west outer gates, drawing rooms, wings, barracks and jails. The ancestral hall consists of screen wall, gate, sacrificial hall and back hall. Yamen is the core of the entire layout. The front gate opens onto the street, and a broad corridor with pillars stands in front of the gate. There is a couplet on the pillars by Zheng Xiaogu, a famous Guangxi calligrapher of the Qing Dynasty. The couplet says, "The territory is defended, people are governed, and those who live in Shiliubao are all your people; the territory is developed and governed through taxation, and several miles of land belongs to our imperial court." On both sides of the gates are memorial archways called East Anteport and West Anteport. "庆南要地" and "粤西边隅" are respectively written on their lintels, indicating the location and position of the place. Mo clan's ancestral hall is 20 meters away to the east of the yamen, covering an area of 1470 square meters. It was founded in 1753 and rebuilt in 1847 after being destroyed in the turmoil of war. Three entrances separate the main entrance, main hall, and rooms housing Mo clan's ancestral tablets. On both sides of the main hall, there are guest rooms with carved, gilded and finely-crafted windows and luxurious decorations. On its east side there is the unique Sanqing Temple, and on its west side there is a continuous row of official residences for tusi's closest family members including siblings, nephews and uncles. Those official residences are equipped with rooms providing services including training grounds and clinics. On the west side of the official residences, there is Guandi Temple. With a rigid hierarchy, residences for tusi's Wei, Liu and Yang clans are arranged near the two temples, and ordinary people's residences and city walls are farther removed. South of the tusi yamen are unique Half-moon Pavilion and Longyin Cave for tusi's meditation and self-cultivation. North of it are pavilions, stone bridges, and pools surrounded by exotic trees and flowers. To the northwest is tusi's solemn family cemetery. The overall style of all buildings is in harmony with that of Tusi yamen.

9.3　House construction and villages

9.3.1　House construction

The construction of Zhuang houses includes selection of site and auspicious day, construction, inauguration ceremony, etc. According to Zhuang customs, each of those processes has its sacrificial rite to guarantee good auspices. The good location should be spacious, sunny and near some land feature. In a valley plain, houses should be built on raised land instead of low-lying areas, where there might be floods. The location should be near sources of water such as rivers, channels or pools for the convenience of water carrying and cleaning business. The houses can be oriented either south or east.

When Zhuang people want to build new houses, generally they avoid busy farming seasons so that neighbors and other villagers can help them. Also they avoid the rainy season so that their houses can be built with solid foundations and construction. They pick a day when there are auspicious omens for people and for good fortune. House construction starts after materials have been prepared and a specific time has been set.

Zhuang craftsmen make roof trusses without detailed drawings. They use the experience of masters and follow strict specifications and proportions. A typical large ganlan house is about 5.33 meters wide, 10.7 meters long, and 8.00 meters high, while a typical small ganlan house is about 4.00 meters wide, 8.00 meters long and 5.33 meters high. These ganlan houses usually have three to five entrances. Carpenters shape timber to specified height and depth according to its size. The external gable walls are supported by four pillars and one beam, and internal gable walls are supported by three long pillars, one short pillar and one beam. The short pillar over the beam supports the ridge purlin. Rafters are supported by fish-shaped or vase-shaped short pillars. Five to seven short pillars stand on each slope, with small beams connecting to center pillars. The whole structure looks like a mountain ridge. Connected by tenons, four pillars, one beam and several short pillars form a complete gable wall. Standing on plinths and likewise connected by tenons, several gable walls (at least two external and one internal gable wall) form the skeleton of a ganlan house. Mortise and tenon joints are removable, and use no nails. Great technique is required. Poorer families use bamboo to make beam columns. They are not able to make tenon joint with bamboo, so rattans or split bamboo is used for connection, with columns buried. Usually the roofs are covered with thatch or fish scale tiles, and the walls are woven using split bamboo. Well-off families use timber planking while wealthy and influential families use red bricks to make walls.

While the house frame is being made, stonemasons construct the foundations. There are some specifications for the foundations of ganlan houses. Generally the front section is 2.5 to 3.0 meters high. The back section is built as a living area for cooking. The plinths are made of patterned blue stones. Wealthy families use a great number of long stones to build stairs with more than 10 steps, while poor families can only use wooden ladders.

After the foundations are ready, an auspicious day is picked for erecting pillars, laying beams, rafters and purlins as they are considered as solemn processes during which ghosts and gods should not be offended. Taoist priests are invited to practice divination for selection of auspicious day and propitious time, and they offer sacrifice, chant, and pray. Also, there are many taboos, for example, beams cannot be set up at noon, as the timing is called "逢午" which suggests the sound of "忤逆" and means the disobedience of offsprings; it might bring general turmoil to a family if chickens and dogs are not left in peace, or chickens fly to the beam. When the selected day comes, the whole village is in a happy mood as if festivals like the New Year have come. Able-bodied persons from different families offer to help house construction. Young people climb up the frame and use mallets to connect tenon and mortise. Laughter, sounds of mallet and cries are mixed in the valley. If the host family is short of money, villagers and relatives will bring rice and meat. When the time for setting up beams comes after the framework is assembled, the decorated beams are raised accompanied by the sound of firecrackers. After mortise and tenon joints go together, people enjoy the feast and toast the family. After people depart, the host family will select good days for tiling, completing the bamboo walls, and finishing the interior, spending several months or even half a year.

The completion of a ganlan house is auspicious. On the day of housewarming, relatives and friends gather to celebrate moving into a new home. It is very important to move shrines, spirit tablets and censers into the new home with solemnity, to butcher pigs and chickens in worship of ancestors, and to invite Taoist masters to chant. Religious rites are solemn and fervent, filled with people's vision and expectations. Then people drink wine with the host, and wish him prosperous and happy family, thriving domestic animals and success.

Last comes the greening of the new home. After moving to a new house, bamboo, fruit trees and other trees should be planted around the ganlan house to beautify the environment and generate income. For a separate house, thorny indocalamus should be planted to form a fence protecting the house.

9.3.2 Villages

With rice agriculture, Zhuang villages formed for agricultural production and development. Typically Zhuang people inhabit the sharp turn of rivers or the intersection of large and small rivers, where the river is wide, water flows slowly, and is backed by hills. People can obtain abundant aquatic life to support life, and can take refuge in the hills when there is a torrential flood. To ensure a life in which there are fish in the water and rice in the paddy field, there should be open, arable and irrigable land nearby for growing rice.

In the Zhuang region, there are high mountains and rolling lofty hills with plentiful rivers. In mountains and river valleys, small and large valley floors are available for reclamation. With favorable land, water sources and climate for rice-farming, Zhuang villages are located in these valley areas. Zhuang people live near paddy fields, mountains and water sources. After the First Emperor of Qin opened Lingnan channels, people in the Central Plains moved to the Lingnan region to avoid chaos caused by war, therefore Lingnan started to be co-inhabited by Han and Zhuang people. Han people usually live near cities and towns with convenient transportation, while Zhuang people create their farming villages at the mouth of a valley, or in the upper reaches of rivers. As the saying goes, "Han people live at street corners while Zhuang people live near water sources."

Strict rules for site selection, orientation and location for Zhuang villages have been followed from generation to generation: near mountains and water sources, facing wide agricultural land in the south with a sunny exposure, and backing on to high mountains providing protection from the north wind.

The size of Zhuang villages varies according to the area of nearby arable land. High mountainous areas with little land are sparsely populated, with small villages. Larger villages are densely distributed through hills and valleys. In such villages, ganlan houses stand on the gentler slopes. Oriented to the south or east, ganlan houses are located on open ground in arable valleys with nearby water sources. The roads are formed naturally between the houses.

Zhuang villagers emphasize afforestation and landscaping. There are bamboo forests around villages, in which Zhuang people surround their ganlan houses with thorn fencing to form a ring-shaped land as their yards. They grow vegetables and fruit trees, such as greens, papaya, ceiba, pomelo, citrus, wampee, longan, banana, peach, and plum. The planting of these plants adds color of green to the ganlan houses and brings much joy to life with the houses surrounded by fruits trees and massive bamboo area.

9.4　Relationship between Zhuang dwelling and medicine

Characteristic Zhuang dwelling culture was developed based on the geographical conditions and climate in the Zhuang region. Ganlan houses were designed specifically to prevent disease and insect and beast intrusion, and to satisfy hygiene needs.

Zhuang people live in southern China where it is hot, rainy, humid, and filled with miasma, insects and beasts. Ganlan houses can help people adapt to the harsh environment and meet their physical and mental needs. These houses have the following features. First, it can help the avoidance of miasma. The Zhuang region was known as "a miasmatic region" with many discussions of its miasma in numerous history books and local chronicles. Miasma and miasmatic region were synonymous with deadly toxic gas and death. In ancient times, it was said that banished officials, men of letters and soldiers were all terrified of the deadly "miasmatic region". Zhuang ancestors emphasized prevention before disease onset and summarized characteristic methods of age-old practices for prevention of miasma. Ganlan houses are one of the method. Second, it can help the avoidance of dampness. The Zhuang region is situated in the hot, rainy and humid subtropical zone. In *On Proper Therapies for Different Diseases Geo-*

graphically, *Suwen*, "The south region, where everything between the heavens and the earth grow and develop, and Yang Qi is exuberant; it is characterized by low altitude, soft water and soil, and fog and dew gathering; the local people are accustomed to eating the sour and fermented bean curd, so they look fine and reddish in skin, and tend to suffer from diseases with spasm and arthralgia ..." Humid and rainy climates give rise to spasm and arthralgia. People are less likely to have rheumatism if they live above ground in ganlan houses with dry air and good ventilation. Third, it is useful for the prevention of insects and beasts. Ganlan houses are built on stilts to prevent insects, snakes and beasts entering. Fourth, it is for hygiene. Separated from livestock in the lower layer, humans live comfortably in the upper layer of ganlan house with good ventilation and lighting, feeling warm in winter and cool in summer. This kind of residential building reflects Zhuang people's ecological aesthetics: learning from the nature and living in harmony with nature.

References:

[1] Qin Cailuan. Discussion on Traditional Zhuang Residences [J]. Study of Ethnics in Guangxi, 1993 (3): 112 – 118.

[2] Chen Liqin. Ecological Research on Zhuang People's Ganlan Houses in Napo [C]. Yuxi: China Forum and International Academic Conference for Anthropology of Art: Collected Papers on Living Art Inheritance and Cultural Sharing, 2011.

[3] Liang Tingwang. Records of Zhuang Customs [M]. Beijing: China Minzu University Press, 1987.

[4] Yuan Shaofen. Research on Contemporary Zhuang [M]. Nanning: Guangxi People's Publishing House, 1989.

[5] Fan Yang, Qiu Zhensheng. Preliminary Discussion on Ancient Zhuang Customs [M]. Nanning: Guangxi People's Publishing House, 1994.

[6] Qin Shangwen, Chen Guoqing. Zhuang History of Science and Technology [M]. Nanning: Guangxi Science and Technology Press, 2003.

10　Zhuang Medicine and Dance and Sports

Zhuang medicine is traditional medicine created and continuously used by Zhuang people, with distinct national, traditional and regional character. Its formation and development are closely related to Zhuang dance and sports, which are also important components of Zhuang medical culture. Over the ages of production and life practice, Zhuang people have developed diverse special traditional dancing and sports activities, which are typically performed in traditional folk activities. These play an important role as traditional methods for health preservation, by promoting qi and blood, removing stagnation, soothing joints, improving constitution, preventing diseases, promoting healthcare, and prolonging life.

10.1　Zhuang medicine and dance

10.1.1　Dance culture

10.1.1.1　Origin of dance culture

Zhuang people like dancing and they are good at singing and dancing. They have created various time-honored dancing arts. In the Pre-Qin Period, ancient Luoyue people created a brilliant and distinctive dance style. It is reflected in the cliff paintings along the Zuojiang River in Guangxi and in bronze drums, and represents the splendid history of Zhuang dance. In the imposing scale of cliff paintings along the Zuojiang River, people are doing half-squats, bending their arms at the elbows and knees. They are lining up vertically, horizontally or in a circle, acting in unison. In different groups of lines, there is a front-on portrait of a tall person bearing swords and wearing a feather hat or high hair bun. There is a starred bronze drum or horn-shaped bell nearby, reflecting typical collective ritual dance and representative movements. Relevant research has revealed the identity of the tall, distinctive and front-on portraits. They are chieftains, sorcerers and leading dancers responsible for sacrificial rites. The nearby bronze drums and bells are musical instruments for the dance. The paintings show that people follow shamans to dance with exciting music accompanied by drumbeats.

Most primitive Zhuang dances were created by imitating animals. According to ethnologists, frog dance is the theme of dances revealed in the cliff paintings along the Zuojiang River. People imitate frog jump by bending their knees and stretching their arms up. Frog dance implies ancient Luoyue people's worship of the Frog God for benefit.

Egret dance is another distinctive ancient Zhuang dance. It can be seen on the bronze drums unearthed in Guigang, Guangxi. Dancers are dressed delicately and distinctively. They wear feather crown and long dress adorned with feathers. The front of the long dress is slightly longer than knee-length, and the back is floor-length. The dancers move their center of gravity back, swing both hands, move legs apart like walking, and coordinate head, breast and body to imitate an egret. It is the distinctive movement in this dance. Two or three performers form a group and there are 8 groups in total. Those independent groups dance together in graceful and consistent steps indicating it is a group dance. Egret dance reveals Zhuang ancestors' egret worship and they hope that they can obtain egret's spirituality to enhance themselves. It is evident that primitive Zhuang dances were essential for human activities and social life, while modern dances are recreational performances.

The Zhuang nationality is one of the first Chinese ethnic groups to grow rice, and primitive agriculture in the Zhuang region features rice-farming. Zhuang live in Lingnan which has warm climate, plentiful rainfall, rolling rivers, good water sources and fertile land, all being good for rice crops. With great affection for dance arts, Zhuang people created various dances reflecting their production and life practice through long time observation. For example, the dances include carrying pole dance, bronze drum dance, rice pounding dance, embroidered ball dance, shrimp-catching dance, tea-picking dance, and bamboo pole dance. The themes of dances are expressed clearly in vigorous, vivacious and ebullient steps and movements. Such dances reveal Zhuang people's farming methods, their industriousness, persistence, and clear distinction between love and hate. Most dances are still popular today.

10.1.1.2　Common Zhuang dances and their categories

Zhuang people are good at singing and dancing, and they live in a sea of songs. Liu Sanjie enjoys a good reputation both at home and abroad. With original and insightful study of dances, Zhuang people have more than 300 types of dances, involving aspects of social life, including sacrificial ceremonies, prayers to gods, expelling of the evil spirits to resolve misfortunes, labor, social intercourse, reproduction, marriage, funeral arrangements, and holiday entertainment. Traditional Zhuang dances can be roughly divided into religious dancing and recreational dance. Religious dances are performed for religious purposes, mainly involving prayer to gods, expelling the evil spirits, and resolving misfortunes. Aimed at entertaining gods, they are the predominant form of traditional Zhuang dance and have a profound impact on social life and ideologies. Examples include Taoist priest dance and bronze drum dance. Recreational dances include those for enjoyment and for artistic performance, as well as Zhuang opera dances. They are frequently performed in festivals or joyous activities. Forms and themes of dance mainly involve the imitation of production and animals. Production dances include shrimp-catching dance, fish-catching dance, rice transplanting dance, harvest dance, and rice pounding dance. Animal dances include lion dance, dragon dance, cattle dance, butterfly dance, rooster dance, frog dance, and turtledove dance.

(1) Rice pounding dance

Rice pounding dance came from the action of pounding rice, which is also the theme of the dance. People dance to the pounding sound with rhythmic beating. They perform the dance during the Spring Festival to celebrate the New Year, anticipating a successful harvest. According to the record of *Strange Stories in Lingnan* by Liu Xun, "There is rice pounding dance in Guangxi. When performing the dance, 10 people stand around the wooden rice mortar holding a wooden pestle. Men and women stand on opposite sides and they use the wooden pestle to beat rhythmically in the wooden rice mortar. The beating sound is like drumming that can be heard several miles away. It is even louder than the sound of pounding clothes while women wash them in the autumn." Rice pounding dance is called "guhlongj" in Zhuang. Most of the dancers are women. They hold a wooden pestle, and stand around the wooden rice mortar filled with unhusked rice. They use the wooden pestle to beat gracefully in the wooden rice mortar. The sound from the pestle is like that of a wooden fish. After repeated pounding, rice is husked.

(2) Carrying pole dance

Carrying pole dance is popular among Mashan, Du'an, Donglan, Yongning, Nandan, and other Guangxi regions. People perform the dance from the 1st to 15th days of the first lunar month. Most performers are women. The number of performers should be even, for example, 4, 6, 8, 10, or 20.

Carrying pole dance came from rice pounding dance and originated from the action of pounding rice. Originally Zhuang people performed it by using the carrying pole to beat the board cover of the rice mortar. Therefore, it is also called "guhlongj" in Zhuang. As the rice mortar was too heavy to be moved, gradually it was replaced by a bench. In modern carrying pole dance, a normally wooden bench, and bamboo carrying pole or simply bamboo pole are used for performing in a variety of ways. The performers stand on either side of the bench, and they pound the bench or beat the carrying poles together. The performers dance to rhythmic pounding of the bench or beating together of the carrying poles. They beat and dance. Two, four or more people beat each other's carrying pole while standing, squatting, in bowed position, or twisting and turning around. The pleasant rhythms can be heavy or light, strong or weak, and fast or slow. The dance is the imitation of actions in agricultural activities, including driving the cattle into the field, harrowing, transplanting rice seedlings, harvesting, threshing, pounding rice and weaving. Loved by Zhuang people, carrying pole dance can improve constitution with concerted actions, graceful movements, flexible and coordinated walking, strong rhythms, clear and melodious sound.

(3) Bronze drum dance

Bronze drum dance is one of the Zhuang dances with a long history. It originated from the sacrifice offering ceremony in ancient times. Playing bronze drum for fun is depicted early in the cliff paintings along the Zuojiang River of the Zhuang region. Later, it was used in recreational and ritual activities.

Bronze drum, the famous Zhuang folk instrument, is used in the dance, which is performed by people in Donglan, Du'an, Mashan and other Zhuang regions during the Spring Festival and harvest celebration. *Records of the Southern Barbarians*, *Book of Tang* says, "People sing and dance while playing the bronze drum and the horn for fun." It is recorded in *Miscellaneous Poems of Lingnan* by a scholar in the Ming Dynasty named Wang Guangyang, "Villagers play the bronze drum and sing in a celebratory atmosphere during days of worship."

Generally there are more than 7 people in the dance team. 4 of them beat the bronze drum, one of them plays the leather drum, one plays the bamboo sieve or rain hat, and another plays the bamboo tube. Two or four bronze drums make up a group. In the group of two drums, two performers play one drum, and there is one male drum and one female drum. In the group of four drums, each of the four performers plays one drum, and there are two male drums and two female drums.

The content of the dance is a representation of agricultural production, for example, opening, spring ploughing, summer planting, autumn harvest, storing of grain in winter, and welcoming spring. Thus, the dance is inspiring and exciting and vibrant.

(4) Embroidered ball dance

Embroidered ball dance is a Zhuang folk dance. It was popular as early as the Song Dynasty among Zhuang people in Debao, Jingxi, Tiandong, Tianyang, Long-zhou, Tiandeng, Daxin, Du'an, Mashan, and other Zhuang regions.

Embroidered ball is a love token for Guangxi Zhuang young people. During the Spring Festival or song fairs in the Sanyuesan Festival, they gather and sing folk songs together to express their love. When a young Zhuang girl falls in love with a young man, she will tie cloth shoes, towel, or other gifts to an embroidered ball made by herself. She will throw it to the young man, singing and dancing. After obtaining the ball, the young man will also return the gift to the young girl, singing and dancing. This custom gradually developed into the embroidered ball dance, which is mainly performed in song fairs as dance and sports entertainment. Its dance movements include spinning, swinging, throwing and catching the ball.

(5) Tea-picking dance

Tea-picking dance is mainly performed in Yulin, Guangxi during the New Year as a self-entertaining folk dance. Typically, one male called tea man and two females called tea women perform the dance with singing, using coin whips, colored fans, handkerchieves, colorful ribbons and other implements. Its major theme is the manifestation of farming processes, and sometimes the plot of love between young men and women is added. Its movements are simple, open and amusing. The tea man shakes his legs, and bends his knees and makes brisk, natural and unrestrained steps. The coin whips can be used as hoes in performing land clearing. The man imitates pumping the bellows with amusing movements while acting out the toasting of tea. The tea women usually perform it with reserved, small and light steps. They do bandy-legged turns and cross steps, and use the fan flexibly making it like dancing cloud and willow catkin. Their elegance and coquetry express girls' artlessness, vivacity and cuteness. They dance with song or music accompanied by drumbeats in an exciting and recreational atmosphere.

10.1.1.3 Features of Zhuang dances

Dance arts emerged with social production and life. With the formation and development of the Zhuang nationality, Zhuang dances became cultural ideology in daily life based on Zhuang psychological quality and cultural connotation. The styles of

Zhuang dances are rooted in the political culture, religious culture and living environment of Zhuang society.

(1) Totem worship

Zhuang dances have distinctively primitive style, as they were formed and developed in the matrix of primitive sorcery and the worship of nature. Zhuang people have attached great importance to sorcery since ancient times, and are known for worshipping ghosts and gods and believing sorcery. It is recorded in *Jiuge*, *Chuyu* and other ancient books that Zhuang ancestors worshipped many gods and believed in sorcery and religions. Shamanic sacrificial rituals were closely related to Zhuang dances. Mother Nature's secrets are boundless, and she is ever-changing. Zhuang ancestors had very low productivity, and failed to explain natural phenomena (e.g., earthquake, flood and volcanic eruption) and even the commonest ones (e.g., sunrise, sunset, wind, rain, thunder and lightning). In particular, they felt mystified by dreams, birth, death, old age and disease. Therefore, based on boundless imagination, they started to believe animism and immortality of soul, and worship many gods. Zhuang people worship deities from nature, social gods, defenders, and many other gods through rituals which varied based on the functions of the gods. When shamans worship gods, they dance and sing to entertain the gods in order to remove ill fortune and pray for good.

Many Zhuang dances were closely linked to totem worship. In the cliff paintings along the Zuojiang River in the Zhuang region, ancient Luoyue people performed frog dance aiming at entertaining the Frog God for benefit. Egret dance on Han Dynasty bronze drums reflects Zhuang ancestors' worship of egrets. They hoped that they would acquire the egret's essence to predict climate, fly over the mountains, soar in the sky, and thus avert misfortune. The origin of bronze drum dance and frog dance is related to Zhuang people's frog worship and imitation. Both dances are usually performed during the Frog Festival.

(2) Reflection of labor

Zhuang people are passionate about labor and they turn production activities into dances. Carrying pole, rice pounding, shrimp-catching and tea-picking dances all imitate the instruments and movements of labor. With cheerful music accompanied by drumbeats, the imitation of typical movements of labor expresses the celebration of festivals and harvest as well as the yearning for a happy life. In carrying pole dance, performers imitate the action of using the carrying pole to beat the rice mortar; in rice pounding dance, the wooden pestle is used to beat in the wooden rice mortar to imitate the process of husking rice through repeated pounding; in tea-picking dance, mountainside tea and tea baskets are chosen to reflect the image of Zhuang girls' picking tea, selecting tea and chasing butterflies on the way home; in hand towel dance, the hand towel, commonly used for wiping away sweat and wrapping the head or things, reflects Zhuang people's rich working life.

（3）Conveyance of emotions

Busy farming, young Zhuang people leverage singing and dancing to express their emotions. Embroidered ball dance is popular, and uses an embroidered ball as a love token. Young men and women sing in antiphonal style, and they throw the ball to the person they like most. The dance originally signified that when young men and women exchanged gifts, they wrapped the gifts with stones in "throwing handkerchief" to ensure the correct direction when throwing them. Afterwards the embroidered ball was used as a love token. Bamboo pole dance is a common dance for young Zhuang people as well during festivals. Cooperation is required for performing the dance, and performers skip swiftly between bamboo poles. Skillful young men tend to be appreciated by girls for their agility. Bamboo pole dance, to the accompaniment of music, has become an effective way to exchange ideas and express emotions as it can enhance people's understanding of beat, coordination and sense of rhythm.

In dance culture, limb movements reveal the modes of production and life patterns. Zhuang dances embody the historical ecology of the Zhuang nationality. With the rising of economy and advancement of culture and politic, people's ideas about divinity began to change, and Zhuang dances gradually became closer to life. Nowadays, Zhuang dances are usually performed during festivals, and are aimed at enhancing friendship, exchanging production and life experience, and expressing emotions. They have enriched the cultural life in the Zhuang region.

10. 1. 2　Influence of dance culture on Zhuang medicine

Dance is one of the basic forms of culture. Zhuang people are good at singing and dancing and they have created diverse folk dance that has made great contributions to the development of Zhuang healthcare and sports medicine.

10. 1. 2. 1　Zhuang dance has promoted the formation and development of Zhuang medicine

In primitive times, there remained a fashion of sorcery in the Zhuang region where there was extremely low social productivity. Believing in ghosts and gods, Zhuang people treated diseases with sorcery. Hunting, sacrificial rites, prayer, medical treatment and many other activities were conducted through dance. Shamans' sacrificial rituals were reflected in ancient frog dance, egret dance and bronze drum dance. Isogeny and coexistence of medicine and sorcery are features of the development of Zhuang culture, and they had a significant impact on Zhuang medicine. However, they can only be studied through customs because of the passage of time, and inadequacy of written records and material objects. In ancient times, Zhuang sorcerers were distinguished by gender — female sorcerers and male sorcerers. When there was sickness or disaster in the host family, the host would invite female sorcerers to ask immortals about the causes of the sickness or disaster. Then the host would pick an auspicious day to invite male sorcerers to carry out religious rites when animals were killed for worship, immortals were urged to depart. And people prayed for the ending of the disaster. And male sorcerers brandished swords, heated up a pot with oil, and drove away evil spirits. Those are the activities of witch doctors. According to Zhuang folk tales, Zhuang people considered Sanjiegong as the God of Medicine as he was able to dispel pathogenic and noxious factors, protect their homes and defend their territories. They built temples for his regular annual worship. In the old society, Zhuang medicine was effective in treating some diseases but in the form of witchcraft medicine. We can see the relevant details in *Miscellaneous Review*, *Lingbiao Jiman* (*Records of the Barbarians of Lingnan*) by Liu Xifan, "The barbarians use herbs to treat trauma, carbuncle and all other diseases requiring surgery. It is often effective, but they also treat those diseases through superstitious activities … I have seen a patient with carbuncle invite a Zhuang fellow to treat him. When the Zhuang fellow came, he asked the patient's family to place in the hall a rooster, a ten-cent silver coin, water and rice. The performer put the ten-cent silver coin into a bag, took off his straw sandals, placed them on the ground, got some water and cast a spell. Then he sprayed water onto the wound, and cut it with a knife, then pus and blood flowed out, but the patient felt no pain. When the pus was drained, topical application of drugs would cure the patient." Witch doctors knew about medicine, they performed witchcraft while giving drug treatment, and treated diseases using witchcraft in the form of dance, particularly among Zhuang people in the outlying mountain area and before the founding of the people's Republic of China. Superstitious sorcery can impede medical development, but sorcery played a positive role in the formation and development of Zhuang medicine in ancient Zhuang region, and featured the isogeny and coexistence of medicine and sorcery.

10.1.2.2 Zhuang dance has promoted the formation of healthcare awareness

Limb movement in dancing is used to express people's emotions, improve their constitution, and promote the formation of Zhuang healthcare and disease prevention awareness. Since ancient times, Zhuang ancestors have been living in Lingnan, a hot, mountainous, wooded and inaccessible region. As conditions for life were harsh, they always sought instinctive ways to survive and keep healthy. In the long-term practice, they gradually realized that dancing could improve physical and psychological health as well as constitution, and make them expressive and flexible. Therefore, in free time or during festivals, people sang and danced. They imitated hunting, labor or animals to express emotions and for enjoyment. Therefore singing and dancing had an important impact on the spectrum of disease in the Zhuang region. Zhuang people have fewer miscellaneous internal damage diseases, particularly emotional diseases, and that is closely related to their preference for singing and dancing.

10.1.2.3 Zhuang dance has promoted the formation of principle of Zhuang medical treatment

Zhuang medicine has a deep understanding of qi, which is highly valued and considered as the original substance constituting the human body. Qi movement is important. It is believed that humans can maintain health only when the qi of the three parts of the human body can remain synchronous, coordinated and balanced. The routines of Zhuang dances involve hands, head, neck, chest, hip, legs and other parts of the body. Dancing helps people feel comfortable, promote qi and blood and regulate qi. Therefore, Zhuang people liked dancing since ancient times and they live in a sea of songs. They sang and danced to make human qi work well and synchronize it with qi of heaven and earth by regulating, stimulating or unblocking it. Gradually, a therapeutic principle of regulating qi was formed, and now it has become an important principle of Zhuang medicine for preventing and treating diseases, and has made a great contribution to people in the Zhuang region.

10.2 Zhuang medicine and sports

10.2.1 Sports culture

10.2.1.1 Origin of sports culture

Zhuang sports are closely related to Zhuang customs and deeply rooted in Zhuang culture and lifestyle. They have become an important part of traditional Zhuang customs, with some of them in the form of customs while others appear as folklore activities. Occurring early in Zhuang people's life, Zhuang sports activities reflect their production practice, social life, ethnic reproduction, and religious beliefs. For example, bullfighting is a characteristic Zhuang sports activity that reveals agricultural production. As a typical rice-farming minority, Zhuang started rice agriculture in the upper reaches of the Hongshui River early in the Neolithic Age. Since ancient times, Zhuang ancestors have been living in Lingnan, a mountainous region. As Guangxi people said, "People of Yao nationality live in the top of mountains; People of Miao nationality live in the middle of mountains; Han people live on flat ground while Zhuang people live in mountains." Zhuang people live by farming and nowadays, they still focus on rice-farming, and have formed a rice-farming culture with profound cultural connotations. Cattle are a major instrument of production, therefore cattle-related sports activities emerged. According to *Buluotuo Poetic Scripture*, Buluotuo created cattle and taught Zhuang ancestors to use cattle to plough fields. As ploughing work needed strong cattle, Buluotuo taught people to select the strong and lively ones through bullfighting. *Buluotuo Poetic Scripture* is the scriptures of Zhuang in the Ming Dynasty. In the book, Buluotuo created everything and was considered as the god of creation, ancestors and religion. According to research, the Ganzhuang Mountain is a site of Buluotuo culture as well as the home of Zhuang ancestor Buluotuo who is also the ancestor of human civilization for native ethnic groups in the Pearl River basin. The age-old bullfighting is still followed today, and it can be seen on wide hillsides or fields during idle farming seasons.

Zhuang people have formed the spirit of exploration and industriousness over the ages of production and life practice. During festivals or joyous activities, they carry out traditional fitness activities, such as throwing embroidered balls, dragon boat racing, catching sky lanterns, and Zhuang boxing. Those activities can improve constitution, build willpower, and prevent diseases.

10. 2. 1. 2 Common Zhuang traditional sports activities

Zhuang people gradually developed its unique traditional sports activities over the ages of production and life practice. These activities are recreational as well as methods for health preservation and physical improvement. Common Zhuang sports activities include throwing embroidered balls, dragon boat racing, catching sky lanterns, Zhuang boxing, sparkler-grabbing, singing folk songs in antiphonal style, lion dance, and shoe plank race. The following paragraphs provide introductions about throwing embroidered balls, dragon boat racing, catching sky lanterns and Zhuang boxing.

(1) Throwing embroidered balls

As one of the traditional folk sports, throwing embroidered balls is popular in the Zhuang region, and has a history of over 2000 years. Ancient Zhuang people cast a kind of bronze weapon in war and hunting, and from this the throwing of embroidered balls was derived.

Nowadays, people play embroidered balls to convey emotion, entertain themselves, and improve their health. Most embroidered balls are handmade colorful balls with round shape, but some of them have other shapes including oval, cubic and rhomboid. Embroidered balls are fist-sized, filled with cotton seed, cereals, chaff or other materials, and adorned with colorful ribbons and red pendants on opposite sides. Zhuang people play embroidered balls at their leisure time for entertainment and as a form of communication. During traditional festivals including the Spring Festival, the Sanyuesan Festival and the Mid-Autumn Festival, groups of Zhuang people hold song fairs, in which young men and women play embroidered balls and express emotion.

Throwing embroidered balls is interesting and simple and shows distinctive Zhuang characteristics. With some modern change, it has been adapted into Guangxi Traditional Games of Ethnic Minorities and National Traditional Games of Ethnic Minorities.

(2) Dragon boat racing

As one of the traditional Zhuang folk sports, dragon boat racing is popular in Wuzhou, Nanning and other Zhuang regions. It is also seen as a traditional Zhuang activity in the Dragon Boat Festival. This can be traced back to the late period of primitive society. There are many theories of its origins, including sacrifice offering ceremonies for Cao'e, Qu Yuan, the Water God or the Dragon God. Introduced into Japan, Vietnam and England, it has become an official Asian Games sport in 2010 Asian

Games in Guangzhou. Now it has been inscribed on China Intangible Cultural Heritages List.

It is held during the Dragon Boat Festival. Having no standard size, the dragon boat is a long and narrow water vessel, the front and back of which is shaped and decorated as a Chinese dragon. There may be dozens of rowers in one boat. The competition rules include ranking according to elapsed qualifying time.

(3) Catching sky lanterns

As one of the popular, unique and traditional Zhuang sports activities, catching sky lanterns is carried out during joyous festivals and harvest celebration. According to Zhuang custom, sky lanterns symbolize auspiciousness and longevity. In ancient times, sky lanterns were used to inform villagers of bandits' whereabouts. Gradually this practice developed into a recreational activity called catching sky lanterns.

People from one village team up with each other to catch sky lanterns. Typically there are dozens of players, most of whom are strong. It is very simple to make a sky lantern. Bamboo is used as the frame, paper is stretched over the frame to shape a bucket, and an oil lamp is placed at the bottom. A sky lantern will fly as the temperature in the lantern rises after the oil lamp is ignited. Players strive to chase the lantern, which is an arduous journey. The sky lantern can be seized when it descends after the oil lamp has burned out. The first team to regain the sky lantern wins.

(4) Zhuang boxing

As one of the traditional Zhuang sports activities, Zhuang boxing is a unique type of boxing with a long history. It can be found in the 2000-year-old cliff paintings along the Zuojiang River in Guangxi. *Annals of Ningming Zhou* says, "The Huashan Mountains are about 50 li away from the city. On its cliffs along the river, there are many red naked human portraits of different sizes holding weapons or riding horses." In typical cliff paintings, the portraits are tall and strong, standing like a pole. Their knees and arms are bent. They can stand staunchly and steadily, with their center of gravity naturally focused on dan tian which means the region in the lower abdomen beneath the navel. It is a typical position in kung fu bearing weapons revealed in the cliff paintings. Weapons such as knives, swords, spears, darts, crossbows and bamboo arrows were presented in the paintings. Zhuang ancestors were so wise that they developed Zhuang boxing, a set of fitness activities based on the depictions of cliff painting. Knives and swords are common instruments used in Zhuang boxing. With dozens of routines, Zhuang boxing features clear, vigorous, athletic and sturdy movements, stable stances, simple form, extensive hand techniques and vocal articulation in the Zhuang language. Contemporary Zhuang boxing has developed different schools and benefited many people.

10. 2. 1. 3   Features of Zhuang sports activities

With rich cultural connotation, Zhuang sports activities are national, traditional, regional, recreational, and diverse. With the development of society, some traditional sports activities became less recreational and pragmatic over time, but more performable and competitive. For example, throwing embroidered balls originally implied the interaction with opposite sex and happy love life, but now it has become a recreational performance. Dragon boat racing came from different sacrifice offering ceremonies for Cao'e, Qu Yuan, the Water God or the Dragon God. Now it has become a competitive sport, in which crews in dragon boats compete on the river to the sound of gong and drum and cheering.

10. 2. 2   Influence of sports culture on Zhuang medicine

Sports in the Zhuang language means frequent activities. Zhuang people of any age or gender are industrious and they love sports. During festivals or joyous activities, Zhuang people carry out traditional fitness activities, such as throwing embroidered balls, dragon boat racing, and catching sky lanterns. Zhuang sports culture influences Zhuang medicine in different aspects.

10. 2. 2. 1   Zhuang sports have promoted the formation of Zhuang medical theories

Containing rich Zhuang medical thinking, Zhuang sports have promoted the formation of Zhuang medical theories. Early in the Pre-Qin Period, typical movements in kung fu have been recorded in the cliff paintings along the Zuojiang River in Chongzuo, Guangxi. Prestigious Zhuang doctor Qin Baolin said that in every tropical year, the heaven, earth and human are on the same macroscopic ray while the sun is in the exact same position along a meridian line in the Zuojiang basin. It is the best time for doing exercises according to macro theories of celestial mechanics. The exercises are called "Zhuang qiankun zhang ziwu gong practice" and have been followed by the later generations. Zhuang boxing originated from the practice.

The practice emphasizes the synchrony of heaven, earth and human qi and has promoted the theory of synchrony of triple initial qi in Zhuang medicine. As a core Zhuang medical theory, the mentioned theory is the unique man-nature theory coming from Zhuang ancestors' basic understanding of the origin of nature and the universe. It is used to explain the connotation, relationship and rules of the heaven qi, earth qi and human qi in the natural world and within the body. It is also an argument for explaining the body's etiology and pathogenesis and for guiding disease prevention and treatment. According to the theory of synchrony of triple initial qi, the space of the natural world can be divided into three parts — heaven, earth and human, and the qi of the three parts is synchronized. Also, the human body is divided into three parts — the upper part as heaven, the lower part as earth and the middle part as human. The qi of the three parts of the human body is also synchronized. Physiologically, humans can maintain health only when the heaven, earth and human parts of the body, and the natural world interact with each other, move synchronously, and emerge naturally; pathologically, all kinds of diseases and ailments will break out if the heaven, earth and human qi do not move in synchrony.

10.2.2.2　Sports activities have enriched the connotation of health preservation in Zhuang medicine

In Zhuang medicine, we can find rich experience and knowledge of disease prevention. Sports activities have long been important for health preservation, and loved by Zhuang ancestors. They realized that physical exercises could unblock tracts, regulate qi and blood, coordinate yin and yang, nourish heart, tranquilize mind, improve constitution, and prevent diseases. Shoe plank race, throwing embroidered balls, dragon boat racing, catching sky lanterns and other traditional fitness activities are popular among Zhuang people. Health improvement through sports activities is a powerful weapon in disease prevention. Physical exercises can build muscles, sinews and bones, remove stagnation, soothe joints, build willpower, boost metabolism, promote the circulation of qi and blood, and improve constitution. Therefore, the body is less likely to be affected by pathogenic factors and human can be in harmony with natural and social environment so that goals including bodybuilding, disease prevention and treatment, and longevity promotion can be achieved. Physical exercises have become an effective method for preventing and treating disease, and they have enriched the connotation of health preservation in Zhuang medicine.

References:

[1] Zhang Shengzhen. A General History of the Zhuang [M]. Beijing: The Ethnic Publishing House, 1997.

［2］Huang Hanru，Huang Dongling. Ongoing Investigation and Organization of Zhuang Medicine ［M］. Nanning：Guangxi Nationalities Publishing House，1994.

［3］Li Kunrong. Origin of Zhuang Bronze Drum Dance ［J］. Ethnic Arts Quarterly，1998（1）：194－199.

［4］Qin Cailuan. Research on Zhuang Dance Culture ［J］. Ethnic Arts Quarterly，1997（3）：123－136.

［5］Song Ning. Connotation and Application of Synchrony of Triple Initial Qi in Zhuang Medicine ［J］. Journal of Traditional Chinese Medicine，2013，54（14）：1183－1185.

［6］Pang Yuzhou，Song Ning. Preliminary Discussion on the Preventive Treatment of Disease in Zhuang Medicine ［J］. Journal of Medicine and Pharmacy of Chinese Minorities，2008，14（7）：5－6.

［7］Li Meikang，Song Ning. Analysis of Thoughts on Preventive Treatment of Disease in Zhuang Medicine ［J］. Chinese Journal of Basic Medicine in Traditional Chinese Medicine，2014，20（8）：1034－1035.

［8］Qin Naichang，Zheng Chaoxiong，Qin Deqing，et al. Investigation and Research on the Hongshui River Culture ［J］. Study of Ethnics in Guangxi，2000（2）：77－79.

［9］Song Ning. Medical Thoughts on Preventive Treatment of Disease in Zhuang Medicine from the Perspective of Murals on the Huashan Mountains ［J］. Journal of Liaoning University of Traditional Chinese Medicine，2008，10（10）：49－51.

11　Impact and Reflections of other Medical Cultures on Zhuang Medicine

11. 1　Impact of other medical cultures on the formation and development of Zhuang medicine

Throughout more than 2000 years of Zhuang medical development, Zhuang people continually summarized experience in disease prevention and treatment, and absorbed medical culture from other ethnic groups.

11. 1. 1　Impact of traditional Chinese medicine on Zhuang medicine

TCM has the greatest impact on the formation and development of Zhuang medicine. On one hand, Han population is the largest immigrant group in Guangxi and on the other hand TCM theories were formed early. Compared with Zhuang medicine, TCM is more advanced, and the absorption of TCM and the convergence of Zhuang medicine and TCM conform to laws of social development. The impact of TCM on Zhuang medicine focuses on three facets.

11. 1. 1. 1　Theory of yin-yang harmony

As one of the core TCM theories, yin-yang harmony involves the unity, opposition, mutual rooting, waxing and waning, and mutual convertibility of yin-yang. According to TCM, all things in the world mutually reinforce and neutralize each other and we can stay healthy only when the body is in a balance of yin and yang. Yin-yang theory has been introduced to Zhuang medicine, but it is not as highly refined or applied in the entire basic theory and system of diagnosis and treatment as it is in TCM. It is interpreted as exuberant yin and declined yang, and exuberant yang and declined yin in sickness, without being associated with the mutual promotion and restraint between the five elements. Generally speaking, yang syndrome is shown in patients with exuberant healthy qi and toxin or in early stages of illness, and yin syndrome is shown in patients with deficient healthy qi and toxin or in late stages of illness.

11. 1. 1. 2　Theory of monarch, minister, assistant and guide

In TCM prescriptions, each herb plays a role in keeping the healthy system running smoothly, including those of monarch, minister, assistant and guide. The status and responsibilities of members in social order correspond to different roles and functions of herbs. In Zhuang prescriptions, similarly, there is the "bohmeh" relationship between herbs. The Zhuang region was far away from the Han administration center in the Central Plains. With simple social order, Zhuang social structure features families under the control of the "dulao". "Dulao" have no administrative power but use their own prestige and cohesion to influence villagers. Therefore family structure is very important in the Zhuang region and "bohmeh", the relationship between major family members, was introduced into the composition of prescriptions in Zhuang medicine.

11. 1. 1. 3　Theory of meridian, collateral and acupoint

According to TCM, the body has 12 regular meridians and 8 extra meridians, which can link upper and lower, exterior and interior, and zang and fu organs, and can help circulation of qi and blood. Acupoints are points on the body where qi and blood converge from zang and fu organs, meridians, and collaterals. When lesions occur in the body, acupoints can be selected based on meridian location and stimulated through acupuncture, tuina and other methods to regulate meridians, collaterals, qi and blood for recovery. In Zhuang medicine, the body has two closed-ended tracts inside the body called "Longlu" (the tract of blood) and "Huolu" (nervous system). The two tracts link the body surface and the links are acupoints. External treatment is used to stimulate acupoints to remove stasis in both tracts and unblock both tracts to prevent and treat diseases. Compared with meridians and collaterals in TCM, the two tracts in Zhuang medicine can better reflect Zhuang people's simple intuitive way of thinking. External treatment in Zhuang medicine has absorbed the experience of acupoint selection in TCM and included some TCM acupoints. For example, when diarrhea is treated with Zhuang medicated thread moxibustion, the special Qizhou acupoint is selected. But for diarrhea accompanied with chest distress and vomiting, Qizhou acupoint in Zhuang medicine and Neiguan acupoint and Zusanli acupoint in TCM are selected.

11. 1. 2　Impact of Taoist medicine on Zhuang medicine

As an indigenous religion of China, Taoism has contributed to great medical achievements with far-reaching influence on traditional Chinese medicine too, as Taoists kept exploring how to become immortal and have prolong life. The influence of Taoism on Zhuang culture is much greater than that of Buddhism and other religions. The impact of Taoist medicine on Zhuang medicine focuses on the following two facets.

11. 1. 2. 1　The unity of heaven and man

"Human beings follow laws and principles of Mother Earth, Mother Earth follows laws and principles of Heaven, Heaven follows laws and principles of Tao, Tao is a nature's way." That is the core theory of Taoism. In Taoist medicine, humans themselves are a microcosm of the natural world. Humans need to follow the laws of nature in order to achieve the unity of man and nature for prolonging life and warding off diseases. In Zhuang medicine, correspondingly, human beings grow with the blessing of heaven and earth qi, and humans themselves are a microcosm. The birth, death, old age and disease of humans are all nourished and constrained by the heaven and earth qi. Humans can maintain health only when human qi, and heaven and earth qi can remain synchronous, or diseases will visit. Thus it can be seen that the spirit of the etiological and pathogenetic theory of Zhuang medicine is shown in the respect, adaptation and understanding of nature. That is intimately tied up with philosophical thinking in Taoist medicine, and is the specific application of "Tao is a nature's way" in medicine.

11. 1. 2. 2　Faith healing

Typically, traditional medicine is intensely philosophical and religious. Faith healing can be understood as treating physical or psychological diseases with patients' religious faith. Immortals are of primary importance in Taoism. Taoist incantations and prayer, who are believed to be able to treat diseases and resolve misfortunes, were popular and had a solid cultural background in the Zhuang region. Zhuang ancestors believed in animism and worshipped many gods. They believed that natural disasters and illness were related to the soul. Therefore, disease treatment by use of drugs and witchcraft was popular for a long time. From the start of the Song Dynasty, medicine was promoted but sorcery was prohibited through repeated issuance of policies to stop the popularity of witchcraft medicine. That removed obstacles for medical development, and Zhuang medicine gradually became independent from witchcraft medicine and started on a path to more rational development. In the first year of Emperor Taizong in the Northern Song Dynasty, Yongzhou official Fan Minzhi banned sorcery, used his own salary to purchase drugs for local people, and cured more than 1000 patients. He asked stonemasons to carve proven prescriptions on the hall walls to make local people realize the importance of medicine and they gradually came to believe medicine. Therefore, people in northern and eastern Guangxi, influenced by Han culture, gradually got rid of the custom of treating diseases by the worship of ghosts and gods. However, witchcraft medicine remained important in western Guangxi until the founding of the People's Republic of China.

11. 1. 3　Impact of Buddhist medicine on Zhuang medicine

Buddhist medicine is a medical system guided by Buddhist theories and based on ancient Indian study of diseases, medical treatment and prescriptions. Ancient Zhuang people had broad contact with foreign countries through the Maritime Silk Road. According to research, Buddhism had spread, across the seas, to Hepu Port, whence it came to Guangxi via the Jiaozhi-Guangxi Corridor. Influenced by Zhuang primitive beliefs, Buddhism became secularized and pragmatic soon after coming to the Zhuang region. According to *Records of Religions*, *Guangxi Local Records*, there were 45 Buddhist temples during the Tang Dynasty and 131 during the Song Dynasty. With the spread of Buddhist culture in Guangxi, Buddhist medicine permeated the Zhuang medical system. The absorption of Buddhist medicine into Zhuang medicine was limited to methods of diagnosis and treatment instead of core theories, which remained greathy influenced by Taoist medicine. The impact of Buddhist medicine on Zhuang medicine also focuses on two facets.

11. 1. 3. 1　Pathogenicity of stasis and external treatment

In Buddhist medicine, a healthy body can be maintained by balancing three energies through diet, exercise, herbal medicine, massage and meditation. Massage is important in Buddhist medicine, according to which health problems will occur if the energy in meridians and collaterals is blocked. If corresponding body parts are massaged, the energy can be regulated and flows normally, and the stasis in tracts can be removed to achieve disease treatment and health care. In Zhuang medicine, when stasis and clustered nodules occur in Longlu and Huolu, qi and blood movement will be blocked, causing various syndromes in various body parts. In Zhuang meridian sinew therapy, the doctor similarly uses fingers to touch and find the clustered nodules that block Longlu and Huolu, and removes clustered nodules through massage, acupuncture or fire cupping to free Bi, treat sinew injury, ward off diseases and relieve pain.

11. 1. 3. 2　Dispelling pathogenic factors through aromatics and treating diseases with aromatic medicine

In Buddhist medicine, the therapeutic effect of aromatic medicine is highly valued, and "aromatics" are believed to be the medium of connection between disciples and Buddha. Misfortune can be removed and diseases can be warded off by burning aromatics, smearing or showering with aromatic medicine, and using aromatics as medicine. During the Qin and Han Dynasties, aromatics were continually introduced into ancient China via the Maritime Silk Road. During the Five Dynasties' period, Li Xun wrote *Haiyao Bencao* based on his own experiences. It provides a record of many aromatics from Southeast Asia and West Asia, such as rosemary and benzoin. The import of plentiful aromatics from other countries enriched the treasure of TCM. *Prescriptions of Peaceful Benevolent Dispensary* in the Northern Song Dynasty contains 788 medical prescriptions, and its first volume in particular contains 89 medical prescriptions, of which 20% are overseas aromatics. There are many aromatic herbs in the Zhuang region that are believed to be able to dispel pathogenic factors and repel foulness. They are extensively picked for disease prevention and healthcare, and are popular among the people. Wearing, fumigation and washing are major external uses of Zhuang aromatics. Wearing aromatics can treat different syndromes, and it was an important way of disease prevention and healthcare in some Zhuang areas until the early 1970s, particularly for children and the infirm. They wore local wild aromatics. Aromatic fumigation and washing are widely applied in the case of many skin irritations. At the end of spring and the beginning of summer when miasma prevails, all families pick leaves of Ai, pomelo, Shichangpu (*Acorus tatarinowii*) and other aromatic herbs that can resolve dampness and promote circulation of qi. People place them under cover and boil them for bathing. In the Zhuang region, people boil pomelo leaves or other aromatics to bathe or wash hands, and to repel foulness. In addition to wearing, fumigation and washing, Zhuang people widely use different aromatic herbs in daily food to promote circulation of qi, invigorate spleen, and remove fishy flavor. For example, Bajiaohuixiang (*Fructus Anisi Stellati*), Rougui (*Cinnamomum cassia* Presl), coriander (*Coriandrum sativum* L.), Laliao (*Polygonum hydropiper* L.), Zisu (*Perilla frutescens* (L.) Britt.), Xiaohuixiang (*Schizonepeta tenuifolia* (Benth.) Briq.), Bohe (*Mentha haplocalyx* Briq.) and Xiangmao (*Cymbopogon citratus*). In Zhuang's sliced raw fish banquet, there are fresh aromatic herbs and seven or eight aromatic spices. Zhuang people also like different kinds of ginger, such as *Al-*

pinia japonica, *Curcuma phaeocaulis*, *Dioscorea zingiberensis*, and *Kaempferia galanga*.

11. 2 Objective conditions for the impact of other medical cultures on Zhuang medicine

Over the more than 2000 years of Zhuang medical development, there have been internal and external changes. Internal changes promoted Zhuang medical development and these changes came from the economic and social development of the Zhuang region, and from improved understanding of nature and the body. External changes changed the trajectory of Zhuang medicine and they came from the absorption and integration of outside culture. Without adequate written records, we cannot be certain when or how complex traditional medical systems have influenced each other. However, it is clear that great influence on Zhuang cultural development was brought by convenient transportation, large-scale migration, and cultural exchanges. The change of cultural forms certainly has served to transform healthcare customs as well as methods of diagnosis and treatment.

11. 2. 1 Convenient transportation

In ancient times, mountains were barriers to transportation, and rivers became vital transportation lines. Crisscrossed waterways in the Zhuang region have long been the major channels for ethnic migration and cargo. In 214 BC, Qin Shi Huang ordered the construction of the Lingqu Canal in order to supply the expedition to Lingnan. The completion of the Lingqu Canal is a milestone in the historical development of Guangxi and brought far-reaching influence on the economic and social development of the Zhuang region. Vessels from the Central Plains came to the Hongshui River, the Nanpanjiang River, the Liujiang River, the Nanliujiang River and the Xijiang River via the Xiangjiang River and the Lingqu Canal. The canal became the main gateway to the sea for the Central Plains and Southwest China as it connected Yunnan-Guizhou Plateau in the west, Beibu Gulf Port in the south, and Guangzhou in the east. In the Han Dynasty, Hepu, Guigang and Wuzhou in Guangxi had developed into important commercial harbors, Hepu in particular became the home port of Maritime Silk Road. Vessels went west along Beibu Gulf in the South China Sea to Sri Lanka via the east coast of

India, forming a sea lane that passed through two oceans and the Straits of Malacca. During the Tang and Song Dynasties, waterways in Qinzhou connected Yizhou, Tiandong, Nanning and became convenient gateways to the sea and overseas countries. Therefore, Qinzhou became an important harbor for domestic and international trade. *Lingwai Daida* has described the prosperous international trade in Qinzhou. Convenient transportation has provided favorable conditions for economic and cultural development in the Zhuang region.

11. 2. 2　Migration and exchanges with other ethnic minorities

In the Paleolithic Age of around 50,000 years ago, Zhuang ancestors lived in South China. In 1965, eighteen human fossils were discovered in Zengpiyan site in Guilin. Six of fourteen skulls have artificial holes on parietal bones. It is similar to the 5000-year-old perforated skulls unearthed in Dawenkou site in Shandong. Is there any correlation between it and the craniotomy of ancient western medicine? Was it a practice derived from prehistoric human migration and communication? It is hard to study these questions without adequate documents. However, the contact between Lingnan or Guangxi and inland areas has been recorded in historical works including *Shangshu*, *Shijing*, *Yizhoushu* and *Mozi*. Since the Qin and Han Dynasties, people in the Central Plains were constantly moving to the Lingnan region to defend the frontier or avoid chaos caused by wars, and as part of the southward movement of the economic barycenter. In *Records of the Grand Historian*, Qin Shi Huang set up Guilin Prefecture, Nanhai Prefecture and Xiang Prefecture in 214 BC, and he sent half a million people to defend the Five Ridges and live with Yue people; in order to reassure soldiers, 30,000 unmarried women were originally requested to sew clothes for soldiers, and finally Qin Shi Huang gave permission for 15,000 women. Ordinary people started to seek refuge in Guangdong, Guangxi, Fujian and other places to avoid the chaos caused by the Mongol invasion of 1273. In addition, more and more other people moved there, including court officials, banished officials, businessmen, and exiled sinners. According to *Book of Han* and *Comprehensive Mirror in Aid of Governance*, eleven people moved to Hepu Prefecture because of crimes from 24 BC to 23 AD. In addition to the southward migration of people from the Central Plains, multi-ethnic cohabitation was formed due to the continuous migration of people of the Zhuang, Dong, Miao, Yao, Dai, Mulao and other nationalities.

Massive migration and communication brought cultural integration and collision.

Because of its advanced state and adaptability, the culture of the Central Plains was soon accepted and absorbed by Zhuang people. As revealed by archeological discoveries in the Zhuang region, many cultural relics of the Qin and Han Dynasties, unearthed in Guangxi, have cultural features of the Central Plains. For example, phoenix is the most common and characteristic decorative image in Chu culture. A pair of bronze phoenix lamps (unearthed in the Han Dynasty tomb in Wangniuling, Hepu) is a tangible evidence that Han culture permeated Guangxi. After the bureaucratization of native officers, many officials established schools in the Zhuang region, and enrolled Zhuang juniors to learn Confucian culture and the Four Books and the Five Classics. Gradually, loyalty, faith, benevolence, righteousness, courtesy, wisdom and other virtues became principles in the Zhuang region, where well-educated scholars emerged, including Ming Dynasty Wei Zhao, Wei Guang, Zhang Xuan and Li Wenfeng, all of whom were from Yishan (now Yizhou) Jinshi (graduates of the highest Chinese palace examination). With uneven development, however, the culture of the Central Plains mainly influenced northeast central and southeast Guangxi, without having great impact on western Guangxi.

In addition, Buddhist culture influenced Zhuang culture as well. Colored glaze, agate, amber, crystal and other relics have been unearthed in the Han Dynasty tomb in Hepu, Hezhou, Guigang, Wuzhou, Guilin, Zhaoping and other cities in Guangxi. Hepu along Beibu Gulf has the most relics. Those relics might have come from India and its neighbors as they belonged to the seven treasures recorded in the Buddhist scriptures. Presumably, Buddhism came to Guangxi via seaways during the Western Han Dynasty, thrived in the Tang Dynasty, and then blossomed slowly. As Buddhism influenced Zhuang ancestors' religious beliefs, they started to believe in animism and perform soul deliverance rites. However, the absorption of Buddhist medicine into Zhuang culture was limited, as Zhuang just absorbed and transformed certain pragmatic contents.

11.3　Reflections on the impact of other medical cultures on Zhuang medicine

11.3.1　Negative impact of other medical cultures on Zhuang medicine

The formation of culture involves the continuous absorption, transformation, and integration of foreign culture. Zhuang medical culture also absorbed, transformed and integrated many achievements from other ethnic medicines in its development. It is true that some idealistic and wrong concepts had a negative impact on Zhuang medical development due to limited productivity and understanding. For example, incantations and prayer in Taoist medicine was combined with primitive religions and had wide impact, which impeded Zhuang medical development for a long time. However, the combination of foreign medical culture and Zhuang medical culture has greatly enriched and developed Zhuang medical culture throughout its development.

11. 3. 2　Shock to Zhuang medicine from other medical cultures

Lacking cultural confidence, Zhuang medical culture easily got lost in the absorption of foreign culture, and lost its unique advantages and features. After the southward migration of people in the Central Plains, some Zhuang people learned and deeply admired the advanced culture of the Central Plains. Under the influence of Han culture centrism, they proactively studied and spread this new culture, while looking down upon their own culture. During the 1950s and 1960s in Shangsi, Ningming, Fusui and other cities of southern Guangxi inhabited by Zhuang, many continued the practice of acupuncture, Nie Sha and other therapies in treating common diseases. However, they believed that their treatment was superstitious and unscientific because of advanced western medicine. Therefore they did not proactively apply traditional treatment any more. The spread and development of their medicine became very difficult because of the lack of generally recognized writing system throughout Zhuang history, and the great difference in local languages. With the permeation of other medical cultures, some medical prescriptions and skills were gradually lost and could no longer be studied as they were recorded in fragmentary pieces by other ethnic groups. It is certain that some therapeutic methods could no longer serve people in the developing society. For example, pottery needles and porcupine's spikes were used by ancient Zhuang doctors as tools for acupuncture, but they are now replaced by more advanced equipment; Zhuang doctors preferred to use wattle-necked softshell turtle, snake, pangolin and other wild animals as drugs, which is now banned by policies that protect wildlife. Therefore, Zhuang medical workers must have a correct understanding of Zhuang medical development and the position of Zhuang medicine in the entire field of medicine, and dialectically view the relationship between Zhuang medicine and other ethnic medicines.

References:

[1] Liao Guoyi. Development of Buddhism in Guangxi and the Relationship Between It and Culture of Ethnic Minorities [J]. Buddhist Studies, 2002 (1): 228 - 239.

[2] Fan Honggui, Gu Youshi. Zhuang History and Culture [M]. Nanning: Guangxi Nationalities Publishing House, 1997.

[3] Zhu Mingsui, Xie Chunming. Records of Religions, Guangxi Local Records [M]. Nanning: Guangxi People's Publishing House, 1995.

[4] Feng Lijun. Exchanges of Traditional Chinese Medicine Between Ancient China and Southeast Asia [J]. Southeast Asian Affairs, 2002 (3): 8 - 19.

12 Inheritance and Development of Zhuang Medical Culture

As an important part of traditional medicine in China, Zhuang medicine is a unique ethnic medicine formed and developed over the ages of production and life practice. In the tide of economic globalization, traditional medical culture is facing unprecedented challenges. Relying on scientific and technological advantages, western medicine has been widely applied all over the world for nearly one hundred years. Zhuang medicine, more than 2000 years old, is influenced by other cultures. We should consider the opportunities and challenges for Zhuang medicine, and help it grow and thus benefit more people.

12.1 Major problems in the inheritance and development of Zhuang medical culture

After the founding of new China, especially since the reform and opening up, much progress has been made in Zhuang medicine under CPC's guidance. Research, clinical and educational institutions for Zhuang medicine have been established. As an important part of Guangxi health system, Zhuang medicine has become more accessible. Zhuang medical culture is further promoted among people through activities such as Wuming song fairs during Sanyuesan Festival, and Jingxi drug fairs during the Dragon Boat Festival on the 5th day of the 5th lunar month. However, there are some depressing problems in the inheritance and development of Zhuang medicine.

12.1.1 Failure to properly understand the position of Zhuang medical culture in historical development

Historically, Zhuang medicine reached a high level of development, and influenced and promoted the development of TCM. *On Proper Therapies for Different Diseases Geographically*, *Suwen*, *Huangdi Neijing* says, "So, the therapy with nine kinds of needles also comes from the south." This is proven by two Western Zhou

Dynasty bronze acupuncture needles unearthed in Matou Township, Wuming District, Guangxi. Zhuang ancestors were experienced in treating summer heat, sha (filthy-attack diseases caused by spotted qi), miasmic malaria, toxin, and other diseases with a series of effective and characteristic methods of diagnosis and treatment. In the Han Dynasty, for example, Zhuang ancestors knew about preventing and treating sha and miasmic malaria with Yiyiren (*Semen Coicis*) and betel nuts. There are documentary records early in the Jin Dynasty about poisons and detoxifying drugs used by Li people in Lingnan. Zhuang detoxifying drugs were highly praised in the Central Plains, including Chenjia Baiyao, hawksbill turtle blood, and Mantuoluo (*Darura stramonium* L.). Medical practice in the Zhuang region was recorded in Han people's classics, and medicinal materials were constantly transported to the Central Plains. Some of them have played an important role in TCM, including Tianqi [*Panax pseudoginseng* Wall. var. *notoginseng* (Burkill) Hoo et Tseng], Rougui (*Cinnamomum cassia* Presl), Luohanguo [*Siraitia grosvenorii* Swinge], Gejie (*Gecko*), Ezhu (*Curcuma phaeocaulis* Valeton), Guangdougen (*Sophora tonkinensis* Gagnep.), Bajiaohuixiang [*Illicium verum* Hook. f.], and longan. On the one hand, Zhuang medical practice has enriched the medical culture in the Central Plains. On the other hand, TCM has integrated with Zhuang medical culture after coming to the Zhuang region, and this has given rise to special Guangxi schools of TCM, and has promoted the enrichment and development of TCM culture. With rich vegetation and flowers in the Zhuang region, TCM Master Ban Xiuwen is expert at treating diseases with different flowers, includ-ing Suxinhua (*Jasminum grandiflorum* L.), Lingxiao [*Campsis grandiflora* (Thunb.) Schum.], rose, and Foshou (*Citrus medica* L. cv. *Fingered*). Influenced by Zhuang acupuncture, Guangxi schools of acupuncture are characterized by acupoint selection, needle insertion and retention of needle. Zhuang medical experience and techniques in treating fracture and tendon injury are used in Guangxi Wei Family's chiropractic school of TCM, and that school has great academic influence in degenerative spinal diseases. Zhuang medical culture at one time sank into oblivion. However, ever since the First Emperor of Qin (Qin Shi Huang) unified Lingnan in 214 B. C. the Zhuang region has been developing along with the rest of China. Many Han officials rejected medical practices and lifestyles in the Zhuang region, where economy and culture were underdeveloped and there were language barriers. Some historical records about Zhuang customs were exaggerated and distorted by biased writers to satisfy the curiousity. Zhuang culture and education were restricted by feudal rulers. As

Zhao Yi wrote in *Yanbao Zaji* （*Scattered Notes*）, "Local people were able to study but not allowed to take examinations, which is to prevent them from becoming officials and improving status." In 1932, Guangxi warlords established "Committee for Improving Customs" in Sanjiang. Local Zhuang people were forced to dress in Han Chinese clothing and they were not allowed to gather and sing folk songs, or stay up late on New Year's Eve. Subsequently, Zhuang people learned little about their history and culture because of underdeveloped cultural education. With deep historical nihilism, some medical practices were associated with ignorance and backwardness, and so Zhuang medical culture made halting progress. Limited by productivity and education, Zhuang medicine was inevitably affected by folk religion and idealism, and disease treatment by drugs and witchcraft was popular for a long time. That kind of treatment emerged with the development of human society as the common psychological course, due to the ignorance of but reverence for nature. Now we should show recognition of the effective results from spiritual and faith healing.

After the founding of the People's Republic of China, CPC has paved the way for the development of traditional ethnic culture, which was conducive to the development of Zhuang medicine. We should comprehensively understand Zhuang medicine and consider the problems in its development. It has positive aspects and achievements as well as negative aspects and limitations. In order to ensure it can adapt to social development and meet people's demands, we should disentangle truth from falsehood in its practice, give play to its strong points and avoid its shortcomings.

12.1.2 Potential loss of considerable and valuable folk experience in Zhuang medicine

With large population and distribution, Zhuang people were governed by "divide-and-conquer" Tusi system for more than one thousand years. The Zhuang region was divided into various sizes of domains for tusi, and different Zhuang tribes developed their culture independently in an uncoordinated way. With complicated geography and landform, medical customs vary with areas. In northwest Guangxi where there are high mountains and thick forests with four distinctive seasons, people have developed a health preservation culture featuring medicated wine and oil tea for dispelling coldness and dampness; In southeast Guangxi where it is hot and humid, people have similarly developed a culture featuring herbal tea, soup and Gua Sha （scraping sha-bruises） for reducing heat and dispelling dampness. Zhuang people have rich cultural treasures in medicine as their clinical experience accumulated over thousands of years. These treasures were not recorded in classics as they didn't develop into systematic theories before the 1990s. There are pressing problems in the investigation and organization of these treasures. The first is the language barrier. There are various dialects in Guangxi as Guangxi people originated from the Baiyue minority and governed by tusi system for more than 1000 years. It is common to find that Zhuang people from different counties or townships cannot communicate with each other. Many folk doctors can only speak of drug or disease names in dialects, which are hard for researchers to translate accurately without a common language background. Secondly, Zhuang folk doctors frequently use secret prescriptions handed down in their families, while many young Zhuang people have left home as well as their own ethnic culture. The aging of folk doctors threatens the loss of a vast amount of unrecorded medical prescriptions, whether proven or unproven.

12. 1. 3　Unsolved problems in Zhuang medical culture

Stable and continuous cultural inheritance relies on a writing system, without which inheritance will likely be distorted or broken. Without a generally recognized Zhuang writing system before the founding of the People's Republic of China, the Zhuang nationality has relied on word of mouth to disseminate for several thousand years. Therefore some contents of Zhuang medical culture are inevitably distorted. Nowadays, many folk prescriptions and techniques can only be read in Han people's classics, while most of them became lost in the mists of time. Today, Zhuang medical culture is being investigated and organized. On the one hand, its contents are questionable as many methods of diagnosis and treatment and prescriptions need further study. On the other hand, most of the organized contents of Zhuang medicine are accumulated experience, therefore the connection between Zhuang basic theories and clinical diagnosis and treatment is ambiguous, and the dialectical rules of development for diseases cannot be deduced by means of strict logic. Zhuang medicated thread moxibustion, Zhuang acupuncture therapy, and other Zhuang medical therapies contain plentiful techniques for many diseases, but they are simply pragmatic. It is essential for the survival and development of all medical forms that the accumulated experience can be developed into theories as general guidance, and that diseases can be prevented and treated effectively using methods of diagnosis and treatment with the support of theories. Therefore, one of the major tasks for a long time has been further investigation, organization and improvement of the theoretical system of Zhuang medicine so as to achieve more effective guidance for clinical practices.

12. 2　Principles for the inheritance and development of Zhuang medical culture

12. 2. 1　Respect the changing rules of Zhuang medical culture

Culture is derived from reality over time. The connotative structure of Zhuang medical culture is shown in Figure 12-1. The outer ring represents material culture in Zhuang medicine, mainly comprising tools for diagnosis and treatment, and utensils for collecting and processing drugs; the second ring represents institutional culture, being mainly methods for diagnosis and treatment, rules of drug usage and healthcare customs; the core is the theoretical system of Zhuang medicine. In a mature medical cultural system, its methodologies should conform to contemporary ethics with its core theories as guidance, and contemporary material conditions as foundations. Its core theories are significant as they were developed from the medical experience of generations of people. Zhuang medical culture keeps changing. In particular, medical utensils, diagnosis and treatment behavior, healthcare customs, and core theories in Zhuang medicine vary with developments over time, people's understanding of life science, social ethics, and improvement of material conditions. Generally, the material part in the outer ring most easily interacts and changes with the external world. The theoretical system at the core is hard to change. Institutional culture in the second ring changes with the material part and contemporary ethics.

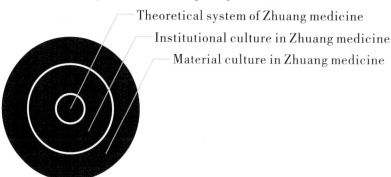

Theoretical system of Zhuang medicine
Institutional culture in Zhuang medicine
Material culture in Zhuang medicine

Figure 12-1　Connotative structure of Zhuang medical culture

Therefore, the rules of cultural development should be followed in the inheritance and development of Zhuang medical culture. For its material part, the achievements of modern society should be maximally utilized as the methods and conditions for improvement and self-development. For methods of diagnosis and treatment, rules of drug usage, methods for collecting and processing drugs and healthcare customs, we should study them to disentangle truth from falsehood and make best use of the progress. The theoretical system at the core has universal significance for Zhuang medicine as the essence and features of Zhuang medicine and the foundations for the sustainable development of Zhuang medicine. We should study the system cautiously and avoid disturbing it carelessly.

12. 2. 2　Steer the development of Zhuang medical culture

Driven by the tide of modern science and technology, western medicine has dramatically changed the whole world and has had unprecedented impact on the development of traditional medicine. Ethnic medicine, including TCM, has been questioned and challenged. In developing and passing down Zhuang medicine, two tendencies in particular should be avoided. The first is idealism. Because of limited productivity and understanding, ancient people could not objectively explain etiology or pathogenesis, and they treated diseases by inviting shamans to worship ghosts and gods to dispel pathogenic factors, as they believed supernatural powers caused diseases. In ancient times, some types of ethnic medicine accomplished great things, but they were dominated by idealism and finally overtaken by other medicine. Their medical experience failed to evolve, the mechanism of syndromes were not investigated and analyzed objectively but they are deduced subjectively instead and attributed to the supernatural. Idealism impeded the development of Zhuang medicine for a long time. Nowadays, it is commonly recognized that it is idealistic to treat diseases by inviting shamans to worship ghosts and gods or dispel pathogenic factors. However, another form of idealism tends to be neglected, in which factors determining and influencing illness cannot be understood correctly. Some aspects are exaggerated and absolutized, causing the separation of theories and clinical practice. The second is nihilism. Nihilists deny ethnic culture, tradition and heritage. They even believe that Zhuang medical culture is imaginary. They thoroughly deny that Zhuang medical culture has existed for over 2000 years, or deny all of it because of its shortcomings in certain aspects. That is a manifestation of the supremacy of western medicine. Therefore, in the organization of

Zhuang medicine, we should retain its essence and features, respect history and reality, and apply rigorous thought, interdisciplinary methods, and absorb achievements in modern science and technologies to construct appropriate research methodologies. And it needs to provide modern explanations for basic Zhuang medical theories, identify the contents that should be reconsidered or abandoned, and build a Zhuang medical cultural system that meets the needs of our times. We should firmly oppose the idea of breaking Zhuang medicine into pieces and then pasting those pieces into the system of western medicine, all in the name of modernization.

12. 3   Methods and approaches for the inheritance and development of Zhuang medical culture

12. 3. 1   Promotion of excellent traditional Zhuang culture

Traditional Zhuang culture is the remarkable result of Zhuang people's hard work and arduous creation over several thousand years. Rice-farming, bronze drum, ganlan and medical cultures are fine traditional Zhuang cultures that have played an important role in human progress and in the spread of civilization. Rooted in traditional Zhuang culture, Zhuang medical culture is an important part of Zhuang people's daily life. With the acceleration of China's modernization process in the 21st century, Zhuang people's lifestyle is changing, traditional Zhuang culture tends to be weakened in their life, and Zhuang medical culture has less opportunity to thrive. The prosperity and development of fine traditional Zhuang culture is associated with ethnic unity and identity, as well as the survival and development of Zhuang medical culture. The prosperity and development of fine traditional Zhuang culture and modernization are not at odds. Modernization is the common experience of social development, and indicates the great cultural change of developing countries for sharing scientific advances in human society. The aim of modernization is to use modern science and technologies to improve people's quality of life, therefore it is not a goal but a method for social development. People live in different environments that suit different cultures. It is essential for us to maintain the diversity of culture just as we do with the diversity of species. Therefore, we should promote the essence of Zhuang people's spiritual culture, such as diligence, thriftiness, goodness, tolerance, respect for nature, solidarity, mutual support, and love of life. The same is true of the customs, systems and festivals that reflect the spiritual culture. Modern Zhuang people's ideal pursuit and social norm can be reconstructed. We should emphasize the protection of forms of ethnic cultural heritage, and promote Zhuang culture including health preservation (e.g., drinking oil tea, wearing sachets, and having medicated bath and going to drug fairs in the Dragon Boat Festival) and health preservation techniques (e.g., Gua Sha and cupping). In this way these can become important ways of health preservation for Zhuang people. For some Zhuang medical cultural projects with great potential economic value, cultural advantages can be transformed into industrial strengths by developing cultural industries.

12. 3. 2 Investigation and organization of Zhuang medical culture

The key to the inheritance and development of Zhuang medical culture lies in whether it can effectively guide people's medical practice and provide scalable and effective solutions for disease prevention and treatment. To this end, the therapeutic effect of Zhuang medicine should be further proven in clinical practice, and its service capability should be enhanced in the healthcare system. Zhuang medicine, without adequate written records, is China's ethnic medical system that remains relatively complete after organization. Current research on Zhuang medicine still needs further improvement and enrichment. Many therapeutic and treatment methods and prescriptions need qualitative and quantitative research based on modern scientific methods. Therefore, Zhuang medical theories can be more systematic, Zhuang clinical diagnosis and treatment can be more objective, and Zhuang drug production and use can be more standardized. The obstacles in linking Zhuang medicine and modern healthcare system will be removed and the service capability of Zhuang medicine will be improved. Take the most characteristic therapy for sha diseases in Zhuang medicine for example. Zhuang people believe that "diseases come from sha". There are more than 100 complex categories of sha diseases in Zhuang medicine. Materials about sha diseases were mainly organized through orally inherited materials. Because of language barriers and different points of view, there are problems concerning of consistent understanding of concepts, non-standard classification of syndromes, ambiguity in the concepts and connotations of disease names as well as in the features of syndromes. These problems have impeded the inheritance and development of Zhuang medicine. For common sha diseases in clinical practice, standardized research should be carried out to explore the concepts and connotations of the disease names, their clinical manifestation and features, their etiology and pathogenesis and rules of treatment based on differentiation. Clinical information databases of sha diseases should be established to continuously improve the diagnostic and treatment methods for sha diseases, to set up diagnostic criteria for common sha diseases in Zhuang medicine, and to develop standardized programs for the diagnosis and treatment of common sha diseases. Certainly, the standardized research for Zhuang medicine is not absolutized. For diagnostic and treatment skills and prescriptions that are not able to be studied in a standardized way or proven effective, we should be careful not to discard them as they are accumulated experience of many generations in Zhuang medical culture. As we have just started to use modern technologies to carry out standardized research on Zhuang medicine, and as medicine is far more complicated than science and technologies, we should leverage scientific methods to explain and improve Zhuang medical culture, rather than to limit or discard it. With the development of science and technologies and the deepening understanding of life science, there will possibly be new research methods, new discovery and new understanding for Zhuang medical culture.

12. 3. 3　Development of Zhuang medical culture education

Zhuang medical culture education should be developed through the following three dimensions.

（1）Improve the level of Zhuang medical culture education

Without a generally recognized Zhuang writing system, the Zhuang nationality has relied on word of mouth to disseminate Zhuang medicine. Since the 1980s, achievements in scientific research of Zhuang medicine were introduced into the course system for TCM by Guangxi University of Chinese Medicine through academic forums, minor courses and other forms. After continuous accumulation and improvement during the past three decades, undergraduate and postgraduate programs in Zhuang medicine have been introduced. However, current educational levels still fail to meet the needs of Zhuang medical development. Doctoral program in Zhuang medicine will be conducive to further improvement of theoretical research, clinical application and promotion, and drug research and development in Zhuang medicine. Therefore Zhuang folk medical theories will be more complete, systematic and scientific.

（2）Expand the coverage of Zhuang medicine education

Zhuang medicine education should not be limited to college education. It should also be expanded to the team development of Zhuang folk medical workers and the development of Zhuang medical culture in medical institutions. Zhuang folk medical workers are the carriers of Zhuang medical culture as well as the genes for its prosperity. Education of folk medical workers should be included in the team management of Zhuang medicine talent to improve their professional skills and capabilities, and to encourage them to pass down Zhuang medical culture through apprenticeship and other methods. Mature diagnostic and treatment skills in Zhuang medicine should be proactively promoted as appropriate techniques in different levels of medical institutions.

（3）Innovate the forms of Zhuang medicine education

As Zhuang medicine education originates from the folk, limited contents of Zhuang medical culture have been organized in textbooks and courses. Centralized training in higher institutions is also relatively restrictive. Therefore, Zhuang medicine education should focus more on practical teaching and field investigation. In the development of teaching staff, folk medical workers with expertise should be employed as part-time teachers and be equipped with highly educated apprentices to carry out research on the inheritance of academic thinking and clinical experience from prestigious Zhuang medical experts, and to enhance the succession of personal medical experience. Meanwhile, colleges and universities should enroll a quota of students who know the Zhuang language or have Zhuang cultural background in order to promote the investigation and organization of Zhuang folk medicine.

References:

[1] Qin Zhuyuan. Some Thoughts on Traditional Zhuang Culture [J]. Economic and Social Development, 2013 (12): 144 - 146.

[2] Fu Guanghua. Discussion on National Assimilation Policy in New Guangxi Regime [J]. Guihai Tribune, 2008, 24 (5): 74 - 78.

[3] Pang Yuzhou, Wang Chunling. An Introduction to Zhuang Medical Culture [J]. Chinese Journal of Basic Medicine in Traditional Chinese Medicine, 2009, 15 (10): 800 - 802.

壮医药实物
Material objects of Zhuang medicine

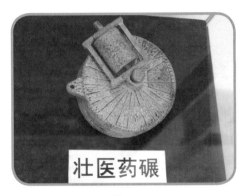

药碾
herb grinder

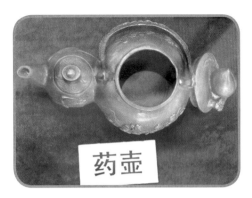

药壶
drug kettle

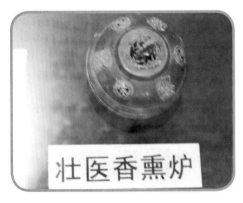

香熏炉
incense burner

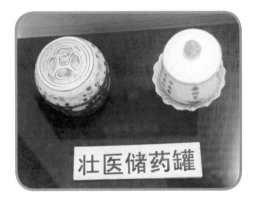

储药罐
drug jar

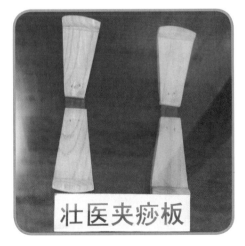

夹痧板
gua sha clips

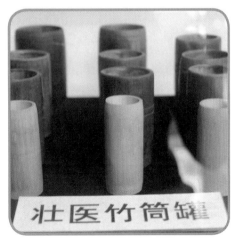

竹筒罐
bamboo jar

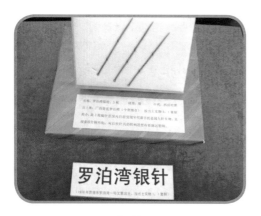

银针
silver needle

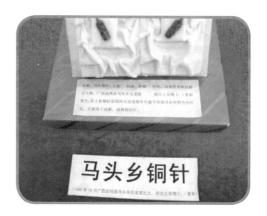

铜针
bronze needle

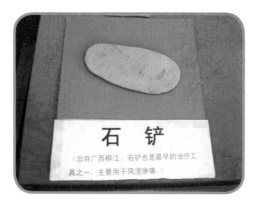

石铲
stone scoop

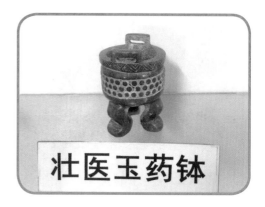

玉药钵
jade drug container

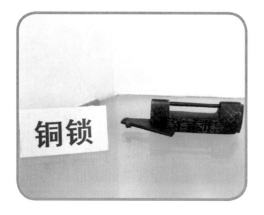

铜锁
bronze lock

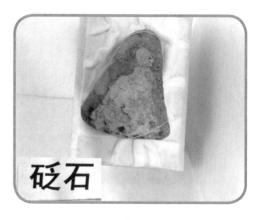

砭石
stone needle

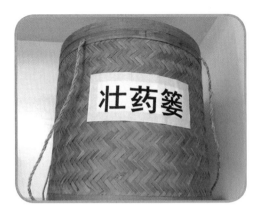

壮药篓
Zhuang drug basket

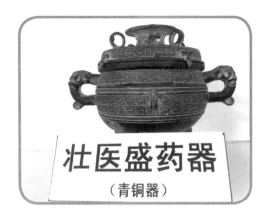

盛药器
drug container

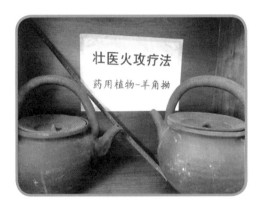

火攻疗法器具
tool for fire attack therapy

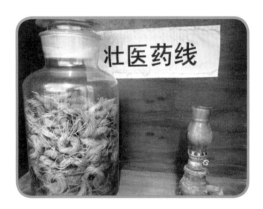

药线
medicated thread

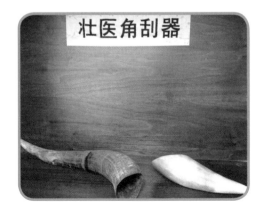

角刮器
horn scraper

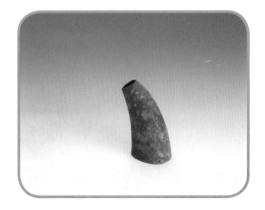

牛角药瓶
horn drug bottle

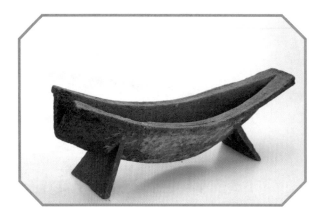

铁制药碾槽（大）
iron mortar (large)

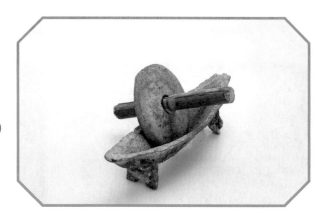

铁制药碾器（小）
iron mortar (small)

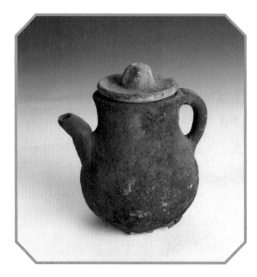

宋·药罐
drug jar from the Song dynasty

哲学宗教文化
Philosophical and religious culture

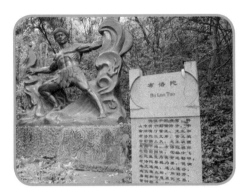

布洛陀像
statue of Buluotuo

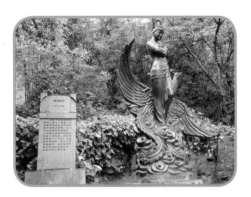

达勒甲像
statue of Muliujia

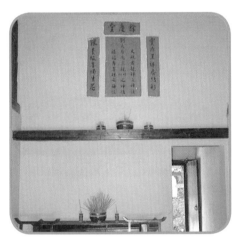

祠堂（局部）
ancestral hall

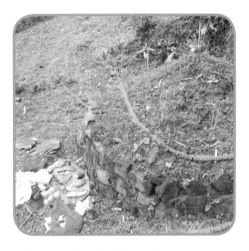

"三月三"扫墓场景
tomb sweeping during the Sanyuesan
festival

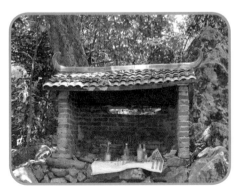

土地公、土地婆庙
Tudigong and Tudipo shrine

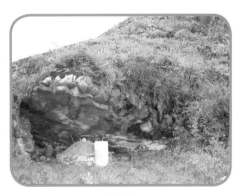

祖坟
ancestral grave

稻作文化
Rice–farming culture

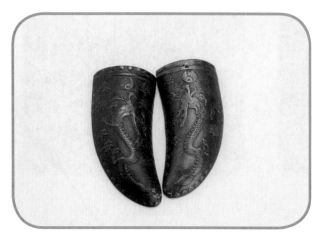

道师公用的铜角
bronze horns for Taoist masters

道师公用刀
knife for Taoist masters

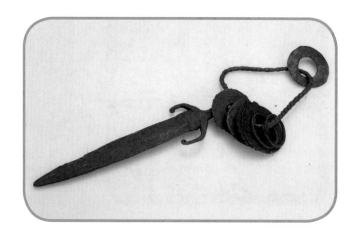

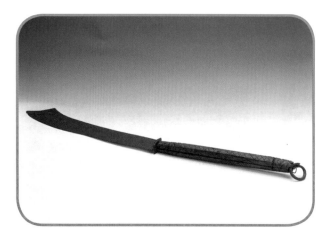

长把砍刀
long broadsword

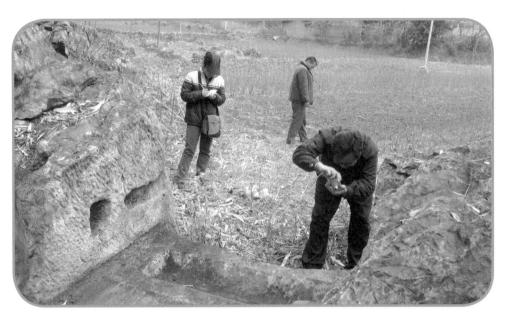

壮族先民因地制宜设置的榨糖作坊遗址考古现场
archaeological site of sugar workshop established by Zhuang ancestors according to local conditions

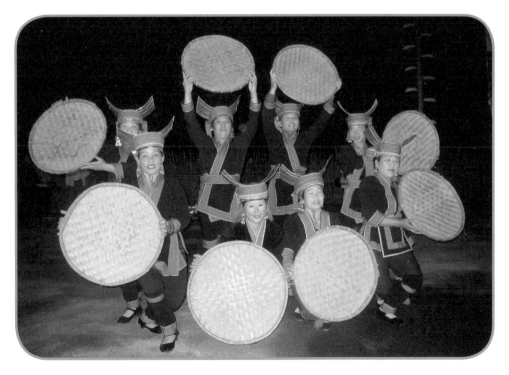

壮族人民表演庆祝丰收歌舞
Zhuang people singing and dancing to celebrate the harvest

习俗文化
Customary culture

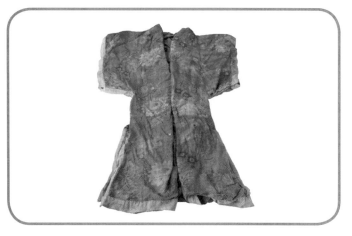

刀工服装
clothes for Taoist masters

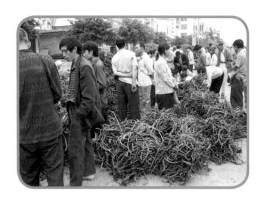

靖西端午药市一角
scene from drug fair of Jingxi City on
Dragon Boat Festival

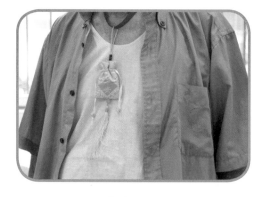

佩药习俗
worn medicine

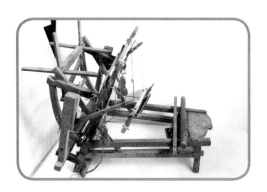

壮锦织锦机
loom for making Zhuang brocade

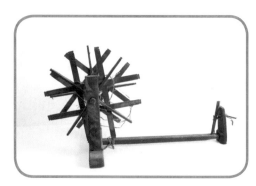

壮锦织锦机
loom for making Zhuang brocade

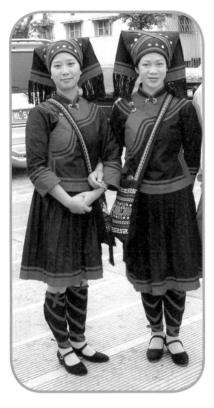

壮族服饰
Zhuang clothing

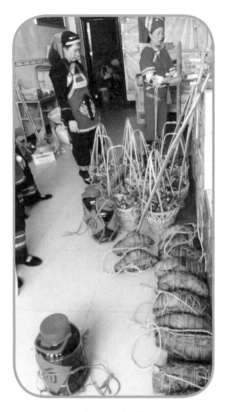

壮族节日的粽子
zongzi during Zhuang festivals

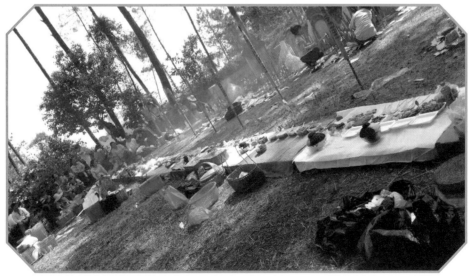

壮族"三月三"祭祖
ancestor worship in the Double Third Festival

歌谣文化
Ballad culture

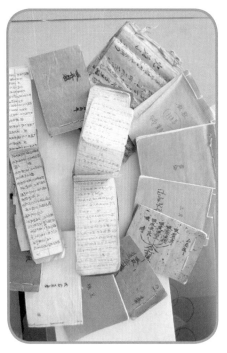

壮族歌谱
Zhuang song music

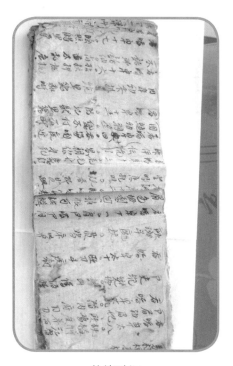

壮族歌词
Zhuang song lyrics

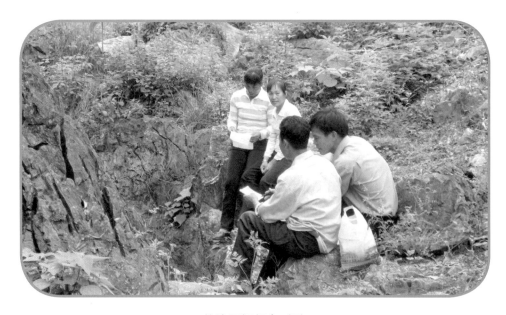

壮族民间相亲对歌
Duige (antiphonal singing) employed by young Zhuang people in matchmaking events

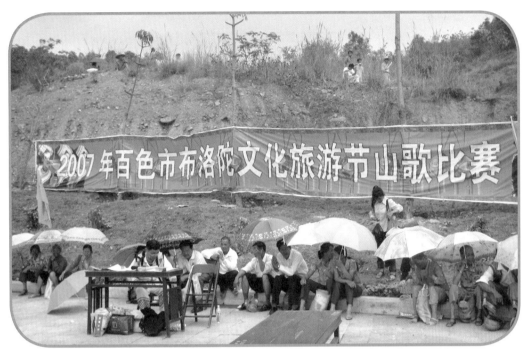

壮族乡村山歌大赛
singing competition for shange (mountain songs)

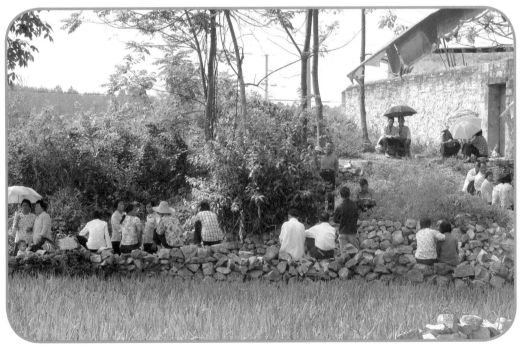

壮族村头对歌
Duige (antiphonal singing) in a Zhuang village

饮食文化
Food culture

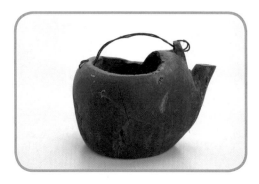

木壶（原名木臼）
wooden kettle

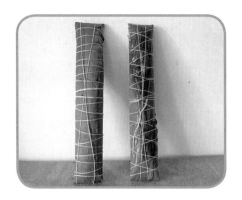

粽子
zongzi

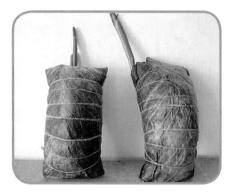

粽子
zongzi

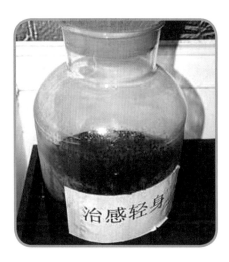

壮药酒
Zhuang medicated wine

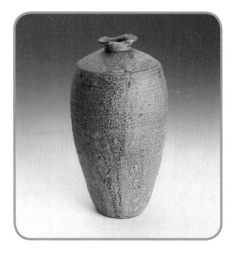

宋·酒瓶
wine bottle from the Song dynasty

人居文化
Dwelling culture

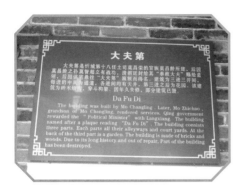

忻城大夫第（局部）
Xincheng Dafu Mansion

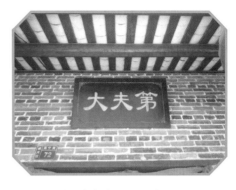

忻城大夫第（局部）
Xincheng Dafu Mansion

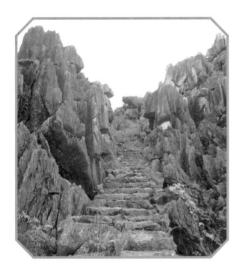

石板道
stone slab path

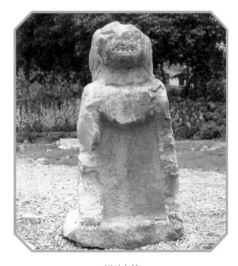

镇村兽
village guardian

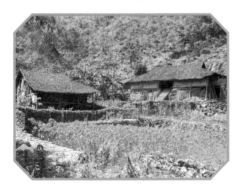

壮族干栏式建筑
Zhuang ganlan houses

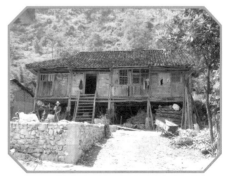

壮族干栏式建筑
Zhuang ganlan houses

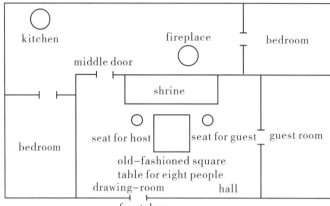

壮族住宅布局
layout of Zhuang residence

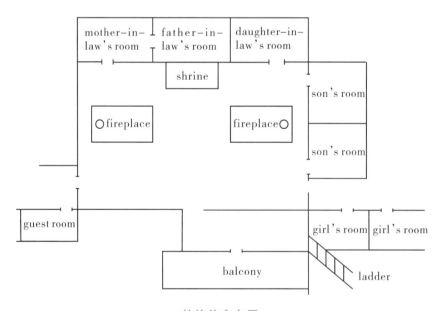

壮族住宅布局
layout of Zhuang residence

舞蹈体育文化
Dance and sports

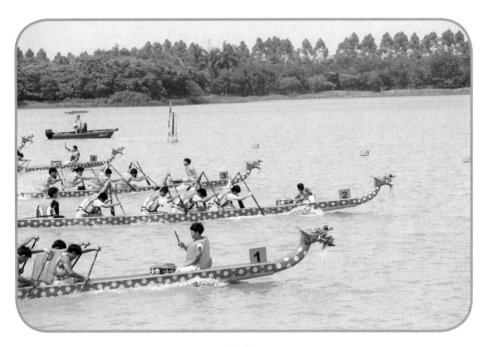

赛龙舟
dragon boat racing

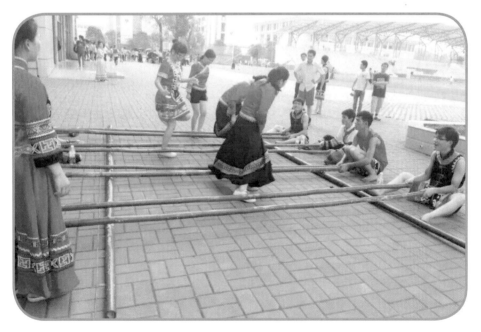

壮族竹杠舞
bamboo pole dance

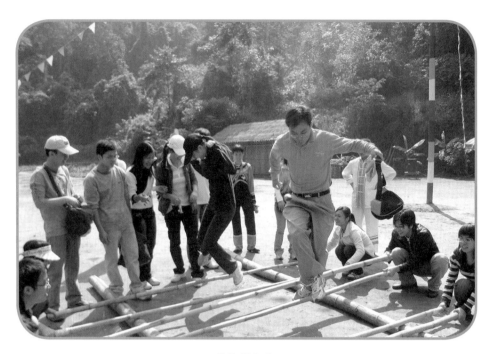

壮族竹杠舞
bamboo pole dance

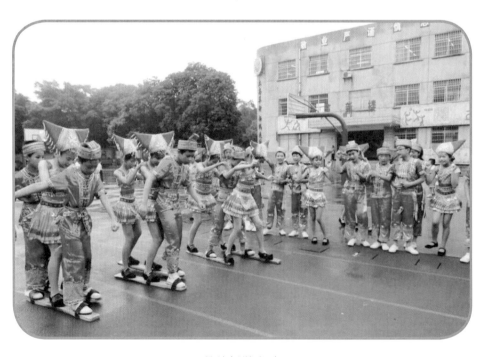

壮族板鞋竞速
shoe plank race